Ace all of life's tests at home, work, and school.
Even learn how astronauts manage stress!

HOW THE

MORE POWER TO YOU

BEST

BY USING YOUR HEAD

HANDLE

AND HEART

STRESS

Dr. Ron Rubenzer

HOW THE BEST HANDLE STRESS

Published by:
Warren Publishing, Inc.
19809 North Cove Road
Cornelius, North Carolina

Author accepts responsibility for accuracy of research.
ISBN 1-886057-85-0

Library of Congress Catalog Number 97-062244

Printed in the United States of America

TO DONNA: MY WIFE, MY LIFE

To Al Pecor —
"North Star" of Truth,
To set your life's compass by.
The "Lighthouse Beacon" to safety
in the foggy, sometimes stormy seas of life.

To my "midnight writer" partners —
Charlotte, Cheyenne, & Scarlett,
faithful from beginning to end.

ACKNOWLEDGEMENTS:

Thank you to those who have helped with this book knowingly or served as examples of one type or another.

Some of the kind and talented people who helped me are:

My brothers, Bernie, Eugene and Phil;

Moms and Dads both here (Doris and Jack O'Dell) and there

(Effie and Bernard Rubenzer), without whom I would not be here;

To brother Tim, truly talented at what he does;

Shirley Mabe and Woody Mansir,

who have led us through troubled waters

with their beacon of good example;

Eddie Townes who found William James' 1899 cornerstone book;

Bill Joyce, always uplifting;

June and Hank Schutzberger, for helping us see the world;

To Marie McCarty, who has shown us the way;

To Eutha Godfrey, who provided delicious "food for thought" and

Connie Hicks, whose humor lightened the load;

Jeanie Biscoe, friend and "encourager," who introduced me to Sandra Redding;

Sandra Redding, book critic and newspaper columnist who connected me with the North Carolina Writers' Network (largest state network in U.S.);

To Dan Jones, NC Principal of the Year, who read and encouraged my work;

Dan Boswell and Diane Barber for keeping me "current;"

To the gifted editor/writer from the North Carolina Writers' Network,

Dr. Linda Hobson;

To graphic designer, Kimberly Cannon;

To Richard Wilson, owner, Wilson Wordworks;

To Cathy Warren, CEO - Warren Publishing, Inc., for making this book a reality;

To the members of the NC-TCCS "Dream Team,"

who are stellar examples of the power of positive leadership,

To the positive, innovative pioneers of the Midwest Center for Stress and Anxiety, Inc.,

having helped over a half-million people cope with stress,

Lucinda Bassett, Founder and Carolyn Dickman, Education Director;

To my New York friends:

Dr. Paul Rosch (M.D.), President of the American Institute of Stress,

who had me join the job-stress panel at his 1997 World Congress of Stress in Switzerland;

To Caroline Sincerebeaux of a NY publishing house, who helped me build & improve a national book-launching platform;

To friends met abroad:

Dr. Richard Rahe (M.D.), one of the world's leading pioneers in stress measurement who helped me norm the ISR in Switzerland;

To special friends in Australia and Denmark:
Rowena Robinson and Mark Lewis respectively;
To those who let me "see the light:"
My Former WTC advanced administrative intern supervisor, Grace Lacy;
United Nations-NYC contacts who involved me in their project,
Mr. & Mrs. Stanton;
My Washington, DC supervisor while on special assignment, Dr. Dorothy Sisk;
The following top leaders in their fields who took time to share their
personal stress management tips:
(Arranged by chronological order in the study's development)
Dr. Jeffrey Parker, A&T University-University of North Carolina;
Dr. Lee Kinard, top Nielson-rated local TV news anchor/
most-trusted man in a million;
Rex Best, two-time Emmy award-winner;
Bill Flynn, top daily morning radio show host of WMAG, High Point, NC;
Dr. Sanford Danziger, M.D., Director of TRP (Totally Responsible Person);
Jose Riba, K.M., Honorary Consulate General of the
Republic of San Marino, Italy;
Dr. Deborah Rozman, Executive Vice President, Heartmath, Boulder Creek, CA;
Also Jeff Goelitz of Heartmath who provided steady encouragement;
Roy Bixby, M.B.A., Human Resources manager, Fortune 500 Corporation Executive;
Judge Charles Biscoe, Administrative law judge who brought
a calm sense of wisdom and humor to this Mt. Everest task;
Rowena J. Robinson, Olympic Tryout competitor,
B. Sc.Ed. PDHPE, Dip. HM, Health and Fitness consultant, Monte Sant'Angelo Mercy College (private school), North Sydney, Australia, who had her entire class help with my research;
Tim O'Dell, nationally renowned sports photographer for Sports Illustrated;
Dr. Linda Hobson, professional writer and
Executive Director of NCWN;
Dr. Lillie M. Jones, Yale consultant,
friend and retired interim superintendent, Guilford County Schools;
To all my Columbia University National/State Leadership Institute professors:
Professor A.J. Tannenbaum, Ph.D., advisor & National Project Leader
for seven universities;
(My Columbia doctoral dissertation team, where this book began 20 years ago)
Professor Harry Passow, Ph.D.,
Professor James Borland, Ph.D., and
Professor Linda Hickson Bilsky, Ph.D;
To the folks at GCS,
who shaped my "views of the rules" . . . forevermore.

CONTENTS

DEDICATION III
ACKNOWLEDGEMENTS V
INTRODUCTION
How To Use This Book IX - XI

Chapter 1 — 1
WHY BECOME STRESS-INTELLIGENT?
BECAUSE STRESS IS THE FLY IN THE OINTMENT

Chapter 2 — 27
WHAT IS YOUR ABILITY TO RELAX "AT WILL"?
AND HOW DOES IT BOOST YOUR PERFORMANCE?

Chapter 3 — 35
ARE YOU SPEEDING?
GAUGES ON YOUR DASHBOARD

Chapter 4 — 47
INDUSTRIAL-STRENGTH STRESS CONTROL?
AN INSIDER'S VIEW FROM THE WORLD TRADE CENTER

Chapter 5 — 57
JOB-STRESS PRESCRIPTIONS

Chapter 6 — 67
"POWER" ATTITUDES

Chapter 7 — 81
BREATHING EASIER

Chapter 8 — 89
WIN/LOSE — YOU CHOOSE:
YOUR FREEDOM TO CHOOSE

Chapter 9 — 105
2001: A CYBERSTRESS ODYSSEY
COMPUTER ANXIETY

Chapter 10 — 115
MORE FREEDOM OF CHOICES
IN THE C.A.R.E. PACKAGE

Chapter 11 — 129
BOOSTING YOUR WILL POWER

Chapter 12 — 141
REFUSE TO LOSE YOUR MIND

Chapter 13 151
MAKE FUN OF STRESS & SMILE
IT MAKES YOU LOOK SMARTER

CHAPTER 14 157
PUBLIC SPEAKING: PUBLIC ENEMY NUMBER ONE

Chapter 15 167
CHILDREN: STRESS CURES AT HOME

Chapter 16 183
WHY KEEP COOL AT SCHOOL?
NINE-YEAR-OLDS TAKING COLLEGE ENTRANCE EXAMS!

Chapter 17 195
SCORING BEST ON ALL LIFE'S TESTS
BY USING YOUR "WHOLE BRAIN"

Chapter 18 225
RELAXATION: THE FOURTH "R" FOR EDUCATORS

Chapter 19 237
THE "RULES"
MEN AND WOMEN AREN'T FROM DIFFERENT PLANETS,
BUT FROM DIFFERENT HEMISPHERES (OF THE BRAIN)

Chapter 20 249
HOW THE BEST HANDLE STRESS:
LESSONS FROM THE TOP

Chapter 21 265
WHEN YOU TAKE STRESS PERSONALLY:
CONQUERING ANGER, WORRY, HEADACHES AND "SLEEPWORKING" (INSOMNIA)

Chapter 22 281
THE YOUNG AND THE REST OF US
THE LITTLE ENGINE THAT COULD - ADJUST

Appendix A 289
ONE-MINUTE ANTI-STRESS FACT SHEETS
(CRIB SHEETS OF THE COMPLETE CHAPTERS)

Appendix B 357
TIME-CAPSULE: HOW TO MANAGE TIME

Bibliography 363

Index 375

How to Use this Book

Read for Need and Speed

This book is designed for the time-starved person on the go. Just as you don't buy everything in a store, but shop according to a list, a list of topics is provided for you in the table of contents and at the beginning of each chapter. Reading each topic takes no longer than fifteen minutes. Take one topic at a time. If the section fits your circumstances and personal needs, read the whole chapter and practice the steps suggested. If a particular topic fills your personal need, then read it. If you have a headache you don't open your medicine cabinet and take every medication there is in sight. Neither does one read the fine print "ingredients section" of all your headache medications while your head is pounding. Similarly, if you have a stress headache you want relief fast, so just go to the headache prescription in this book in Chapter 21. If you want to find out the only clinically proven herbal remedy to improve your memory, go to Chapter 22, under the section, "Using it or losing it — your memory."

Stress Is the Fly in the Ointment

This book proves stress is the fly in the ointment, so to speak. This book provides a crisp list of 21st century reasons why you should not let stress harass you anymore. Only practical, proven tips are provided to reduce your stress and improve your effectiveness. This book clearly shows how children may be the unwilling victims of greatly increased test stress.

Chapter 16 explains why even nine-year-olds are now taking college entrance exams at the cost of test-anxiety sickness. Later in the book, ways to reduce your child's home and school-stress are clearly explained. The key to dramatic test-score improvement is also uncovered. If you want to know the 21st century "Rules for the opposite sex" which even Einstein did not know, just go to Chapter 19. A cure for the common complainer is provided in Chapter 8. Chapter 11 reveals the world's oldest form of medication. If you are interested in naturally boosting your brain-power during testing or working you will find, "Food for thought," in Chapter 17. Find out what a top MIT scientist has to say about brain foods. Discover how humor makes you "seem" more intelligent in Chapter 13. Chapter 10 targets in on how to deal with nasty people, which is a top source of stress, even for astronauts. Read Chapter 1 to discover the identity of one of the world's most successful corporations that requires psychological counseling for "just plain rude" employees. The best Harvard Medical School study on the mental/physical health link is showcased in Chapter 1. The centerpiece of Chapter 1, the power of positive leadership, is framed in a "poster format" for your immediate use. A quick and easy LEAD-

ERSHIP REPORT CARD© "self-test" is also provided, to help set your compass heading if needed. Information on the best true measure of leadership is provided. In Chapter 4, the author's firsthand insider's view from the WTC about workaholism is revealed. The latest results of the first major scientific stress-study ever done on survivors of 9/11 are reviewed. In Chapter 1, the extremely important issue of gifted-genius under stress is explored. In Chapter 20, those individuals who are at the "top of their game" share their tips on how to enjoy life while still achieving.

Basically, your life's emotional weather forecast will be mostly sunny, with a 20% chance of whine. This book is the umbrella to keep you safe and warm when life starts "whining" on you. At any given time, depending on the conditions, one out of five people wants to rain on your parade.

How the Book Is Organized

The book is organized according to different types of stressors — from job, to school, to family, to yourself. The best way to control stress is to control the cause. This book emphasizes providing you with coping-tools to dismantle major causes of stress, from those we have no control over (9/11 — World Trade Center bombings; job loss; aging) to those where we have more control (our attitudes).

There are as many cures for stress as there are causes. This book offers hundreds of simple, effective and fast stress busters based on experience with thousands of individuals, from kindergarten to cardiac rehab. You are already doing many of these things!

One-Minute Anti-Stress Skill-Builders Are in the Appendix

These Anti-Stress Skill-Builders offer readers self-diagnostic-prescriptive activities. Each Skill-Builder Checklist can also be used as a lesson plan, a study guide for individuals in high school and college, or homework sheets for those in stress-control coaching or employee assistance program (EAP) settings. Again, these "quick note" prescriptions are designed for home, work, school, seminar employee assistance programs, or stress-control coaching settings.

How Do Astronauts Manage Stress?

The answer to the question, "How do astronauts manage stress?," sheds light on "down-to-earth tips" you can apply. No one's job is more 24-7 than that of an astronaut! No one else's job concerns the daily fear, "Am I going to return from this alive?" This book reveals their space-stress coping secrets. With the historical discovery of "life-supporting ice" on Mars (March 2002), there will definitely be future flights to Mars, requiring at least two years for the round trip.

The No Bore or Baffle Clause

Every effort has been made to neither "bore nor baffle you." It's a delicate balance between too much information or information that is so rare that you will never use it. Like a top shelf of a tool box, I have provided three proven tools that will do many things. Of course, more complex situations require more complex tools, and these specialized tools are provided directly to you or you are given a quick reference you can contact. For example, to help with the rudeness-rampage in this country, a quick 2002 reference is provided to a whole corporate program devoted to treat workers on the job who are "terminally rude."

The Fine Print

"In God we trust, everyone else needs references." For detailed documentation of what is covered in the text, a "fine print" section is offered in the "Bibliography" which includes over 200 references spanning a century. Because references are often considered "speed bumps" when trying to read, most references are at the end of each chapter or at the end of the book. In total there are about 315 references.

Speaking to Both Brains

November, 2000 research revealed that females read with both left and right brains, while men use primarily their left brains. The left brain is mostly verbal, the right brain is mostly visual and emotional, and so this book features words and stories to provide a holistic approach to learning. The sometimes-humorous "Bob and Delia Story" throughout the entire book provides a continuous look at life's stressors through male and female brain perspectives based on true-life stories.

The "Best of" Series

A "best of" feature is found in most chapters, highlighting the best national programs, best human resources or best books on a particular topic. The intent of the "best of" list is to provide you with materials that can be used in building a platform to launch your personal stress-management program or even a system-wide program requiring funding. The "best of" materials have all been road-tested and are ready-made, ready to be implemented immediately. The "best of" section usually features a phone number and when available, an Internet connection. For example the Midwest Center for Stress and Anxiety, Inc., which has helped a half a million people cope with stress through self-help materials, is featured in Chapters 6 and 7. The best computer-assisted-biofeedback program is provided by the Heartmath program, appearing in Chapter 3.

Hopefully this book can be a one-stop center to help you find what you need in terms of reasons for managing stress and how to manage stress, without actually creating more stress. Extreme stress-management systems can load you down with more stress than they relieve. There is also a "For Further Reading" section included at the end of each chapter, featuring professional grade references on facts presented in each chapter. So welcome to low stress reading. Remember, just read what you need.

1

WHY BECOME STRESS-INTELLIGENT?

BECAUSE STRESS IS THE FLY IN THE OINTMENT

The top 21, 21st century reasons why you should not let stress harass you anymore.

Do you want to be *stress-intelligent?* That IS the question.

Intelligence means the ability to adapt *(Merriam Twentieth Century Dictionary)*. People who are stress-intelligent are more adaptable to life's twists and turns according to a 2002, Harvard Medical School study.

We know enough now about stress so you have a choice to be intelligent about it if you want. Consider the alternative to being stress-intelligent. The road map to this first chapter is divided into three major sections:

I. FOR IMPROVED QUALITY OF LIFE,

II. FOR THE CHILDREN: GREATER SUCCESS AND SAFETY,

III. AT THE WORKPLACE.

Section I, IMPROVED QUALITY OF LIFE, applies to everyone.

Section II, FOR THE CHILDREN: GREATER SUCCESS AND SAFETY, talks to all parents, grandparents, educators and those with children at home or school or at home-school. Nine-year-olds are starting to take the college entrance exam, SAT, and it is making them physically sick from test stress.

Don't tell me to relax — if I weren't "wired" together so tightly, I'd fall apart.

The story is the same for many of us, only the details are different.

Bob was scheduled to be a keynote speaker in New Orleans at 9:00 A.M. for an audience of 1,000. His plan was to leave home at 5:00 A.M. for the airport. He called a cab and it was on its way. Suddenly his cat brought in a half-live squirrel he'd been chasing around the house in the predawn hour. Bob had to catch and remove the squirrel before he left for the speaking engagement.

At the same time Bob noticed that the ceiling in the den was swelling; a water pipe had broken in the crawl space. With the cab waiting in the driveway to go the airport, Bob grabbed his work gloves and a laundry basket. He cornered and captured the cat and the squirrel and threw the squirrel outside. Then he took a broom

Section III, AT THE WORKPLACE, is important if you are working under stressful positions.

Consider if you will, each numbered topic under each major section as a street sign. If you don't need to go down that street (topic), skip to the road(s) that will lead you where you want to go.

Battle-tested Advice

Ironically, most stress-management consultants are not in the job trenches any more, and rarely get shot at. This book was written in the trenches, where one could hear the bullets whistling by while being shot at. Many people now live in a territory where they "shoot first" and ask questions later. These warning shots gained new "proper perspective" after 9/11. The author worked at the World Trade Center in New York City, but fortunately changed his career path in time. The first major scientific study of the disastrous psychological fallout for survivors of ground-zero is featured in Section 1.

The top 21, 21st century reasons why it is important to be "stress-smart" follow.

handle and poked it into the den ceiling. The water gushed through the hole, emptying the water that had gathered. He turned off the water source, grabbed his suitcase and jumped into the running cab.

Trying to accentuate the positive, he took several deep breaths while in the cab. After arriving at the airport, he ran to the plane, being the last passenger boarding the New Orleans flight. Sitting on the plane Bob chuckled to himself, "This is great material for a stress-management speech."

We don't have much choice about what happens to us, but we do have a choice about how we think about what happens to us. Each of us has free will, and no one can steal it from us.

Section I — For Improved Quality Of Life

- The pursuit of happiness is your birthright.
- An extremely high, fivefold increase in anxiety-disorders in NYC inflicts the 9/11 ground-zero survivors. We must regain our quality of life. 9/11 changes U.S. language and emotional landscape forever.
- Stress is fattening, and it's not just in your head. One in four adults is a victim of "stress-belly."
- According to Harvard Medical School, "The good don't die young." Optimists are healthier and outlive pessimists.
- Energy crisis: when you are too tired to get out of the way or play. Breathing boosts athletic performance—from passing out to surpassing state records.

- Life is 44% more stressful in the U.S. than 30 years ago, so you have to be thick-skinned yet tenderhearted. Treatment for depression has increased at an alarming rate (fivefold) over ten years.
- Stress robs a dozen years off lifespan. Unwarranted feelings of stress are neurochemical lies. Being treated like a dog, ages you like one (seven years for one).
- Making strong men faint: The "nocebo" effect proven hazardous to your health. Cortisol slows physical healing.
- IOS, "Information overload stress," is on the rise. Or genius under stress.
- How 30 seconds of insight on the "Rules for the sexes" can spare you 30 years of stress.

Section II — For the Children: Greater Success and Safety

- Use love not fear for effective teaching, according to the greatest educational mind – ever.
- Fifteen-percentile point test-score increase, or a whole letter-grade improvement results from learning test-taking skills for students. (The U.S. Senate passed a bill on June 14, 2001, requiring 3rd through 8th grade students to take math and reading tests.)
- Children are smarter than ever, but stress still stupefies through performance anxiety. Stress is the single greatest cause of impaired learning in school. Test stress is making children sick earlier.
- Safer schools and reduced drug abuse.
- Reduction in extreme stress-reaction behaviors, including copy-cat shootings, suicidal bombings, and even running away from home.
- Increased need to reduce stress over our "ever-increasing" catastrophic events such as the 9/11 suicidal bombings.

Section III — At the Workplace

- Conquering your urgency addiction, while remaining "nimble."
- The 4-10-02 shooter's stress syndrome: recognizing the warning signs in others who are about "ready to snap like a twig." Dealing with the nasty twenty percent.
- High-risk male stress syndrome: The triple threat to aggress under stress.
- P.S. Avoiding a nervous breakdown when your computer has one.
- Dealing with CSA, Computer-separation-anxiety, as millions of obsolete computers are permanently separated from their users.

As indicated earlier, proceed only if you feel the need to read more. Again, think of the 21 items as headlines in the newspaper. You can select and choose the "news" you are really interested in. Otherwise move on to Chapter 2 on measuring your RQ.

Section I — For Improved Quality Of Life

1. The pursuit of happiness is your birthright.

A subtle anxiety invades our families after the September 11, 2001 suicide bombings of the World Trade Center and Pentagon.

The inborn need for happiness is so deeply woven into our humanity that it was made a Constitutional right (i.e., the right to life, liberty and the pursuit of happiness). The very foundation of our country is the idea that pursuing happiness is a worthwhile national and life goal. We can reset our compasses in that direction by not working hard to deal with stress, but working intelligently; thus the term stress-intelligence. Again, remember the definition of intelligence, the ability to adapt, even to any condition.

People are less happy today than thirty years ago. The percentage of people claiming to be happy has decreased from 40% in 1970 to 30% in 2001. Trying to be happy today is an uphill battle. There is also an alarming increase in teenage depression.

Rudeness rampage

People are much ruder today than ten years ago. Most people polled on a 2002 Internet survey strongly feel that rudeness is on the rise. Defending yourself against these onslaughts can drain you. Rudeness hurts business so much that one of the top places to work in the country, SAS of Cary, North Carolina has a corporate code that abusive, rude behavior is against company policy. Those violating the rudeness code are provided assistance in locating a psychologist who does counseling. *What is the cure for the terminally rude (Don't try this on your own)? Force equally rude, bossy people to be in the same room, with no way out. They'll soon learn a lesson in manners.*

Desk rage, road rage, school rage . . . rage is the rage today. Much of today's unhappiness comes from the collision of too little time with too much technology.

2. 9/11 fallout — We must regain our quality of life.

Even after eight weeks, an extremely high, fivefold increase in serious anxiety disorders inflicts the 9/11 ground-zero survivors according to a March 28, 2002 report by the New York Academy of Medicine. This study is the first of its kind that scientifically examined the skyrocketing rates of post-traumatic stress disorder (PTSD) and depression in New York City. 9/11 changes U.S. emotional and language landscape forever.

According to Dr. Carol Waryas, (Ph.D., CCC-SLP), the terrorist attacks on September 11, 2001 were so psychologically shocking that the Psychological Corporation sponsored a workshop, entitled "Conference for New York: Harmony and Healing," to help professionals affected by events of that day.

Even for those not directly involved with the horrific suicide bombings of September 11, 2001 and the anthrax scare thereafter, a subtle state of increased anxiety has blanketed our entire country even down to the family. Fear of flying has cut revenues almost in half at this point. Our hypervigilent state cannot be maintained forever. We'll never get used to the fear around us, but we can adjust to the level that it doesn't affect our health and longevity.

---

3. Stress is fattening, and it's not just in your head. One in four adults is a victim of "stress-belly."

The March 2001, *Harvard Health Letter* states that stress level contributes to obesity. All weight reduction programs should include stress management, in addition to modifying your eating patterns and monitoring the foods that are available. Genes more or less determine your tendency to gain weight. Studies cite genetic inheritance plays a role in obesity from 40% to 70%. You can blame your genes for being fat, but you determine if those "fat genes" express themselves on the scale. We can't control our genes. We can control one of the proven culprits in weight gain—stress.

How can stress make you fat enough to develop a "stress-belly"? Cortisol, the stress hormone, signals the body to store abdominal fat and increase insulin level. It is claimed falsely that grapefruit is a fat burner, but studies at Wake Forest University and Yale found that the stress hormone, cortisol, is truly a fat maker, triggering our bodies to convert calories directly to fat rather than burning those calories off in a normal fashion. As many as one out of four Americans carries around stress-produced fat. This fat usually goes to the belly and that is a heart risk. A comical but unfounded term for beer over-drinkers is the "beer-belly." Indeed, scientific evidence supports the development of "stress-belly", because stress-produced fat goes to the abdomen like a magnet. The good news is with diet and exercise, "stress-belly" fat is the first to go. A diet without a stress-management program is doomed to failure, though. Not only is getting fat upsetting emotionally, but gaining as few as ten pounds can increase diabetes, hypertension and heart attack risk. Again, the good news, is that "stress-belly" fat is the first to go when properly dieting.

Stress-eating comforts us and actually stimulates the physical urge to eat. Eating distracts us from the unpleasant by getting our mind on something pleasant in the present rather than focusing on the fearful future. Finally, food was used by our family (grandmothers, especially) to express their love, so of course, we turn to food when we feel low or not particularly loved. There is even a commercial to the effect that says, "Nothing shows lovin' like something from the oven," which helps bond the connection between food and affection in our society. We start off our day wanting to consume, as evidenced by the jingle, "The best part of getting up is something in your cup." To confuse our love affair with food, our advertisers have put a famous female pancake-maker on a strict diet; Aunt Jemina is now almost anorexic, whereas she used to look like a lovingly plump grandmother who sampled her own cooking.

We often overeat because we are celebrating or thinking we deserve a treat. We also turn to food for comfort when we are upset, feeling down, mad or nervous. Many people eat out of boredom. When you get mad, write a letter, then destroy it. Punch a pillow. When our energy tank feels like it's on empty because of physical or psychological effort, food seems to help us regain energy, improve concentration and makes us feel more alert. Take a break (catnap) rather than eating to fill your energy reserves. Food works as an "emotional pain killer." Alcohol, in addition to being an emotional painkiller, increases your appetite, tempting you even more to overeat.

Gaining weight from stress is not all in your head. Through a complex chain of events, when you are stressed your body also produces extra insulin which boosts your appetite, and actually localizes the development of fat cells in the stomach area. As indicated earlier the "fight-or-flight" hormone, called cortisol, increases your desire for high energy foods that are packed with calories contained in high fat foods, or high calorie foods. Also, your switch that keeps you from overeating is deactivated under stress, increasing your desire to overeat.

---

4. According to Harvard Medical School: "The good don't die young." Optimists are healthier and outlive pessimists.

A 2000 study of 800 people discovered that highly-pessimistic people tend to die younger than their positive-thinking counterparts. A study in a 2001 issue of *Health Psychology* revealed that people who are easily stressed out or irritable are at increased health risk for infections, especially hepatitis B.

Harvard answers the question: Why become stress-intelligent?

A cornerstone article from Harvard Medical School on dealing with the 9/11 trauma, also clearly states that optimists outlive pessimists.

The question of cancer

The jury is still out according to a May 2002, Harvard Medical School article on the immune system and the mind. Cautious optimism should be used in using stress management as a complementary (definitely NOT an alternative) treatment of cancer. Faith healing alone has its limitations, and a better bet is to have faith in your doctor to heal cancer. To quote this very important Harvard "study of studies," they summarize that "Evidence on how states of mind affect the risk of cancer in human beings is limited and conflicting" (p. 1). Having a positive attitude in general may make one more likely to get regular and early checkups, which will reduce cancer.

Stress hormone, cortisol, kills

Medical experts state that when under great stress, cortisol causes cortical convulsions in your heart. That is, cortisol gets your heart ready for "fight or flight." If you don't run or fight under stress, cortisol, directly courses through your heart, making it beat wildly, erratically and sometimes lethally out of rhythm. Chronic cortisol flooding of your cortical system kills by making your heart skip a lot more than one beat.

How long would your car engine last if you pressed your right foot, full throttle on the gas pedal and at the same time pressed the brake pedal to the floor? You are doing the same thing to your irreplaceable engine (heart) when you stress yourself out. You are all "revved up but no place to go."

Bob was enjoying driving with his wife down the road to the end of Harper Valley Island. It was a beautiful day and the highway was surrounded on both sides by water on this finger of land jutting out into the ocean. Suddenly, from behind, a car practically rode up on Bob and Delia's car even though Bob was obeying the speed limit. It was obvious that the tailgaiter was fuming with road rage. Honking his horn and flashing his lights about two feet behind Bob's car, this enraged driver was obsessed with passing Bob. Momentarily Bob experienced a "stress flash," becoming very upset over the unwarranted flashing lights and honking horn on his car's tail.

Delia pleaded for Bob not to get involved. Not wanting to spoil their vacation day drive, Bob decided to try to be thick-skinned but tenderhearted. He did his best to "suffer these fools gladly" and calmed down, allowing the enraged driver to pass. To Bob's delight this same car was pulled over for speeding about five miles down the road. Bob said to himself, there is some justice. But people like this often convert road rage into road deaths.

5. Energy crisis: when you are too tired to get out of the way or play.

We all experience our personal energy crisis when we deplete our good stress-energy (eustress) too early in the day. If we sleep well we start each day with a full tank of stress-energy. Just like driving a car at ninety-miles per hour instead of an even fifty-five in a fifty-five miles per hour speed zone, sooner or later you will be on empty or get pulled over by the authorities for speeding. The REDS program in Chapter 11, "Boosting Your Will Power," gives specific activities to Relax, Exercise, Diet and Sleep (REDS) to avoid a personal energy crisis. The REDS program is designed to help you have more energy and a cleaner running engine.

Breathing boosts athletic performance — from passing out to surpassing state records

Rachel Mercury, although making it all the way to the state level for her 100- and 200-yard dashes, found she was having anxiety attacks when the state level competition began. Eventually she was disqualified from running in the state competition because she had passed out cold, twice, on the track. One of the visiting coaches in the crowd observed her great bursts of speed until she passed out on the track. Believing she held great promise, he took Rachel under his wing and analyzed what she was doing wrong. Under the great stress of competition, this junior high school student had been holding her breath through 80 yards of the 100-yard dash, until she passed out. She actually forgot to breathe! A month later, the insightful coach had Rachel run for him in Virginia. He told her all she needed to do to improve her game was to breathe while running. She practiced relaxation breathing as he suggested, and the next year Rachel captured the state title for the hundred-yard dash, breaking all previous records. For her performance-enhancing breathing secret, read Chapter 7, "Breathing Easier: The Key to Stress Management is Right Under Your Nose." To help you keep running in the rat race of life, just simply breathe more deeply and mindfully.

Anyone can notice a difference, but it takes a genius to make a difference.

Example: Cave-man says to cave-woman, "It's really getting cold in here." Cave-woman says, "Try this fire I discovered."

---

6. Life is 44% more stressful. Be thick-skinned but tenderhearted. Treatment for depression has increased at an alarming rate (fivefold) over ten years.

The kitchen is hotter than ever, so the need to keep cool is greater now than ever. Life stress has measurably increased by 44% over the last thirty years, according to Richard Rahe, M.D., one of the leading pioneers in stress measurement. Over ten-million Americans are plagued by an anxiety disorder. According to a Harvard University survey, social anxiety disorder is a common stress disorder and the most prevalent psychiatric problem after depression and alcoholism. Only 20% suffering from this anxiety disorder get help, according to a National Anxiety Disorders Screening Day survey. Being thick-skinned but tenderhearted is important in keeping an even keel. By being stress-intelligent you will learn "to wake up and smell the coffee AND to stop and smell the roses." Both are parts of life. You will often see young-thinking optimists display on their cars, "NO FEAR." Sadly, you will see others' cars with the saying, "FEAR THIS," prominently displayed.

Over the last thirty years, surveys reveal the percentage of people being happy has gone down from 40% to 30%. Road rage, "going postal," and school violence have become all too prominent in America's landscape.

A 2002 study reveals that those treated for depression have increased almost 500% in just ten years (1987-1997). The number of those treated for depression went from 1.7 million in 1987 to 6.3 million in 1997.

Now hospitals are feeling the tension in the form of ward-rage. Nurses are burning out at an alarming rate. Over 43% of 43,329 nurses polled in a study stated that they felt overwhelmed by their work. This 1998-99 study revealed that 50% of these nurses had been victims of verbal abuse because they were in the wards around the clock. One of three nurses in the survey under age thirty planned on quitting within one year. Forty-one percent of U.S. nurses expressed job dissatisfaction. Job dissatisfaction among nurses affects the quality of services provided. Almost 45% of the polled nurses indicated that indeed the quality of care in hospital settings went down over last year. On a more personal level, having a stressed-out nurse give you a shot or remove a catheter can result in very unpleasant consequences for you, the patient. Give nurses a break, don't verbally abuse them. Appreciate what they do.

Nearly one-half-million workers lost their jobs in the first quarter of 2001. Of all health-threatening stressors, job loss is number 8 out of 43 life changes that can lead to physical illness according to the best measure of stressors to date, Holmes-Rahe Social Adjustment Scale. Laid-off workers go through a severe grieving process that is very stressful, often leading to anger, depression and physical illness. Job survivor stress often plagues those remaining in jobs because they wonder why they were spared and they are burdened with the extra workload legacy left by the newly unemployed in the company.

You could almost interpret the phrase, using your "head" and "heart," for more power to you as being positively hard-headed yet tenderhearted. You have to be thick-skinned to accept unconstructive criticism at work, but you still have to be tenderhearted to have work friends, which will make your job more satisfying. Under stress it is human nature to just become thick-skinned until you get to the point that you are numb, even at home.

But use your free will to balance thick-skinned with tenderhearted. Both are necessary for satisfaction.

7. Stress robs a dozen years off lifespan.

Experiencing three major life-stressors in one given year will prematurely age a 55-year-old by 13 years. A 55-year-old man, experiencing the death of both parents and surviving a near-fatal health problem within a year, would have aged 13 years in terms of biological indicators and health risks (cardiovascular).

Being treated like a dog ages you like one (seven years for one year)

Stress makes you dog-tired. A workplace joke is, "I'm treated so much like a dog that this job is even aging me like a dog; one year here ages me seven years."

Former President George Bush's wife, Barbara Bush, experienced her hair turning white almost overnight upon the death of their child. Allegedly Aristotle Onassis' hair turned white almost immediately upon his son's untimely death.

Unwarranted feelings of stress are neurochemical lies

Unwarranted feelings of fear and anxiety are lies in terms of reacting chemically to non-existent dangers. When brain chemistry goes awry, even through overuse of caffeine or alcohol, your mind will find reasons to justify your fearful feelings. Panic is sometimes a reaction to alcohol withdrawal. Indeed, your fearful feelings can produce fearful thoughts. This is called the "somatopsychic" effect, where your body affects your mind, according to Dr. Richard Rahe, speaking at the 1997 World Congress on Stress in Switzerland. A clear demonstration of the body-over-mind effect is the use of psycho-pharmaceuticals (a fancy word for drugs) to alter moods and thoughts, to put one to sleep for surgery, to deaden pain, etc. Some drugs used to calm one down simply retain serotonin longer in the brain cells. Serotonin is the calming natural neurotransmitter. Exercise works so well because it releases more endorphins (natural pleasure transmitters).

When we have an infection, the body (somato) affects your mind (psych). The same infection in one part of your body can travel through your bloodstream to your brain. Once this infection-carrying blood courses through your brain, it can cause great difficulties with concentration, mood, decision-making and reasoning. The point is that a flu in your stomach will affect your thinking because the same blood is circulated to your brain as to your stomach. So if you are sick, take a sick day, and especially don't take any tests.

If you overreact to reality you may be a victim of your own chemical imbalance. See your doctor if you can't sleep. Natural loss of testosterone, estrogen, melatonin, etc., can trigger unwarranted, unwanted negative, performance and health-robbing feelings. Again, see your doctor, because the principle of body-over-mind may be operating.

8. Making strong men faint: The "nocebo" effect proven hazardous to your health. Cortisol slows physical healing.

Everyone has heard about or witnessed the burly he-man fainting while getting stressed out in the "shot line." Their bodies acted on their mind's fears, tripping a circuit breaker in their brains, causing them to faint, which is the ultimate in a flight response. Negative health outcome expectations can be harmful if not fatal to patients. This is what is called the "nocebo" effect, which is the opposite of the health inducing placebo effect. This "nocebo" effect was observed by an eminent physician. While the placebo effect actually improves a disease, by the same token a "nocebo," or negative expectation (I'm not going to get well) actually delays healing or promotes illness. A far-removed version of the "nocebo" effect would be Voodoo, where people who believe they are cursed are supposedly much more likely to succumb to a host of illnesses. It has been discovered that cortisol, a stress hormone, actually retards healing of physical wounds.

It should be noted also that a denial of symptoms due to the fear that something is wrong, can also be harmful. Always contact your physician about concerns you have about symptoms. A fear of doctors can really be harmful to your health.

9. IOS, "Information overload stress," is on the rise.

We get faxed, e-mailed, conference-called, voice-mailed, paged, cell-phoned, and palm-piloted at a dizzying rate from almost anywhere on earth at any time. "Information overload stress" occurs when we feel overwhelmed by all the information we feel we need to process. We feel inseparably connected to invisible electronic umbilical cords, feeding us more information than we can possibly digest.

IOS — it's a crime in New York

It is now illegal to drive your car and talk on your hand-held cell phone at the same time. IOS, "Information overload stress," is causing too many car accidents. It carries a one-hundred-dollar fine and it is predicted that most states will follow suit. So keep your hand-held cellular phone in your trunk, so you have to stop to use it.

Actual warning label for use of wireless phone while driving. "Do not engage in stressful . . . conversations" (p. 7).

IOS can even lead to depression

A new study by Dr. Larry Rosen, a psychology professor at California State University, advises high-tech professionals to cut back on their computer time. High-tech workers are even at risk for anxiety disorders and clinical depression, because they often sacrifice human relations to stay on the cutting edge. People in high-tech jobs often feel frustrated because they will always be behind the technological advances. Dr. Rosen's new book, *TechnoStress,* helps readers cope with feeling frustrated because they are in a field that is a bottomless pit. In other words, these people are experiencing IOS, "Information overload stress." Fifty percent of high-tech workers in Finland report sleep disorders and physical pain resulting from stress.

But we might ask ourselves the question, "Twenty-five years ago we lived without being tethered to all these communication links, so why can't we let go a little now occasionally, maybe on Sunday morning or on vacation?" We were all born wireless.

Even computers get IOS

Even computers suffer from IOS, "Information overload stress." What happens when you information overload a computer? It gets sent off to another state for a lobotomy. You lose all your files and the memory is wiped clean. It just could be the stressed-out operator's fault, "hypering" around, bringing more files to the computer desktop than the machine is designed to handle. More about this below, under "P.S. How not to have a nervous breakdown when your computer has one."

The 21st century

We are so overwhelmed by information, that information overload is considered the trauma of the 21st century. We drown in a sea of data if we don't know how to calm down and prioritize. Another related trauma is CSA, Computer-separation-anxiety. CSA is simply the panic that computer abusers, who spend more time with their computers than people, experience when having to give up their computers, even for vacation or to have dinner with their families.

IOS in people: gifted/genius under stress

How can being gifted or a genius be stressful? It can be described in one word, isolation. Solitary confinement is the most dreaded punishment even in prison, reserved for the worst. The implications of extreme talent (perhaps one in a thousand as Benjamin Franklin was) in having friends are obvious. Like all of us, they have the need to connect with others in a meaningful way. The problem is that sometimes they spend much less time cultivating their "hearts" compared to their "heads," and can lack social support which is so important in stress management. They may have only one or two good friends.

The point of this detour to gifted/genius and stress is that sometimes they have a need for help in the social-emotional area that can be greater than average. Don't ration your compassion to only the obviously handicapped person.

What a real genius thought was job-stress

The author, when visiting in London, noticed that this genius, named "Einey" (for story convenience), would often listen and actually think before he talked. This made Einey appear almost slow or inattentive in his conversation, which would often annoy those full of fast, but senseless, chatter. But because what Einey said had "life or death" consequences in his job as an atomic bomb scientist, he only spoke after he thought. For example, when asked about job-stress, Einey said, "One time an atomic bomb-tower evaporated, at a safe distance, just after one of my own men shook the wires of the A-Bomb in that tower . . . The A-Bomb would not detonate remotely so I had to send someone to physically shake the shorted wires which should have detonated the A-Bomb." Einey got half a smile on his face and said, "Is that what you mean by job-stress?"

The city "on the edge"

A true story about a "genius city" and stress follows. The "highest IQ" city in the USA, composed of nearly all-eminent scientists, also had a very high drinking rate. This city was truly "on the edge."

A common stress-management pattern for some males is to drink rather than think, even if they know better.

---

10. How 30 seconds of insight on the "Rules for the sexes" can spare you 30 years of stress.

Since about every other person is the opposite sex, it would reduce stress greatly if we could "get inside their heads" just for a moment to know what we are supposed to do. Two extremely important and valuable books are presented in Chapter 19 for the sexes. Rather than learning from the school of hard knocks, learn from the experts (the opposite sex) since they have finally reduced their secret wishes down on paper. Good luck.

Section II — For the Children: Greater Success and Safety

---

11. Greater success: The father of American psychology advises: Use love, not fear, for effective teaching.

The greatest educational mind of the last two centuries in America was William James, the father of American psychology. Along with Wilhelm Wundt, William James is considered the cofounder of the entire field of psychology. In his 1899 Harvard lecture-series on teaching William James said, "The teacher who succeeds in getting herself loved by pupils will obtain results which one of a more forbidding temperament finds impossible to secure" (p. 45).

Set your professional compass to the proven North Star, by using love to teach, if you really want the best performance out of others, or yourself. Use good stress (eustress) to win cooperation. After a century, we've proven that William James was right all along.

In the long run, on the average, it is better to be positive than negative. That is, use a carrot rather than a stick. When one uses a stick more than a carrot to motivate, employees will be thinking about two other things other than working. If abused, workers will be constantly thinking how they can either take the stick away (sabotage, whistle blowing or just plain "going postal") or how they can avoid the stick (quitting). Under the thin disguise of corporate culture, which in some places is just a nicer way to say corporate cruelty, superiors berate subordinates in front of their peers, use threats of firing or try to rule by humiliation using such phrases as, "This is the worst report I have ever seen; your work is the poorest of anyone's in the whole department, you are going downhill fast; you are no spring chicken." Sadly, some supervisors treat their pets more kindly than workers. When workers get fed up they start fighting back indirectly. Abused waiters put ingredients definitely not designed for consumption in people's soups. Angry workers often just wait for the chance to get even with their superiors, as happened on April 10, 2002, when the stressed-out policeman shot his boss, three people and then, himself.

The Power Of Positive Leadership

Dr. Ronald L. Rubenzer © 2003

William James' (father of American psychology) universal principle of positive leadership can be applied in all teaching situations, from obedience training to higher education. Below is a 21st century edition of these North Star principles for successful navigation through still or dark and stormy waters.

- You can lead a horse to water, *and* you *can* make him drink *if* you make him *thirsty* first (Try salty foods).
- Create a *thirst for knowledge* and most everyone will come eagerly to drink out of the "fountain of youthful curiosity."

Inspire leadership and the *need to succeed* by using:

- *Hope* over despair,
- *Humor* over humiliation,
- *Praise* over punishment,
- *Politeness* over pushiness,
- *Compliments* over criticism,

- *Soothing* over a shrill voice,
- *Treats* over threats,
- *Desire* over dread,
- *Good cheer* over fear,
- *Fun* over frenzy.

12. Fifteen-percentile point test-score increase, or a whole letter-grade improvement results from learning test-taking skills for students. (Scruggs and Mastropieri, Purdue University, 1992).

The U.S. Senate passed a bill on June 14, 2001 requiring **all** 3rd through 8th grade students to take math and reading tests. With this landmark legislation all children will have to take tests for at least five years. Since testing is now a federal requirement, your child may as well do well. Attached to this bill is additional aid given to low-performing schools during the first year. What does this mean to the student? If a school does not show enough progress after two years, students would be free to go to another public school. If the school still didn't show improvement after three years, federal funds could be used for transportation to another school or federal funds could be used for tutoring, (Espo, D., Associated Press, Washington, DC, June 15, 2001). Since many parents select their housing based on what the neighborhood schools offer, it would make sense for schools to teach test-taking skills to keep parents happy and ease their child's transition from school to another. Many schools already offer test-taking skills, but parents can also do much to help.

13. Children are smarter than ever, but stress still stupefies through performance anxiety. Stress is the single greatest cause of impaired learning in school.

Children are smarter today than ever, according to a 2000 Yale study. But children are not wiser. Wisdom is what gives us balance and perspective in life, and stress-intelligence is a special form of wisdom. Making students learn more, faster and earlier, without teaching them stress management will set children up for anxiety and depression. Depression among teenagers is, in fact, on the rise. In his 1998 book, *Teaching with the Brain in Mind,* Eric Jensen boldly states that the single greatest contributor to our students' impaired learning is stress. Chronically high-stress hormones kill brain cells in the hippocampus, which is the memory "organ" of the brain. You cannot learn if you cannot remember.

Test stress is making children sick earlier

Even nine-year-olds are starting to take the SAT, and it is making them physically sick from test stress. Children that young make a real "test-stress-mess"; they throw up more.

Such early testing makes insecure children even more insecure. They are put in the test pressure cooker much earlier than even a few years ago. 172,000 pupils in eighth grade or less took the ACT or SAT college entrance exams, which is almost 20% higher than in 1996.

---

14. Safer schools and reduced drug abuse.

D.A.R.E. (Drug Abuse Resistance Education) programs point to stress as one reason children use drugs. Reducing stress reduces the risk of drug use. According to the American Institute of Stress, "Teenage suicides have increased by 20% over the last decade." Increased suicides are primarily due to higher tension than ever before. Intense testing pressure will begin now as early as third grade since federal legislation requires all 3rd through 8th graders to take reading and math tests.

Drug abuse among our youth is on the increase, which is often a short-term attempt to relieve stress and boredom associated with increased demands for test performance. Any child suspected of having a mood disorder should, of course, be seen by a doctor just as if the child had a broken arm.

Even sadder is the self-prescribed use of calming or performance/motivation drugs by teens to supposedly give them the winning edge at school. "Stress-smartness" is a healthy alternative to being "caffed to the max" with more than three cups of coffee a day, or using "nitro-fuel-injection"-type substances to seemingly improve school performance. By way of poor example, some adults are so hooked on drugs that even when they know they are going to be drug tested for a job interview, they still can't resist the urge.

President Bush's Character Education initiative

To make schools safer, President Bush, in March of 2001, attempted to mandate Character Education in all schools. Character Education initiative in the schools depends on stress management. One of the major components of Character Education is self-discipline. Learning to self-calm will go far in improving classroom behavior, student success and satisfaction in school.

---

15. Reduction in extreme stress-reaction behaviors such as copy cat shootings, suicidal plane bombings, and even running away from home.

On Sunday, January 6, 2002, a suicidally depressed 15-year-old ninth grader flew a private plane into a Florida business building, killing himself. A written note on his person indicated that he was in support of the 9/11 suicidal plane bombings of the Pentagon and World Trade Center.

Almost a quarter million of New York City's 1.1-million school children are still experiencing extreme stress symptoms from 9/11. These symptoms include post-traumatic stress, separation anxiety and generalized anxiety. There are over a million runaways/homeless youth in the United States. Running away is the flight part of the "fight or flight" syndrome.

16. Increased need to reduce stress over ever increasing catastrophic events such as 9/11 suicidal bombings.

Dr. Arthur Levine, one of the world's leading educators and President of Columbia University's Teachers College, indicated that children should be taught about the value of diversity. To make some sense of the 9/11 suicidal bombings to children, he articulated specific lessons to be learned and taught from catastrophic events. Chapter 18 addresses this further.

9/11 is so important it became the "new word" for the year, and the most important word (phrase) to be added to our language since 1990, according to the American Dialect Society. Obviously 9/11 is always going to be part of our American landscape, so we have to learn to deal with the increased stress it creates for everyone.

Although at the beach six thousand miles from home and job responsibilities, Bob had to continually call his voice mail. He anxiously checked his e-mail, wishing that he could get his e-mail at the 10,000,000-baud rate instead of the hotel's 100,000-baud rate, saving seconds in his communication efforts. While impatiently driving to the beach, he had written sticky notes to himself, which don't stick very well when applied with sunscreen on your hands.

Later that night, sleepless in Samoa, half-baked ideas raced through his head about how he was going to get a leg-up on his work problems. He felt secure in his stress, believing that putting everything on the front burner, thinking about many things at once, he would not be wasting his time on vacation. Sadly, Bob returned from his vacation more stressed than ever, facing another fifty weeks of the rat race without relief.

Section III — At the Workplace

17. Conquering urgency addiction: Enjoying a more pleasant and productive life, yet still being "nimble."

You may be addicted to urgency if you can't let go of your unpleasant feelings of urgency after years of not letting go. An urgency addict panics at the thought of relaxing and having "nothing to do." The clinical term for this urgency addiction is relaxation-induced anxiety (RIA). These people must always be "in charge," in communication, and "all over everyone," constantly telling others what they should do in every situation.

Still being "nimble"

Like in a classic western gun duel, there are the quick and the dead. It is the same in business. The key to business survival today is being "nimble" (as in be nimble, be quick). It is the ability to shift gears, at will, from being relaxed to being quickly energized for change. We have to be loose as sand. The inability to shift out of the "nimble" gear is when problems begin, according to the January, 2002 issue of *Harvard Mental Health Letter*. Years of being "nimble," without ever relaxing, may make you successful with the downside of having an anxiety disorder. An anxiety disorder is basically the inability to slow down at will.

Sleeplessness, headaches, agitation, ulcers, high blood pressure and lack of friends are common results of urgency addiction. Imagine if you will, a 21st century version of the Mad Hatter in *Alice in Wonderland,* a nervous wreck screaming, "I'm late for a very important date." It never ends and people avoid these folks like the plague, not wanting to be infected with their unwarranted, suffocating sense of urgency.

Go placidly amid the noise and haste, and remember what peace there may be in silence. St. Paul's Church, Baltimore, 1692.

Becoming stress-smart will put you back in control of your stress. Stress is simply energy, and stress management is just "energy conservation." "Stress-smartness" puts you back in the driver's seat.

---

18. The shooter's stress syndrome: recognizing the warning signs in those who are about "ready to snap like a twig."

"Policeman shoots boss, three other people and then shoots himself" was the very upsetting news blared across the nation's radio stations on April 10, 2002. Sadly, this was yet another reminder of the toxically-high level of stress people are experiencing.

The shooter's stress syndrome refers to the fight part of the "fight or flight" syndrome. The shooter's syndrome is the lethal discharge of pent-up stress. The formal psychological term is the "diathesis stress syndrome," where stress becomes so great a person is pushed over the line from neurosis to psychosis. So called "crimes of passion" could be examples of "diathesis stress syndrome." It is said that neurotics build castles in the air, but psychotics live in them. When someone goes "psychotic" they are living in a different world, sometimes driven by voices, visions or compulsions to do things they would never do otherwise. Under stress the chance to aggress becomes more rewarding compared to when these same individuals are relaxed. The "diathesis stress model" (being pushed beyond personal control by stress) is receiving more press than ever. Medical attention is always required. Extreme stress can be caused by physical illnesses.

Murder-suicides, students shooting students, desk rage, road rage, tickets for aggressive driving, on-the-job violence and drug abuse among youth are on the rise. We have to stop the madness in our own backyards by being stress-intelligent. We need to consciously be part of the stress-solution, and not part of the problem.

One ex-employee stated that his job was more stressful than Vietnam! This man was "ready to snap."

To "burnout," you first must be on fire, so increase your stress smoke-alarm sensitivity

You need to increase the sensitivity of your stress smoke alarm so you can detect stress smoke-signals before you set yourself on fire and "burnout." Early stress smoke-signals are irritability, impatience, gaining weight from stress-eating, rising blood pressure from blowing your top, sleeplessness, headaches, stomachaches, vague illnesses, difficulty in concentration and decision-making, over-doing of or avoidance of usual healthy pleasures.

Your three-alarm fire stage includes mood disorders, unfounded but terrifying fears, waking up in cold sweats, and the feeling that you are about to lose it or being told by everyone that you're on edge.

Who can you turn to if you have questions about stress?

The clearinghouse for information on stress is the American Institute of Stress, (AIS). [See "Bibliography."] Professor Paul Rosch, M.D., the President of the American Institute of Stress, is one of the world's leading authorities on any aspect of stress.

The most authoritative guide for mental status assessment is the DSM-IV, *Diagnostic and Statistical Manual IV.* The DSM-IV is the reference that most mental-health professionals use in diagnosing emotional problems. Compiled by experts, DSM-IV actually uses decision-making "trees" in specifying emotional problems. Always contact a mental-health professional if you have any questions about someone's mental status.

The "burnt out" phase could include stress-related insomnia, high blood pressure, stroke and temporary strokes (transient ischemic attacks or [TIA's]) heart attack, ulcers, and other serious illnesses due to decreased immune system functions, or feelings of hopelessness. Being stress-intelligent will increase the sensitivity of your natural stress smoke-detector so you can recognize and cool down the smoke-signals of stress before they become a raging fire that will burn you out.

Dealing with the nasty twenty percent

Sadly, one to twenty percent or one out of five people are nasty according to counseling psychologist, Dr. Jay Carter. His book, *Nasty People,* is a must read if you are going to work with people and remain calm.

---

19. High-risk male stress syndrome: The triple threat to aggress under stress.

Males are much more likely to aggress under stress. Compared to females, males are much more prone to implode (heart attack, stroke, high blood pressure, insomnia) or explode (angry outbursts, physical/verbal aggression) due to testosterone overload during stress.

Anxiety often turns to angry aggression in males because of the additional mixture of testosterone to the stress hormone cocktail (adrenaline and cortisol). This is a reason, not an excuse, for the much higher incidence of fighting and bullying for males. This higher risk for the rapid anxiety-anger conversion in males signals a greater need for stress management.

Under stress, both sexes secrete stress hormones, cortisol and adrenaline, a double threat. UCLA researchers, however, discovered that males release a third hormone, testosterone, which often increases aggression and hostility.

Thus far, the media reports almost exclusively male aggressors in shootings and other physical attacks or violence, such as the suicide bombings of the World Trade Center in New York. Women are much more likely to try to gain friendships and support others under stress because females do not get the testosterone aggression surge under stress. The meaning of this new UCLA study is that males need more intervention in terms of learning self-calming, or aggression-redirection techniques before they implode (get sick) or explode (get angry or fight) from stress. The specific male stress syndrome is a reason for aggressive behavior in males than females but not an excuse. It just highlights the additional need for male stress/anger management (sports, relaxation breathing, counting to ten before acting or speaking).

---

20. P.S. Avoiding a nervous breakdown when your computer has one.

Bob was writing down to the wire on an article on computer-stress management, when his computer decided to have a breakdown. Bob apparently stressed out his computer with "Information overload stress" by having more files than his computer could handle. Ironically, Bob had just mailed in the final payment on his computer the day before his trusty computer crashed. Fortunately, because of his sense of "functional paranoia", he had also made backup copies of what he was working on. He sent the article off, and then, although tempted to use his laptop as a boat anchor, he went to the store where he had purchased his computer. Jack, the cheerful young man behind the service department desk, smiled reassuringly telling Bob not to worry because he had been working with computers since he was ten-years-old. He even suggested this computer problem would be a good sequel to the article Bob was writing on dealing with computer stress. Of course, the computer could not be fixed at the store's location but had to be sent across the United States because it had a "tier-two type" error. The computer needed a brand new hard-drive. In other words, Bob's computer had a lobotomy. All previous memories were wiped out.

Forty-million people per day face the chance of the same thing happening to them. How did Bob avoid a nervous breakdown just because his computer did? The following suggestions may be helpful.

Always get an extended warranty. All Bob's computer hard-drive replacement, shipping, etc., were covered by his extended warranty. Bob had always kept up his installment payments.

Order the special issue (April 9, 2001) of *Time* magazine, entitled "Tech-Support Heaven," which claims that it can help you with any problem you'll ever have with your computer. It is clearly written in non-techy talk. Another reader-friendly article is *Consumer Reports,* "This @!*# Computer. How to Handle Ten Common Gripes." (March, 2001, p. 65).

As your computer's memory fills, get a CD burned for a permanent record of your most important documents. Bob luckily had done this a week before his computer crashed. Ask about saving things to a zip drive if your computer has the capacity. Save anything you are working on floppy disks and label your disks so you don't have to find your "needle in the haystack" document.

Take comfort from your friends to whom this hard drive failure has occurred. Chances are you know someone whose computer has been "lobotomized." If computers in general really stress you out see your employee assistance program (EAP) and/or look in the Yellow Pages for APA approved professionals. Millions suffer from CyberStress, and 50% of adults have no use for computers, even though they have to use them. This other half will learn to adjust to computers out of necessity. Because of the current fear of flying blanketing the U.S. because of the 9/11 bombings, the age of tele-video conferencing may well be heralded in, so people can conduct business without congregating in potentially targeted areas. See the Chapter "2001: A CyberStress Odyssey" for helpful computer-stress-management tips.

---

21. Computer-separation-anxiety (CSA) sweeps the nation as 55-million computers are separated from their owners.

It has been estimated that 55.4-million obsolete computers were retired and either thrown out or used for spare parts by the end of 2001. Many computer fanatics get so upset at the thought of leaving their computers behind that they even take them on their vacation, honeymoons, picnics. Humor them, because the day will come when they have to let go. CSA, Computer-separation-anxiety, is an artifact of the computer generation, and does not really exist "by the book," but it is truly amazing how upset people addicted to their computers can become.

SUMMARY

We have looked at the top 21, 21st century reasons to become stress-intelligent, that is, to manage your stress by working smart, not hard. Each one of the 21 reasons for the need for stress management is expanded and professionally referenced. A 2002, Harvard Medical School article answers the question, "Why become stress-intelligent?" The reason is to live longer! In an 1899 Harvard lecture-series by the founding father of American psychology, William James states in no uncertain terms that using love of learning rather than fear, helps us learn better. The two T's of today's rage epidemic, too much technology and too little time, are discussed. People are much ruder than ten years ago. A top company with an anti-rudeness code is discussed. Basically those who can't be courteous are sent by management for counseling. This chapter provides very important information on the abnormally high, fivefold increase in serious anxiety disorders among the ground-zero survivors of 9/11. The New York Academy of Medicine was the first to do a scientific study of the emotional fallout of the 9/11 bombings at New York's World Trade Center. The most important reasons provided were to help you in your pursuit of happiness, to naturally improve performance, to avoid others' stress hurricanes (the nasty twenty percent) and to teach you the early smoke-signals of stress overload. A new, very useful stress-profile instrument (Nowack) for use by EAP, wellness programs and human resources, is presented in the "For Further Reading" section. Character Education, being aggressively promoted by President Bush to improve school safety, depends on stress management. A major component of Character Education is self-discipline, and the ability to self-calm clearly falls under self-discipline.

The newly-explained male stress syndrome is presented. Males, because of the addition of testosterone to stress-hormone secretion, are likely to turn anxiety to aggression. Self-calming techniques are therefore even more important for males than females because of the increased risk of hostile reactions to stress by males. The American Institute of Stress in New York was discussed as one of the legitimate clearinghouses on any questions about stress. "Words of wisdom" written a week after 9/11 about what lessons can be learned and even taught to our youth are touched upon by the President of Columbia University's Teachers College. We looked at "how to avoid having a nervous breakdown when your computer does." You were provided with five hard-earned tips on how to deal with your computer after it has had a lobotomy (complete memory erasure). How to deal with CSA, Computer-separation-anxiety, was highlighted. CSA, which swept the nation as 55-million obsolete computers were "put out to pasture" in 2001 alone, is a humorous by-product of our computer obsessed population, as people are forced to retire their antiquated PC's. The recent fear-motivated desire for tele-conferencing may well require all business persons to feel comfortable with "high-tech" meetings and computers.

Our next chapter will help you measure your RQ and learn why and how a high RQ helps you in life to enjoy success and satisfaction. This RQ test was developed in Switzerland at the 1997 World Congress on Stress.

FOR FURTHER READING

Note to the "want-to-know-more" reader. The Internet service WorldCat, (short for World-Catalogue), provides complete information on practically every known book (including a photo of the front jacket) in the world's libraries. It is the world's best ReSearch Engine. This service even tells you if you have a specific book in your local library. All you need is a library card, and a password from your reference librarian.

American Psychological Association (1994). *Publication manual of the American Psychological Association* (4th ed.). Washington, DC: Author.

American Psychiatric Association. (1994). *Diagnostic and statistical manual of mental disorders* (4th ed.). Washington, DC: Author.

Basset, L. (2002). *Life without limits.* (New York: HarperCollins Publishers [Cliff Street Books]).

Benson, H. (Consultant) (1996). *The medical advisor.* (Richmond, Virginia, Time Life, Inc.).

Browder, S.E. (2001). The power: *11 ways women gain unhealthy weight and how you can take charge of them.* New York: John Wiley.

Charles, C.L. (1999). *Why is everyone so cranky? The ten trends complicating our lives and what we can do about them.* New York: Hyperion.

Consumer Reports. (2001, March). *This @!*# computer. How to handle ten common gripes.* Consumer Reports 65. Author.

Gabor, Don, (1994). *Speaking our mind in 101 difficult situations.* New York: Simon & Schuster.

Goleman, Daniel, (1995) *Emotional intelligence.* New York: Bantam Books.

Harvard Medical School, (2002, May). *The immune system and the mind...*Cancer. The *Harvard Mental Health Letter* 18. (11), pp. 1-3.

Harvard Medical School, (2001). *How women handle stress: Is there a difference?* The *Harvard Mental Health Letter* 17. (10), p. 3.

Hatfield, E.; Cacioppo, J.T.; & Rapson, R.L. (1994). *Emotional contagion.* Cambridge [England]; New York: Cambridge University Press; Paris: Editions de la Maison des sciences de l'homme.

Houck, C. (2002, April). *Stand up to rudeness.* Good Housekeeping. pp. 98-101.

James, William. (1899). *Talks to teachers on psychology: and to students on some of life's ideals.* New York: Henry Holt and Company.

Jensen, E. (1998). *Teaching with the brain in mind.* Alexandria, VA, Association for Supervision and Curriculum Development. Phone (703) 578-9600 for reprints. Website: <http://www.ascd.org>; E-mail <member@ascd.org> pp. 52-53.

Lacy, G. (1979, May). *Developing defensible differentiated programs for the gifted and talented.* The Education Department of New York; Office of Urban School Services, 2 World Trade Center, New York, NY.

Miller, Michael, M.D. (2002). *The benefits of positive psychology.* The *Harvard Mental Health Letter.* 18, pp. 6-7.

New York Board of Education. (2002, May 2). *N.Y. school survey finds much anxiety six months later.* (Greensboro, NC. *News and Record,* A-12).

New York Academy of Medicine (2002, March 28). *Stress disorders rise in New York following attack.* Author.

Nowack, Kenneth. *Stress profile.* Contact <www.wps.publish.com> or 1-800-648-8857.

Olfson, Mark. (2002). Significant jump in number treated for depression. *Journal of the American Medical Association,* Jan. 9.

Rubenzer, R.L. (1979, May 2). *I.E.P. - The consultant's view. Gifted/Talented Education.* (NY Ed. Department, Office of Urban School Services, 2 World Trade Center, New York).

Schlessinger, L. (1994). *Ten stupid things women do to mess up their lives.* New York: Villard Books.

Tannen, D. (1990). *You just don't understand. Women and men in conversation.* New

York: Morrow.

Tawa, Renee (2002). Use of term 9/11 sparks minor war of words. *Los Angeles Times,* pp. 1-11.

Waryas, C. (2002). Dear VIP: The Psychological Corporation (TPC)* is proud to have sponsored author Elisabeth Wiig, Ph.D., at the Conference for New York: Harmony and Healing. *Clinicians' Forum*™ 12, 1. (*The Psychological Corporation® San Antonio, Texas.)

Zaslow, J. (2002, March). When little kids take big tests. *Time* (New York, NY), 159, 10, p. 71.

2

WHAT IS YOUR ABILITY TO RELAX "AT WILL"?

AND HOW DOES IT BOOST YOUR PERFORMANCE?

She is wound up tighter
than a cuckoo clock
And sadly
She goes off every fifteen minutes.

In this chapter we will explore six major points.

- What is an RQ, and why is it important?
- Marilyn vos Savant, with the highest-recorded IQ, advises relaxing to overcome performance anxiety.
- Going from "Mensa to Densa" in one stress attack: How RQ and IQ are linked.
- Clinical studies prove relaxation improves thinking and test performance.
- What is your RQ? Take the test.
- According to world-class artist, Bob Timberlake, you have to slow down from the rapid pace of life to achieve your best.

What does this test have to do with anything?

Bob opened the test booklet and was amazed to see that the questions apparently had nothing to do with the course he had just taken. He drew a blank like a computer screen going out during a power outage. Regaining his composure, he went back to the test, starting with the simplest question on the page (What's your name?). He figured answering this question might "boot" his brain back up. It did, and through the maze of decoy questions he began to answer the questions. He scored well enough on the test to be considered for promotion. The test was designed to test his frustration tolerance. It was an RQ test, a measure of his ability to stay calm under pressure.

1. What is an RQ (RELAX-A-BILITY QUOTIENT)?

Your RQ, or relax-a-bility quotient, is the portion of time you can relax under stressful situations. The more often and deeply you can relax under tense situations the higher your RQ. For example, if you have a hair-trigger temper and people and small animals better stay out of your way, you have a low RQ. If you don't get mad every time a driver dangerously cuts in front of you, you have an average RQ. If you can calm yourself while waiting in endless lines you probably have a high RQ. If you can accept rude, tense and even hostile people with a sense of humor you definitely have a very high RQ. Like IQ, your RQ can be boosted through studied practice, and the good news is, building your RQ requires you to have more fun, to enjoy life and relationships.

Why is your RQ so vitally important?

Benefits of a high RQ:

Enjoy better relationships. High RQ improves your relationships because you are more likely to listen patiently, accept and accurately act upon what an upset person is actually saying and feeling. Low RQ people impatiently prejudge, make snap decisions and brush people off. High RQ people have more friends and get along better at work. A full 20% of the workforce is considered to have a low RQ.

Become more promotable. Workers who are more relaxed and approachable are more desirable as leaders. Co-workers feel more comfortable communicating and cooperating with outwardly relaxed leaders. Tense, impulsive, irritable administrators are tolerated, breeding defensive workers who do the minimum to get by. Workers may spend more time planning escape routes (resumé writing) than getting the job done.

Enjoy better health. Having a good RQ is so important that leading health insurance companies spend millions promoting stress management. And why? Because both you and the insurance companies win. Relaxing makes you healthier and the insurance companies wealthier. The insurance companies benefit from your making fewer unneeded visits to the doctor. Some visits to the doctor are for real stress-illnesses that can be prevented and controlled by stress management. Medical treatment of diseases can be improved by learning to relax. Also, you may be more likely to go for your yearly physical because you are more relaxed about visiting your doctor before a crisis occurs. Stress symptoms can indicate the need for medical attention, so always see your doctor first for best treatment of anxiety. Being stressed out about seeing your doctor can be truly hazardous to your health.

Excess stress can upset the delicate balance of our disease-fighting mechanism. We all have "germs" that are kept under check by our immune system. Diverting energy from our disease-fighting defense shields increases our susceptibility to colds and flu.

---

2. Marilyn vos Savant, with the highest-recorded IQ, advises relaxing to overcome performance anxiety.

Marilyn vos Savant, who possesses the world's highest-recorded IQ, stated that performance anxiety is "as common as losing your sunglasses," and the best cure is to relax. An example of performance anxiety is when you forget frequently used numbers (important dates, social security number, etc.) under pressure. In a column read by millions every week, "Ask Marilyn", a woman poses the following question:

"Is there a medical term for forgetting frequently used numbers (such as your bank PIN number, Social Security number, important dates and combinations to safes) when you're under a lot of pressure? Two times recently, I have forgotten important numbers that I've known forever. I'm highly educated and well organized, and it scares me when this happens."

Marilyn responds:

"Not to worry! This discomforting little annoyance is as common as losing your sunglasses. The problem is a form of 'performance anxiety,' which is a psychological term, not a medical one. There's nothing wrong with you that a little relaxation wouldn't cure." (As read by 80 million in "Ask Marilyn," *Parade,* February 4, 2001, p. 15, and used by permission of *Parade Magazine* and Ms. Savant.)

Obviously improving your RQ (relax-a-bility quotient) will cure instances of performance anxiety that can occur in everyday life or on tests.

---

3. Going from "Mensa to Densa" in one stress attack: How RQ and IQ are linked.

"Stress stupifies." Stress puts us in the senseless chatter mode. The more tense we get the less well we can think. We can be thrown from the high performing Mensa IQ mode into the Densa IQ mode with one panic attack. If we have trained ourselves to have a stable RQ, we can stay in the higher thinking mode when we need it the most (tests, interviews, etc.).

Today's children have higher IQ's than ever before, according to a 2001, Yale study. They are smarter than ever but not wiser in dealing with life. Stress-intelligence is part of wisdom, and this cannot be left to chance, so stress management should be taught in the schools.

How your RQ boosts your IQ to think faster and better: Relax-a-bility helps you score high both during practice and "show time." Stress science has been applied during training for the 1996 Olympics to enhance performance under pressure. A high RQ protects your IQ under pressure by reducing the "mind blanking" effect of test/math anxiety. The bottom line result of your relax-a-bility under test pressure is better test scores.

"Scared silly" is simply "neurotic stupidity." "Neurotic stupidity" is an ancient term for going blank under pressure.

The true key to success under stress is to *over-prepare* and *under-react.* Formal schooling helps us over-prepare, but only you can learn to under-react emotionally, keeping cool through improving your RQ. Relaxed readiness is the oil in the machinery of your success. Relaxed readiness can be learned just as you learned to drive at the speed limit, even if you do not find it easy at first.

The higher your RQ, the more likely you will actually enjoy the rewards of activities that most people avoid because they consider the tasks too stressful. Our society most highly rewards those who can perform under pressure in athletics, entertainment, debating, and emergencies. High RQ individuals can perform under "stress marathon conditions" to reach peak performance with seeming ease and even enjoyment. Formal education does not teach how to improve our RQ's at this point, but the move toward developing what Dr. Daniel Goleman calls "emotional intelligence" is a 21st century survival tool.

---

4. Clinical studies prove relaxation improves thinking and test performance, raising test scores by lowering test anxiety.

A 100-point gain in taking the SAT was realized by students whose test anxiety level was clinically reduced, according to a Columbia University study conducted by Dr. C. H. Faigel.

In another study it was also shown that the ability to wait (self-calming under stress) at four years of age was related to scoring 210 points higher on the SAT in high school compared to other high-schoolers who could not self-calm or wait at the age of four. Self-calming students were also more popular and better liked than impulsive students.

In a clinical study conducted at Columbia University, it was also discovered that students, scientifically taught to reduce their test anxiety, improved their performance on both IQ and creativity tests.

The performance-boosting effect of reducing excess stress is supported by a bedrock foundation of studies spanning decades.

---

5. What is your RQ ? Take the test.

Your relax-a-bility quotient or RQ, is simply how well you can relax when it counts the most, under challenging circumstances. You will enjoy the personal, professional and health benefits of being able to relax by increasing your relax-a-bility. Following are the "to do's" of relax-a-bility. Take the brief quiz on page 32 to determine your RQ. The more "yes'es" you have, the higher your RQ. The higher your RQ the longer and better you will probably live, if you also maintain a healthy lifestyle.

6. You have to slow down to achieve your best.

According to world-class artist, Bob Timberlake, you have to slow down from the rapid pace of life to achieve your best. Anyone interested in performing his or her best, even at a world-class level, must learn to relax suggests internationally-famous artist, Bob Timberlake (p. 1, Spring 2002).

Mr. Timberlake's work is so outstanding that one of his paintings became a U.S. postage stamp. Mr. Timberlake is held in such high esteem internationally, that the First Flight Centennial Society has commissioned him to serve as the official artist for the Wright Brothers' commemorative flight painting. His painting of the historical Wright Brothers' first flight on December 17, 1903, will be available around the time of the centennial celebration the week of December 13-17, 2003, at Kitty Hawk, N.C.

To summarize the "need to relax to succeed," Mr. Timberlake said, "Out of necessity, you have to slow down from the rapid pace of life . . ." (p. 1).

Bob Timberlake's surprise visit: A lesson learned by Bob and Delia.

Bob and Delia were visiting one of the largest "upscale" furniture stores in the world. A good friend of Delia's was the top salesperson at this fantastic furniture store. This friend let Bob and Delia roam around the store, after hours. He assumed Bob and Delia would not need supervision because they were both over twenty-one. Bob and Delia came upon a new line of furniture by their favorite and world-famous artist, Mr. Timberlake.

Bob, quickly tiring from shopping (as usual), looked for the first "display bed" on the fifth floor of the furniture store. Resting on the top of the display model of the bed Bob said to Delia, "Why don't you put your feet up for a minute and rest on this bed with me?" And by the way, isn't this part of the brand new Timberlake Collection?

Both Bob and Delia were lying back on this bed talking in a low tone. Delia said, "Isn't this Timberlake line great?"

Bob and Delia heard a third, deep, calm voice saying, "I am glad you approve." It was the artist himself, standing at the foot of the bed.

Possible lesson to be learned: "Don't say anything unkind in public, you never know who is listening."

Now let's take a look at your relax-ability, or your relaxation quotient if you will. The more "yes'es" you have the better. A key to success in any field is the ability to show grace under pressure.

YOU HAVE A HIGH RQ (RELAX-A-BILITY QUOTIENT)

1. If you maintain a positive, can-do attitude, even on Mondays, and you usually do not complain much. [YES] [NO]

2. If you look forward to enjoying healthy pleasures daily. [YES] [NO]

3. If you generally feel in control of your life and trust that the future will turn out positively. [YES] [NO]

4. If you worry little, but work a lot, to patiently solve problems without feeling overwhelmed or impatient. [YES] [NO]

5. If you can relax enough under pressure to fully concentrate on what you are doing (phone calls, public speaking, taking tests, conflict, deadlines, and evaluations). [YES] [NO]

6. If you can accept, act and adjust appropriately to rudeness, mistakes, conflict, criticism and major changes. [YES] [NO]

7. If you know how and when to vent pent-up stress, resentment and anger (not ranting/raving at bad drivers, not unleashing fury at innocent loved ones, pets, etc.) [YES] [NO]

8. If you sleep with ease and generally feel energetic. [YES] [NO]

9. If you are generally headache/stomachache free. [YES] [NO]

10. If you can self-calm when faced with frustration, frenzy, or fear, using humor to keep your cool. [YES] [NO]

11. If you can fully live separate personal/professional lives, not dragging shop talk home. [YES] [NO]

12. If you can "get-ready, get-set, and flow," powering-up your "second wind" to flexibly meet surprises and challenges. [YES] [NO]

What your RQ score means

Only Mother Teresa would probably score perfect on this test. A score of 10 "yes'es" on your RQ test is excellent, the same score the famous Dr. Richard Rahe obtained at the 1997 World Congress on Stress in Switzerland. Your "no" responses are merely relaxation targets to aim at, one at a time, for a few weeks, until you can relax under these events. Improving your RQ requires you to work at "taking it easy," which you may have to actually learn. Suggestions in this book are designed to coach you into "taking it easy." Having a high RQ is simply the ability to enjoy complete "head rest" momentarily so you feel rested and recharged at will. Relax-a-bility is a hallmark of the happy, healthy and successful.

SUMMARY

In this chapter we looked at what an RQ is, why it is important to improving performance, and how panic can shift you from high performing to low performing mode. How having a stable RQ can affect your useable IQ under pressure was also explored. You found out that 20% of the workforce will have a low RQ, being irritable and even nasty. Finally you were given the opportunity to take an RQ test yourself. The higher your RQ, the better you are able to relax under pressure. One of the top artists in the country, Bob Timberlake, said about the need to relax to succeed " . . . out of necessity [to be an artist], you have to slow down the pace of life."

The world-record holder for the highest IQ, Marilyn vos Savant, says that the best cure for performance anxiety is a little relaxation or, in other words, cultivating a high RQ. The next chapter looks at possible stress symptoms and how you may need to slow down before you get pulled over (by your doctor).

FOR FURTHER READING

Goleman, D. (1995). *Emotional intelligence.* New York City: Bantam Books.

Timberlake, B. (Spring & Summer, 2002). Bob Timberlake selected as artist for First Flight Centennial Society. *Bob Timberlake Gallery News*. 25, 1, p. 1.

Vos Savant, Marilyn. (2001). "Ask Marilyn." *Parade,* 2-4, 15. Used by permission of *Parade* Magazine.

3

ARE YOU SPEEDING?

GAUGES ON YOUR DASHBOARD

*For lasting "in-depth" change you must **know** yourself, **motivate** yourself and **commit** yourself.*

Let's look at different ways of measuring your stress. We'll go from looking at individual stress symptoms to stress management fitness to a survey which looks at similarities and differences between men and women with regard to stress. The seven main topics of this chapter are:

- Are you speeding? Take the ISR (Inventory of Stress Responses) before you get pulled over.
- "Squeaky-Wheel," "Old Faithful," "Mt. St. Helens," "Paddling Duck" — What's your stress-style?
- Gauging your stress-management fitness.
- What are your stress triggers? A short survey.
- For the purists or test anxious. Buros *Fourteenth Mental Measurement Yearbook* — The ultimate authority on tests.
- And the stress survey says . . . What 500 adults say about causes, costs and cures for stress.
- Sex and stress: Males tend to respond to anxiety with aggression, females with compassion.

1. Are you speeding? Take the ISR (Inventory of Stress Responses) before you get pulled over.

To keep your car on the road, you occasionally glance at your dashboard gauges. Likewise, to keep yourself on the stress-control road, you need to glance at gauges to see whether you're running too fast, too hot, or just plain running on empty. Knowing that you may be overreacting can benefit you in terms of your relationships, your job performance and your health. Taking the following brief ISR will help you gauge whether you are running hot or too fast.

ISR (Inventory of Stress Responses, developed 1997, Switzerland, World Congress on Stress)

Dr. Ronald L. Rubenzer ©

Always see your health professional for suspected emotional difficulties. Many physical problems present themselves with emotional symptoms.

Simply answer YES if any part of each question applies to you. Add up the number of YES answers, and place this score in the space provided. See the end of the inventory for the meaning of your YES score.

If you feel too pressed for time to take this survey, you REALLY need stress management!

1. Do you often feel angry, impatient or aggravated at yourself or others? EXAMPLES: You blame, complain, nag, boss, argue a lot or have anger hangovers (stay mad overnight, hold grudges). [YES] [NO]

2. Do you usually get very upset when you have to wait for things or people? EXAMPLES: You are impatient standing in line, waiting at stop signals; You often interrupt or finish people's sentences, complete their work or become quite upset when people are late. [YES] [NO]

3. Do you expect others or yourself to do everything perfectly? EXAMPLES: You get uptight when things don't go as planned or have a lot of regrets about bad mistakes ("You should have done better"; "Why didn't you?"). You never seem to get things "clean enough," organized or planned enough. [YES] [NO]

4. Do you often feel "pushed around" by life, overwhelmed by all you have to do? EXAMPLES: I have to do everything, everyone else tells you what to do, or you never have enough time to catch up. [YES] [NO]

5. Do you like to do most things fast? EXAMPLES: You usually finish eating before everyone else, like to drive fast, or are very interested in taking shortcuts to get things done. You are almost always early for things. [YES] [NO]

6. Do you often have sweaty palms, headaches/stomachaches, irregularity, heart palpitations, shortness of breath, vague pains or feel tired? EXAMPLE: You've had an exam revealing no medical reason for your complaints. [YES] [NO]

7. Do you worry a lot about things that often turn out OK? EXAMPLES: Most of your fears are exaggerated or never happen; You spend sleepless nights worrying. [YES] [NO]

8. Do you often make mistakes, forget or lose things because you're so busy? EXAMPLES: You're accident prone, clumsy, or feel your

memory is not as good as it used to be. [YES] [NO]

9. Do you binge when under pressure? EXAMPLES: You overdo one or more of the following: eating, smoking, drinking, sleeping, watching TV, shopping, talking on the phone, gossiping. [YES] [NO]

10. Do you put off things or avoid certain situations? EXAMPLES: You're afraid you'll be embarrassed or you'll panic under pressure. You get very nervous over such things as math, tests, being evaluated by your boss, working with computers, public speaking, crowds, high places, making phone calls. [YES] [NO]

11. Do you have nervous habits? EXAMPLES: You chew your nails, clear your throat, have tightly clenched fists, lock your legs and arms. You run your hands through your hair a lot, walk very fast, gesture a lot when talking, sigh, frown, or clench your teeth. [YES] [NO]

12. Do you feel you are in a rut or are just generally frustrated? EXAMPLES: You feel bored with the same "old routine," experience little joy or excitement in life. [YES] [NO]

Total YES score _____

What your ISR (Inventory of Stress Responses) YES score means. *This survey was designed to look at symptoms only and should not be used as a clinical instrument. See your mental-health professional for clinical assessment using DSM-IV criteria or a validated, reliable scientific instrument.(e.g. State-Trait-Anxiety Inventory). The higher your YES score, the more life's pressures are getting to you. The lower your YES score, the better you are at handling your stress. Stress management helps you lower your unpleasant stress reactions so you'll enjoy life more. Only Mother Teresa would probably have a score of no "yes'es." The fictional, funny sheriff from Mayberry R.F.D., Barney Fife, would be a good example of someone with a YES score on the ISR of 12. The average score is about 9. As in golf, you should aim to have a lower score. Most importantly, don't stress-out over your stress score.*

Why should you check with your doctor if you have many stress reactions?

The reason for checking with your doctor is that some, non-life-threatening, but medically treatable problems show themselves through stress symptoms. The "yuppie flu" or chronic fatigue syndrome (CFS) mimics many stress signals such as problems with: memory, sleep, night sweats, panic, and irritable bowel syndrome. Although avoiding stress is a recommended treatment for CFS, some normally stress-relieving activities such as exercise may actually worsen CFS. Even ADD or ADHD that has many symptoms like an anxiety disorder (fidgeting, poor attention, etc.) could be misdiagnosed as an anxiety disorder or vice-versa. Treating an anxiety disorder with ADHD prescriptions will make the anxiety disorder even worse. ADD or ADHD occurs only in about 6% of the population, but anxiety disorders are much more common.

If you would like to see if you exhibit stress-induced ADHD symptoms, ask your local mental-health professional for the scale by Conners'-CAARS-Self-Report: Screening Version (CAARS-S:SV) Adult Rating Scales 1999. This self-report scale asks 30 easy-to-understand questions. The best cure for distress-distraction consists of regular exercise and time management.

"He is here but not all there."
The bottom line — distress distracts.

As usual Bob was rushing around in his hurried state, doing ten things at once, but doing none of them well. Bob justified his scattered behavior saying, "I am multi-tasking." Even Einstein claimed he could only do one thing well at a time. When Bob was asked by a close friend how he felt that day, Bob said,

"I am here." His close friend cleverly responded by saying, "You're here but you're not all there." The obvious implication being that Bob's mind was someplace else, and not on the task at hand. Many of the symptoms of ADHD (distractibility, hyperactivity, impulsivity) are actually transient stress states.

2. "Squeaky-Wheel," "Old Faithful," "Mt. St. Helens," "Paddling Duck" — What's your stress-style?

Knowledge lets me do by choice what others do out of fear. -Aristotle

Four response styles. Which one is best?

How we respond to stress can be characterized in four ways: the "Squeaky-Wheel," "Old Faithful," "Mt. Saint Helens," and the "Paddling Duck." The "squeaky-whining wheel" type relieves stress at your expense by constantly whining and complaining, no matter what. Like a subway train, if they're moving they're screeching. These often angry, hair-trigger tempered, "Squeaky-Wheelers" are stress carriers. They carelessly unload their stress on others.

Some individuals are like the "Old Faithful Geyser" of Yellowstone, which blows off steam, regularly and safely. By contrast, "Mt. St. Helens" reactors explode with a volcanic reaction of epic proportions. When the last straw is put on this person's back, he might even go through a period of what seems like temporary insanity. This person may just say, "I quit," walking off the job or dramatically leaving the scene. This type is very rare.

Another type of stress-style is when we feel like a "Paddling Duck," appearing calm and even on the surface, but frantically paddling underneath.

The faith-fueled ride is more like "rowing your boat, gently down the stream;" the fear-driven ride is more like a tortuous "tilt-a-whirl" (wildly up and down, backward and forwards, spinning round and round).

Relaxers vs. stress carriers

The "Old-Faithful" response style may be the healthiest and most sociable, because blowing off steam harmlessly and regularly provides needed relief and a sense of self-control over stress. These people don't get to the point where they can't control their stress. They go through regular periods of release and renewal. Runners and other exercisers may fall into this group. Most of us may be "Paddling Duck" types. Both "Old Faithful Geyser" and "Paddling Duck" types may have a relaxing effect on others. "Squeaky-Wheelers" and "Mt. St. Helens" types are stress carriers because they can infect others with their stress.

You can control only how you respond in situations, and not how others act. Give yourself credit for doing your best, no matter what the other person may do. If you are dealing with adults, in a nonwork situation, it is not your responsibility to control their behavior, even if you wanted to. Children, however, often need and respond to adult control. It is your responsibility to control your stress responses that may indirectly win you respect, or a "reputation." Even Napoleon recognized the need to start with self-control, when he said you must control yourself before you can control the world.

---

3. Gauging your stress-management fitness.

Like your fuel gauge, the following Stress-Management Fitness scale measures your "coping" fuel supply. The steeper or faster your daily activity road is, the more fuel you will need to make it. Your car has an optimal speed that lets you cruise with minimum use of fuel. Maintaining your stress-management fitness level will put you in cruise control, providing you with smooth, available energy when you need it. You may feel as if you are running on empty, but the survey following will provide you with practical "what-to-do-tomorrow" tips to renew your energy reserves.

SELF-QUIZ STRESS-MANAGEMENT FITNESS
Dr. Ronald L. Rubenzer©

Feeling frazzled? Rate your personal stress-management fitness. Add up your YES answers. See the end of the inventory for the meaning of your score.

1. Do you exercise at your training rate (SEE YOUR DOCTOR!) for twenty minutes at least three times weekly? [YES] [NO]
2. Do you practice a ten-minute relaxation method three times weekly? [YES] [NO]
3. Do you limit caffeine drinks (two or less servings per day, including tea)? [YES] [NO]
4. Are all your medications caffeine and stimulant free? (check with your doctor, read labels) [YES] [NO]
5. Do you limit alcoholic beverages (two or less drinks per day, including beer)? [YES] [NO]
6. Do you get at least seven hours of sleep-per night? [YES] [NO]
7. Do you read or listen to motivational material daily? [YES] [NO]
8. Is most of your self-talk/ communication with others positive and encouraging? [YES] [NO]
9. Do you limit your bad news reviews to summaries and watch few, if any, violent/negative TV shows weekly? [YES] [NO]
10. Have you quit smoking or have never smoked? [YES] [NO]
11. Do you practice "time management" (goal setting, organizing your work)? [YES] [NO]
12. Do you have one half-hour personal free-time daily? [YES] [NO]
13. Are you assertive? (Do you know how to make your needs known in a positive manner? Can you deal with difficult people effectively if required?) [YES] [NO]
14. Do you have a good sense of humor (above and beyond sarcasm)? [YES] [NO]
15. Do you have good communication skills? [YES] [NO]

Total YES score _____

The higher your YES score, the more stress-management fit you are. Your NO responses point to areas you can develop to turn your unpleasant "nervous energy" into powerful, productive energy.

4. What are your stress triggers?

To personalize your stress-management prescription, take a few minutes to complete a short Stress Trigger Inventory. This inventory will pinpoint what triggers your overreactivity at work and at home. As stated earlier, knowing what baggage is throwing you off balance is the most important step in regaining your balance.

STRESS TRIGGER INVENTORY

"IT MAKES ME SO MAD!!!

"THAT REALLY TICKS ME OFF!"

"I GET SO EXCITED."

These familiar phrases show the power of our "learned" negative and positive stress reactions. Although our stress reactions seem like automatic "knee-jerk" reflexes, we LEARNED HOW TO REACT to most situations. Consider being pulled over by a policeman. No matter how you feel emotionally you try to act civilly even though you don't feel civil at all. To help you decide if your "conditioned stress reactions" are helpful, neutral or harmful, simply conduct this Stress Trigger Inventory. Every stress reaction (pleasant or unpleasant) costs you mental and physical energy. Constant overreacting strains your body and mind, resulting in "pain in the neck," fatigue, hampered performance, exhaustion and even illness.

1) **LIST** — YOUR TOP 2 OR 3 STRESS TRIGGERS that usually make you feel "stressed" (e.g., nervous, frustrated, angry, threatened, or overwhelmed). Fill in your answers on a piece of scrap paper.

STRESS TRIGGER EXAMPLE : Dealing with those other jerks' bad driving on the way to work.

2) **STATE** — HOW YOU REACT, thoughts, feelings or actions. (e.g., "expressive" language, clenched fists, arguing, taking it out on others, worrying, daydreaming, headaches, holding grudges, stress-eating/drinking).

HOW I REACT EXAMPLE: I almost always get mad when someone pulls in front of me in traffic. I shout "heated terms" even though they can't possibly hear me.

3) **ESTIMATE** — COSTS (consequences) of your stress reactions. Common consequences include: feeling upset/tired, making mistakes, getting speeding tickets, having trouble concentrating at work, weight

gain from stress-eating, getting headaches/stomachaches, developing a "bad attitude," arguing with co-workers, gossiping/spreading rumors, self-medication with caffeine/alcohol, taking it out on others.

COSTS OF MY STRESS REACTIONS EXAMPLE:

I come to work upset and feel in a bad mood even before I start work. Sometimes I overreact to someone reminding me "again" about that project deadline. I have another cup of coffee and an extra doughnut to "soothe my nerves" and to reward myself for putting up with those jerks on the road. I dread the drive home all day.

Take a breather here. This is only a survey! Don't let thinking about your stressors upset you. Remain calm. You are in control! Think of your stress triggers as indicator lights on your car. Don't panic. Just fix them.

For now only concentrate on tackling two or three stress triggers. It takes time to change lifestyles or workstyles. You will use these target stress triggers in your stress-management plan.

Think also about the survey as it relates to being on the job and your personal life. For example, top stress triggers in your personal life might include money worries; not having enough time; breaking an old habit (e.g., quit smoking); starting a new habit (dieting, improving attitude, time management); sliding back into bad habits; aging or being "too young;" being overweight/out of shape; educational advancement; pessimism; single adulthood; social life, relationships; lack of goals or meaningful accomplishments; health complaints/worries; frustrating gap between what you know you should do and what you are doing; perfectionism (never being satisfied with your own achievements); fear of not doing enough or missing out. Costs of how you react on the job could include disrupting good working relationships; missed opportunities due to resisting learning new skills; coming home upset; worrying about uncompleted things due to procrastination; guilt; having to take work home that could have been completed at work; disappointing evaluations, sick days due to flu, colds, irritable bowel syndrome (IBS), etc.

---

5. For the purists or test anxious: Buros *Fourteenth Mental Measurement Yearbook* — the ultimate authority on tests.

Knowledge can relieve stress, especially for the test anxious. An objective, respected source of test reviews is available.

The most scientific assessment of tests of all types, including any tests dealing with anxiety, is offered online by the Buros Institute. They have been reviewing tests for over 60 years. So before you buy or take any kind of test, just click on to <http://www.unl.edu/buros/>. At your library, just ask in the reference department for the Buros *Fourteenth Mental Measurement Yearbook* (MMY).

---

6. And the stress survey says.

To evaluate stress needs, the author conducted a self-report survey of several hundred individuals. Over five-hundred adults were given a stress survey to answer three questions: What are stressors shared by men and women? What stressors are unique to each sex? How do men and women handle stress? These questions are important because it is comforting to know that you are only human if your worries are shared.

Jobs and shortage of time and money surfaced as major stressors for both men and women. The gender gap widens beyond these three life-stressors.

Stresses between the sexes

Women were more likely to be concerned about childcare and dual career pressures than men. Women also expressed a need for more sharing of home chores and better communication from men. Men care about children, women care for children. Men were more likely than women to be stressed as a result of competition at work and on the road.

In handling stress, most people said they either read or watched TV to relax. Walking and yard work came in next as stress relievers. To relax, women were more likely to engage in soothing, noncompetitive activities such as bathing, crafts or naps. Men were more competitive in how they relieved stress, engaging in sports, watching sports or driving a car, for example.

---

7. Sex and stress: Males tend to respond to anxiety with aggression, females with compassion.

Males are more likely to respond to anxiety by becoming hostile or aggressive because testosterone is pumped out during the stress response. Testosterone flooding for males is in addition to the production of cortisol and adrenaline. Both men and women pump out cortisol and adrenaline under stress, but women are much more likely to comfort and support under stress. Males, because of the extra stress hormone, testosterone, may become more aggressive under the same circumstances.

You may ask, so what if there are differences in what stresses out men and women? Insensitivity to what stresses out the opposite sex can create real stressors that have a life of their own. Workaholics may give their all at work, coming home battle-fatigued and needing to quietly retreat. Others may find communicating refreshing and energizing after work. Much relationship stress can be avoided just by being aware that stress is often belief-based, that is, stress is based on what we believe is stressful, whether anyone else thinks so or not. Thus if you think you are stressed, you are stressed. Considering that someone else could be stressed out by something that we don't mind or even enjoy, is a first step in reducing relationship stress.

K.P. as both pleasure and punishment

Kitchen policing (K.P.) is an objective event, yet the same exact activity can be used to create or cure stress. Bob, who went to private schools and eventually the military, was taught that kitchen work (K.P) was punishment for bad behavior. But those brought up "playing house and garden" were taught that kitchen and yard work were pleasurable rewards. So be sure that before you "reward" someone with the chance to do kitchen work, that they also feel it is a pleasure, not just a punishment for bad behavior. It is a major mistake (but human nature) to assume that everyone thinks like we do.

By the way, the author of the famous "Harry Potter" series of books said she did not do serious housework for four years while she was writing her book, according to a TV special in March of 2002.

Closing the communication gap

Two eye-opening books in demystifying the opposite sex are: *You Just Don't Understand*, by Dr. Deborah Tannen (Ballentine Books, 1990) for men and women; and, *Ten Stupid Things Women Do to Mess Up Their Lives,* by Dr. Laura Schlessinger (Villard Books, 1993) for women.

For the "conversationally impaired"

Don Gabor, professional speaker, offers solid tips on how to become a conversationalist and overcome fear of speaking. His book, *Speaking Our Mind in 101 Difficult Situations,* offers numerous conversation starters. (Stonesong Press, Fireside/Simon & Schuster, 1994).

SUMMARY

For lasting "in-depth" change, you must *know* yourself, *motivate* yourself and *commit* yourself.

In this chapter, we looked at how to know if you are having an excessively high level of stress symptoms by taking the quick ISR (Inventory of Stress Responses). We explored four different stress styles and examined why some people are stress carriers. We assessed your stress-management fitness through the Self-Quiz Stress-Management Fitness. In the Stress Trigger Inventory we looked at what pushes your buttons. Information on the best test review authority, Buros, was provided along with a website address for this clearininghouse for all types of tests, including stress tests. To diagnose basic stressors, a stress survey of men and women was conducted. Suggestions for dealing with some of the differences between the sexes were reviewed. Secretion of an additional stress hormone for men, testosterone, provides an explanation (not an excuse) for why males tend to respond to anxiety with aggression. This may be why males enjoy the chance to observe and/or participate in sports, a socialized form of aggression. The next chapter deals with the number one stressor listed in the above survey — job-stress.

FOR FURTHER READING

Bing, S. (2000). *What would Machiavelli do? The ends justify the meanness.* New York: Harper Business.

Bing, S. (1992). *Crazy bosses: spotting them, serving them.* New York: Morrow.

Buros Institute. (2001). *The fourteenth mental measurements yearbook* (MMY). Lincoln, Nebraska, University of Nebraska Press. p. 1530.

Conners, K.C., Drew, E., & Sparrow, E. (1999). *Conners' adult ADHD rating scales* (CAARS). North Tonawanda, New York: Multi-Health Systems. 1-800-456-3003.

Freeze-Framer™ emotional management enhancer. Call Heartmath, 1-800-372-3100 or email: <info@heartmath.com>.

Interfax Daily, (2001, March 2). Vol. WZ1V7951, Call (336) 397-0000 for a Free-Daily humor fax. Baton Rouge, LA.

Lancaster, H. (1992). *The Wall Street Journal,* Tips for workplace humor: See Lehmann, M.B., *The Irwin guide to using the Wall Street Journal - 6th Edition.* New York: McGraw Hill.

Peale, Norman Vincent (1992). *The power of positive thinking.* New York: Simon & Schuster.

Waitely, D. & Reni, L.W, (1985). *Joy of working, The 30 day system to success, wealth & happiness on the job.* New York, NY: Dodd Mead.

Weil, M., & Rosen, L. (1997). *TechnoStress: coping with technology @ work @ home @ play.* New York: J. Wiley.

4

Industrial-Strength Stress Control

An Insider's View from the World Trade Center

Many would rather quit than fight.

Let's explore some reasons why we need industrial-strength stress management at work and measure our job-stress management habits through these topics.

- An insider's view from the World Trade Center about workaholism.
- Many would rather quit than fight: 79% have been treated rudely; 42% verbally abused; 29% screaming mad; 23% brought to tears; 10% witnessed physical violence.
- The "job-ready" get more out of work, while the "job-stressed" get out of work more. It has been estimated that up to 5% of absences are due to stress. Workers who are appreciated and prepared will naturally be on the job more if they are finding satisfaction and success with the work.
- Staff infections — how negative emotional contagion infects the whole staff.
- "Anti-trust" corporate culture triggers work slowdown.
- The mean shall inherit the earth: Welcome to Business 101.
- Effective job-stress management habits — rate yourself.

1. An insider's view from the World Trade Center about workaholism.

After three challenging years of doctoral work at New York City's Columbia University, Bob finally heard the message, "You have been accepted at the World Trade Center for an internship." He was even further thrilled when he heard, "You will be doing your advanced administrative internship with the New York State Department of Public Instruction on the 54th floor of the WTC." The joy Bob felt was like a high school football player being drafted into the NFL. Bob had now entered the big league in his field. Everyone was "high energy" at the WTC, and Bob had ten cups a coffee per day, just to keep from being trampled by the workaholic stampede. The pace was so fast that people were even impatient with how slowly the elevators climbed up the 100 plus floors. The solution was installing an express elevator to "rocket" peo-

ple up to the fortieth floor, non-stop, at what seemed to be a hundred miles per hour. You almost needed a safety belt to hold you in place during the express elevator ride. Bob would often have lunch at former "Windows on the World" at nearly the top of the WTC. In awe he would look out over the Hudson River and think to himself, "These twin towers will last as long as the Egyptian pyramids." Most people shared his opinion. The WTC was so tall that when you dropped paper towels down the trash shutes you could hear the wind howl. Some said that the twin towers swayed almost a foot on windy days, but the structure of the building was ingeniously engineered to have some give in it. Bob was so proud of his WTC office that he took his wife there several years after his internship was completed.

Fortunately for Bob, his career path took him away from what he thought was the high point of his work life. Having moved to the South, he was stunned when the TV showed the North, then the South Twin Towers slammed into by 767 airliners on 9/11/01. He knew some of his friends and colleagues there were vaporized in Tower 2 at the Office of Urban School Services. Every bit of work he had "slaved over" during his time at Tower 2 of the WTC was turned to dust, as if he had never been at the twin towers at all.*

A lesson to be learned? Perhaps to be careful what you wish for, because Bob often regretted not having taken the job that was his at the WTC. His obsession with work and achievement was greatly toned-down when he saw the "workaholic's temple" destroyed, and with it many of his youthful accomplishments and "driven" memories.

*Excerpt from Grace Lacy's (May, 1979). *"Developing Defensible Differentiated Programs for the Gifted and Talented."* The Education Department of New York; Office of Urban School Services, 2 World Trade Center.

---

2. Many would rather quit than fight: 79% of workers have been treated rudely; 42% verbally abused; 29% screaming mad; 23% brought to tears; 10% witnessed physical violence.

If rude people are stressing you out more than ever, relax, because you are only human.

Rudeness is rampant at work according to a 2002 poll, and much worse than it was a decade ago. The best corporate anti-rudeness program in the United States is provided by SAS, an extremely successful company in Cary, NC. This innovative program helps find and direct rude people to a psychologist for counseling, according to John Dornan, SAS's spokesman. He can be reached at (919) 677-8000.

Loud, annoying and blaming words will eventually be returned in kind

A recent, 2001 Opinion Research Corporation International survey revealed these alarming statistics quoted above. The study researchers, Dr. Robert E. Hales and Diane Hales, revealed that workers are beginning to act out more by pounding their fists on desks, slamming doors, swearing in their workspaces and even stealing other workers' food from the refrigerator. Some workers, feeling powerless and overwhelmed, will even start fighting back. In work wars, the employee may win a battle, but never the war. Instead he or she ends up being cited with insubordination and getting fired.

3. The "job-ready" get more out of work, while the "job-stressed" get out of work more.

Many sick days are mental-health days, when workers feel they just can't take it anymore. Also, absences due to diarrhea from irritable bowel syndrome are increasing. It has been estimated that up to 5% of absences are due to stress. Workers who are appreciated and prepared will naturally be on the job more if they are finding satisfaction and success with the work. To "be nimble" (as in Jack be nimble, Jack be quick) is the key to job survival.

You can run with the lemmings without jumping over the cliff with them.

Bob felt great after his weekend at the beach. He vowed that the main jerk at work would not get under his skin and spoil his mood. By 8:30 A.M. Monday, Bob had forgotten about the refreshing weekend he had had, and was feeling tense and uptight already. He had inadvertently stepped into "whine country" where colleagues were complaining about everything. Going back to his cubicle he reminded himself of the great weekend he had had, which helped him reset his attitude.

4. Staff infections — how negative emotional contagion infects the whole staff.

Have you ever wondered why you can feel on "top of the world" and then suddenly feel irritated or frustrated when "exposed" to certain situations? Negative emotions from others are contagious, and within 30 minutes of "exposure" we can become infected with negative attitudes. Difficult people often have difficult lives, plagued by fear, frustration, frenzy or fatigue. These people are often rude, rushed, and critical.

Learning to identify and deal with difficult people through assertiveness training is extremely important to your mental health. If you know you are going to be read the "riot act," at least you can put your "riot act" gear on ahead of time.

An entire staff can be spoiled by one "bad" apple with a negative attitude. A highly negative person is one who brightens the room by leaving it. Unfortunately these people are present in ever-growing numbers at work, on the road and in our lives. But with industrial-strength stress control we can avoid or reduce the impact "infections" have on us personally. The Columbia University School of Business motto was "unwarranted optimism" (that is you have a 40/60 chance of being successful). This has been the core of many successful businesses. The practice of "focused energy" is also a mainstay of Columbia. A good test of one's ability to focus energy when needed is to try to study while riding a subway in NYC.

Rising above "emotional ambushing"

"Emotional ambushing" is simply any unexpected surprise that registers on your stress Richter Scale. You are irritated or rocked momentarily. "Emotional ambushing" is any real or imagined threat or change that is thrust upon you from "out of the blue." On the job, "emotional ambushing" includes news about downsizing, rightsizing, major increases or decreases in job responsibility/scheduling, conflicts, or criticism. Being "emotionally ambushed" in even small doses can have cumulative effects if we don't rescue ourselves regularly.

In business there is no such thing as an even keel. The one who can regain his or her balance the best after the boat is rocked will win success and satisfaction. Furthermore, we often drag home the effects of "emotional ambushes," extending our workday far beyond what is needed. A common but painful type of ambush is when someone is called an idiot. Dr. Deborah Tannen, a communications expert and author of *You Just Don't Understand* (Ballentine Books, 1990), suggests that you can fight rudeness with humor. The following piece pulled out of cyberspace, may be of some guidance.

What to say the next time someone calls you an idiot?

To be technical, when you see the title of a book such as, *Quantum Physics for Complete Idiots,* by Professor Martin Hornrimmer (Greensboro, NC. *News and Record,* 4-10-02, B-1), it is a joke. The distasteful term, "idiot," according to *Webster's New Twentieth Century Dictionary* (1979), p. 903, lower left-hand corner), actually means an adult with an IQ of 24 or below, who will only peak mentally to a two-year-old level as an adult. I do believe we can use the term "Densa candidate" which is less offensive, as in, "I'll bet you're a good 'Densa candidate,'" (which is completely opposite of the esteemed society of people with IQ's of 130 [98th%] and above. So next time you see a book that has the term idiot in it (such as *Idiot's Guide to Stress Management*), you will know it's a trick, and in bad taste. And next time someone calls you an idiot (or you call yourself an idiot) you know it's just not true and you can correct them. You can say with confidence, "Oh contraire my friend, I know I am not an idiot. I beg to differ with you even further. I can't be an idiot because I can understand your sarcastic message AND I can even read. Most tabloids are written at the fifth-grade reading level, and I was able to read tabloids in my twenties . . . so there. Be careful next time you call someone an idiot!!"

---

5. "Anti-trust" corporate culture triggers work slow down.

Workers who are not trusted slow down because of irrational fears of making mistakes, or they do the absolute minimum out of resentment. Many times micro-management turns into micro-scopic management where one's performance is put under the electron microscope on a faultfinding mission. Despair eventually overcomes hope to ever hit the mark of excellence. The saying, success breeds contempt, does have merit, so if you happen to be successful, keep it among loved ones and your fans.

Stress strangles productivity, according to a landmark study conducted by Professor Christine Pearson of the University of North Carolina School of Business. Individuals who feel targeted for incivility spend less time working and are less committed to the job. Lowering job-stress will raise productivity and boost the bottom line.

Under stress, most individuals report irritability, followed by worry, headaches and insomnia. Clearly, one cannot perform well when burdened by these symptoms. Bottom line performance and reputation of an organization are obviously impacted by irritable, tired employees who may be plagued by stress-related headaches and insomnia.

Proven benefits of job-stress management

As opposed to the "job-stressed," the "job-ready" are better at accepting change, cooperating, communicating and resolving conflicts. The "job-ready" are less likely to be overwhelmed by overwork, and are less prone to overreact because they can concentrate more on thinking rather than being distracted by negative feelings generated by stress. The "job-ready" get more job satisfaction, while the "job-stressed" have more sick days. The "job-stressed" are absent more and are more absent-minded.

---

6. The mean shall inherit the earth: Welcome to Business 101.

It is a business fact, "The mean shall inherit the earth," according to Stanley Bing, a writer for *Fortune* magazine. He found that top survivors in the business environment have two major traits in common. They are very strategic, always planning ahead, and they are amoral (not immoral). They care little about softer human emotions (kindness, friendliness, do unto others...) and only care about how they can further themselves by any means that is not illegal.

In the long run, on the average, it is better to be positive than negative.

The hurting and healing power of words

And words can never hurt me . . . Wrong!

Words wound. Words have the power to heal or hurt. Words transcend time and space. If you believe, "Words can never hurt me," you are exposing your "jugular vein" to those emotional vampires who are just waiting for a free lunch. These mosquitoes live off the lifeblood of others. These mean people have learned that one way to make you a bleeding heart is to use wounding words. The double-edged-sword they love to use is the "hired-fired" sword. But again, some folks are hardboiled or Teflon coated, and when they are told you're fired, they'll say, "Says who?"

Your immediate bloodline of 2,000 great grandparents, going back let's say 40,000 B.C, knew the "power of words" or symbolic communication. To get a grip on the power of words consider this — words are a major meaningful link to your ancestors. Your talking "Adam and Eve "great...grandparents" go back about 2,000 generations. A handprint in the ancient cave-man days loudly and clearly says to you personally, "Bob, your great, (add 2,000 greats here) Grandpa Leroy was here." If you wrote a single name for each of your immediate fore-bearers in your family *Bible* (births only), you would completely fill the first four pages of your family *Bible*. You would start with, "Our Adam and Eve Smith begat . . . Leroy who begat, Billy-Bob, who begat . . . who begat . . . Again, you would probably fill about four pages just with the "who-begats." If you are twenty now, having actually been born before the existence of the PC in 1980, only the last four "begats" or generations would take you back to your immediate Civil War great grandparents. (To trace back to the civil war military records regarding who served, contact <www.nara.gov/genealogy/civilwar.html> for the address of the National Archives in Washington. There is a small fee.)

The urge to use words is as biological as the urge to eat. We have a physical part of our brain called the language acquisition device (LAD) which makes us talk. This LAD in our brain, makes us babble, as infants, in all sounds of all languages. Each language group rewards (Let's say American English) only those sounds of that language group, so you narrow down the sounds you use. So, watch the words you use.

When someone says to you, "They're only words," then our greatest documents are only words: the *Bible*, *Koran*, Magna Carta, Declaration of Independence, Constitution, amendments to the Constitution, all laws, all religions and most sciences. The most life-changing words you will ever utter are, "I do."

The healing power of words, even only those by word-of-mouth

It has been speculated that even the Christian *New Testament* was preserved for at least a whole generation, only by word-of-mouth with nothing being committed to writing for nearly thirty years. Some historians believe that the first Gospels were only written down many years after Christ's death. It can be argued that few word-of-mouth accounts, such as the *New Testament*, have had more power to help and heal millions for the last hundred generations.

Corporate cruelty can backfire

Some administrative dinosaurs still use Theory X (Employees can't be trusted, must be punished and controlled, must want to live to work). Hopefully the next generation of administrators will apply the more effective Theory Y approach. To build and earn trust from workers, compliment them in public, but correct them in private.

When one uses a stick more than a carrot to motivate, employees will be thinking about two other things instead of working. If abused, workers will be constantly thinking how they can either take the stick away (sabotage, whistle blowing or just plain "going postal") or how they can avoid the stick (quitting). Under the thin disguise of corporate culture, which in some places is just a nicer way to say corporate cruelty, superiors berate subordinates in front of their peers, use threats of firing or try to rule by humiliation using such phrases as, "This is the worst report I have ever seen; you remind me of that crazy guy I had to fire; your work is the poorest of anyone's in the whole department; you are going downhill fast; you are not the man I hired, you are no spring chicken." If you were constantly getting comments like these, it would be well to save six months wages and start looking for another job. Sadly, some supervisors treat their pets more kindly than workers. When workers get fed up they start fighting back indirectly. Abused waiters put ingredients definitely not designed for consumption in people's soups. Angry workers often just wait for the chance to get even with their superiors. This author worked as welder in a factory. Disgruntled workers would often take ice-picks to deflate unfair supervisors' tires.

Rather than give up your humanity and personality to get ahead, you need to build yourself up so you can rise above, yet function in the business world that believes the "mean shall inherit the earth." Being in good shape will help you shake off the influence of the business world like a dog shaking off water. You can survive the business world if you are thick skinned but tenderhearted, as mentioned before. Bing's book, *"What would Machiavelli do?"*, is a "tongue-in-cheek," but accurate, view of how very thick skinned business types think. Hopefully you will never have to become amoral to survive the 21st century job scene, but at least you will be able to be more strategic, by learning how the other half thinks as detailed in Bing's book.

GE cutting the bottom ten percent

During the week of May 7, 2001, it was revealed that General Electric has adopted a policy to motivate employees. If you are performing at the bottom ten percent in your job, you are automatically fired. Needless to say, worrying about your performance may bring about the thing you are worried about — getting fired because of stress-induced mistakes, fatigue and irritability.

Forgiving the unforgivable, the most stressful, unnatural thing you will do

In nature it is estimated that every one out of a hundred of any animal will have brain damage, that is, faulty wiring. Likewise, there are those in our society who actually take pleasure in the pain they inflict. They may feel they can control people through fear, or possibly they just gain pleasure from other's pain. They want to be the feared little Hitlers. Avoiding these toxic people may be the best approach to avoiding the inborn stress of interacting with these damaged individuals. But if you cannot avoid these people, try to forgive them, even if they are unforgivable, and they don't want your pity or concern. In fact they may feel that forgiveness is a weakness. Using phrases, like "This meeting is really going to hurt," is a red flag to anyone of normal mind. Negative people will search obsessively for the dark cloud that may be suggested by the silver lining.

Negative people are just a "toxic waste of space."

---

7. Effective job-stress management habits — rate yourself.

By taking this brief "Job-Stress Management Habits Checklist," you can quickly access if you are doing your part in practicing habits known to reduce your job-stress and improving your effectiveness on the job.

EFFECTIVE JOB-STRESS MANAGEMENT HABITS CHECKLIST

Do you consistently?

1. Foster a "we attitude" rather than a "me attitude." [YES] [NO]
2. Know/do what your supervisor wants. [YES] [NO]
3. Encourage communication/trust. [YES] [NO]
4. Practice clutter management. [YES] [NO]
5. Employ consistent (daily, weekly) time management. [YES] [NO]
6. Walk at break/take legitimate breaks. [YES] [NO]

7. Use a relaxation technique (Wall Street professionals do)* [YES] [NO]
8. Deal with difficult people/conflict effectively. [YES] [NO]
9. Use problem solving/conflict resolution. [YES] [NO]
10. Engage in professional development. [YES] [NO]

GRADE YOURSELF (SIMPLY ADD UP YOUR YES SCORES)

A YES SCORE of 9-10 = GRADE A, Model employee, leader. A YES Score of 7-8 = GRADE B, Keep up the good work. A YES Score of 5-6 = GRADE C, Need improvement. A YES Score of 3-4 = GRADE D, Re-examine priorities. A YES Score of 0-2 = GRADE F, Retrain, get help.

*On February 7, 2001, CNN, with an audience of 22 million, recognized the *Freeze-Framer*™ program by HEARTMATH as so effective it significantly reduces stress in teachers, students, and even policemen. Call Heartmath, 1-800-372-3100 or email: <info@heartmath.com>. This enjoyable, but highly accurate and effective biofeedback product makes relaxation training fun and fast in almost any setting, (business, school, stress-control coaching setting or home).

SUMMARY

In this chapter we looked at important reasons why we need "industrial-strength" stress management on the job. A stark lesson about the futility of workaholism was taught with the destruction of the World Trade Center, where "Bob" worked as a youth.

The 21st century sources of job-stress are closely examined. A disappointing 79% feel that people are ruder than they were ten years ago. An alarming 25% of workers are constantly mad, 29% have screamed at co-workers, 23% have been brought to tears, 10% have actually witnessed physical violence. Many workers would rather quit than fight these incivilities. The job-satisfied get more out of work, while the "job-stressed" get out of work more (more absences). If they do stick with the job, they often gain weight, become insomniacs or even start fighting back. Stress contagion from other negative people is a primary cause for job-stress. Job-stress reduces our effectiveness. The best anti-rudeness program in the United States is featured in this chapter.

The "mean shall inherit the earth" in the business world is another strong reason why industrial-strength stress management is needed. Some top achievers are coldly strategic and amoral (not immoral). Under the heading, "And words can never hurt me," it is demonstrated how the "mean" can use the double-edged-sword of words to control employees (e.g., you're hired/fired). Also the healing power of words, even unwritten "words of mouth" can have tremendous healing power. Trying to forgive the unforgivable is briefly addressed. A survey was provided to help us identify whether we are doing our part to promote personal effectiveness that will reduce job-stress. This section covered important reasons why we need job-stress management. The next chapters will provide job-stress prescriptions.

FOR FURTHER READING

Hales, D., & Hales, R. (2001). "Is work driving you mad?" *Parade* Magazine 3. 18, pp. 8-9.

Houck, C. (2002, April). "Stand up to rudeness." *Good Housekeeping.* 98-101.

Interfax Daily, March 2, 2001, Vol. WZ1V7951, Call (336) 397-0000 for a free daily humor fax. Baton Rouge, LA. In Baton Rouge call 1-888-967-1720 or in North Carolina call 1-866-828-2424 for more information.

Peale, Norman Vincent, (1992). *The Power of positive thinking.* New York: Simon & Schuster.

Weil, M., & Rosen, L. (1997). *TechnoStress: coping with technology @ work @ home @ play.* New York: J. Wiley.

5

JOB-STRESS PRESCRIPTIONS

"WHEN UPSET HIT RESET"

Don't let anyone push your buttons, especially your panic button. When they hit your panic button, hit your "reset button."

"HIT RESET" TO AVOID A "STRESS-MESS": All Bob ever needed to know about stress he learned from his dog.

Bob felt confident that he had picked up a couple of stress-control tips by surviving the streets and schools of bustling New York City. On top of that, he even had the rare opportunity to study stress with all the clinical and diagnostic tools available at an Ivy League university. He had also taught courses on stress management, but he really didn't know about stress until he and Delia adopted a 70-pound standard poodle. Bob had bought this poodle as a security measure to protect Delia while he was away from home at night teaching.

What does having a giant standard poodle have to do with learning stress management? Charlotte, the poodle, taught Bob the basics of stress management, the hard way, through "stress-mess" therapy.

In the Big Apple, Bob quickly realized he'd be crushed into applesauce if he didn't out shout and out gesture others. Try getting a cab in New York City by using a normal tone of voice, with your hands at your sides. After living in highly energized New York City for several years, he moved South, and married Delia, a Southern girl. In the South, people, for the most part, were polite, using charming accents and low tones to very effectively converse. Although having been away from New York for years, Bob still shouted and waved his arms when communicating, often prompting people to ask, "Where are you from?" Bob did not know better, until Charlotte changed Bob's stress-charged behavior faster than any conventional therapy ever could.

Ranting and raving one hectic Monday, Bob was accusing everyone of having taken his car keys, because they weren't where he thought he had put them. He was "hypering" around as usual, getting ready for his long drive to work. (Remember, in NYC this behavior was normal, and actually "admired.") Brushing by Charlotte, Bob noticed that she was crouching with her tail between her legs. Next came the unpleasant duet of the "stress-

mess" projecting out of both ends of Charlotte at the same time. This set Bob off even more, since he was definitely going to be late, with a classroom of sixty college students waiting to take their final exam. He not only couldn't find his car keys, he now had to clean up the dog's "stress-mess" and call the vet. His wife had already left for work so she couldn't help during this emergency.

Bob first cleaned up Charlotte's "stress-mess" and found his keys (where he had actually put them). Next he called the college and instructed his assistant to have his students read the next chapter in the stress-management book and "relax" until he could arrive. He loaded nervous Charlotte into their car, hauled her to the vet, and said, "I'll bet she's been drinking out of the toilet again." At day's end, Delia picked up Charlotte from the vet, who reported that no physical reason for their dog's getting sick could be found.

The following Saturday, Bob and Delia were looking forward to trying their new boat on the lake. They were meeting their equally excited friends at the lake. Bob, being a landlubber, thought he was all prepared for their first boating venture. His thoughtful wife had even bought the "required" life jacket for Charlotte, which was no easy task, and it was even harder trying to get Charlotte into the life vest. As they were just pulling out of the driveway, Delia kindly asked, "You did charge the battery to start the boat?" Bob slammed on the brakes, opened the car trunk, and checked the battery indicator that was "dead as a doornail." Immediately, he threw his new "Captain's hat" on the ground and began ranting and raving just as he had earlier in the week. Well, poor Charlotte again reacted to Bob's Type A behavior with her "stress-mess." Being a "trained behaviorist," Bob thought, "There seems to be a pattern here. When I rant and rave, Charlotte gets sick."

After Charlotte settled down, Delia and Bob ran her to the veterinarian. He confirmed that Bob's ranting and raving behavior was causing Charlotte's "stress-mess." There were three choices. Either Charlotte or Bob would have to go, or Bob could learn to talk in low, soothing tones (at least around Charlotte). To this day Bob tries to talk calmly around his dog.

Your pets probably pick up more stress than you think. So give them and yourself a break, and lighten up! To avoid the "stress-mess," Bob finally learned to "hit reset" to convert his unpleasant R&R (ranting and raving) to healthy R&R (rest and relaxation). On-the-job situations can trigger ranting and raving in just about anyone sooner or later, but if you remember to "hit reset when upset," you can regain your composure and gain respect.

To help you get a feel for job-stress management skills, let's look at the following set of skills to include in your "tool box."

- Don't complain — train.
- The 20/20 rule: "When upset, push reset."
- How to prevent "job rust out."
- Tips to reduce job-stress — goal setting.
- Dealing with Mondays: Hardly a fun day but …

---

1. Don't complain — train.

When pressure is mounting, don't complain, but train yourself to improve your stress fitness. Even though your job-stressors are real (e.g., problems with control, conflict, change, complaints, computers), only you control how you really react to these problems. Stress fitness empowers you with the strength to rise above your stress. As with golf, you will be aiming and training to have a "lower score" on your stress scorecard.

Learning stress skills may be as awkward as learning how to write with your opposite hand, because stress skills involve training the right side of the brain, in contrast to the almost totally left brain training emphasized in our jobs, schools and society. Learning to passively accept, and let go, are right brain stress skills that we have to learn to balance out overly left brain emphasis on control.

---

2. The 20/20 rule: pushing your own "reset button" rather than your panic button.

We are so easily "blindsided" by stress because it is partially an instantaneous, involuntary response. By learning a few basics about how stress works, we are better able to "Nip it in the bud" before it gets out of control. Like emergency braking a roller coaster car at the very beginning of the ride, a full-blown "stress flash" can be halted, if stopped within the first twenty seconds of our noticing it. That is, you can hit your "reset button" before you go into a stress attack.

Just as you practice a fire drill before a fire, it is useful to practice your reset drill when you are not upset. Before the next "stress-storm" you might want to learn by heart the motto, "Don't forget, reset when upset." Right now, before doing anything else, repeat this saying to yourself, "When upset hit reset."

Your ten-minute reset-recess

Even federal judges in court call for recesses. Certainly you can take a ten-minute recess to reset yourself so you are calmer and more productive. It takes about ten minutes to reset yourself.

Try the ABC approach to your reset drill. That is, rehearse a single "Attitude, Breathing technique and Choice" to groove-in your reset habit. You don't go shopping for a garden hose when you have a brushfire in your backyard. It's best to have the equipment you need when the fire starts.

Your 20-second reset drill could consist of a favorite attitude affirmation ("Just for now I'll relax" or "This too shall pass"), a little deep breathing — four or five deep belly breaths; and what choice you will make when you are upset and you need to reset. A sometimes helpful choice to help you reset is to quietly accept (just for now) what is going on. This reset drill emphasizes working from the inside out (inner attitudes, breathing, outer choices). This ABC approach is the foundation of managing job-stress and is covered in the next chapters. Although in-depth relaxation probably takes at least twenty minutes, ten minutes just to clear your mind and ten minutes to really relax your body, your reset drill can be effective in as little as three minutes, if you practice daily.

The 20/20 rule: The term, "stress flash," is used to reflect the instant reflex a stressor triggers within us. In less than the blink of an eye, a perceived threat triggers emotion, followed by thinking, and within 20 seconds followed by action. This action can release stress hormones that can keep you very hot or cold for 20 minutes. You will be hot if you become angry, you will be "cold and clammy" if you become anxious. How we think and even rethink about the perceived threat within the 20-second window of opportunity will gauge how frustrated or fearful we feel for about 20 minutes.

A useful reset or "Nip it in the bud" technique is to give the incoming stressor a rating between two and ten, take a few deep breaths, and then choose your action. Helpful choices include controlling, accepting, enjoying the humor in it, or avoiding the situation. As stated above, your first immediate escape route is to choose, for now, to accept the situation. Then later try to get control of the problem, see the humor in it or start preparing to retreat.

3. How to prevent "job rust out."

"Job rust out" is far more common than the dramatic job "burnout" we often hear about, but rarely see. "Rust out" means forcing ourselves, year after year, to plod along in boring, meaningless or highly stressful jobs. Relaxation and "working smart" provide the oil to prevent your "rusting out" on the job.

- Practice real PR (patience and relaxation) when faced with impatience from yourself or others. Remember, "Easy always does it."
- Try to do one thing at a time, "This one thing I do." You won't feel as overwhelmed and what you do will be done better.

- "Knowledge is power" over your job. Know your job, what is expected, when and how you will be evaluated.
- Seek positive co-workers. It only takes a QUARTER (25%) of a group to bring DOWN (infect) the entire job place with a negative attitude, so beware of the QUARTER DOWNER principle.
- Write it down. Trying to remember many important details creates stress. Remember the Chinese proverb: "The palest ink is better than the best memory."
- Schedule your work; work your schedule to avoid getting swamped with unfinished work. Schedule the next day's activities before you leave work. Time management is the best antidote for a pressure-cooker work environment. It increases your sense of control.
- DeRail unpleasant people by being *relaxed, assertive* and an *intensive listener.* If you get an unpleasant phone call, turn the phone slightly away but so you can still hear it. Take the attitude that you are not merely a sponge soaking up their complaints, but that you can "transform" their problems into projects.
- Limit or even eliminate "pity parties." If you must have a gripe session, make it brief and try to come up with at least one possible solution.
- Try the TGIE (Thank goodness I'm employed) approach and really try to like your job.
- Take your breaks. If feasible, take a short walk away from your workplace during your break, or sit comfortably and relax your hands, shoulders, neck, forehead and jaw muscles while breathing deeply and slowly. Also, slowly "decaffeinate" your coffee breaks. (Try a half-caffeinated, half-decaffeinated blend for a week and then decrease the caffeinated portion weekly thereafter. Sudden caffeine withdrawal causes stress).
- Expect delays and have projects you can do while waiting.
- Do it now. Procrastination consists of excessive perfectionism, "I need just one more day," and lack of planning.
- Keep your eyes on the prize. Have pictures/reminders of past vacations, future trips, loved ones, etc., to help bring about peaceful moods. Reward yourself weekly for doing a good job. Take two of these principles a week, practice them, and reward yourself at the end of each week. Go through all twelve principles.
- REMEMBER: DON'T WORRY — WORK.

4. Tips to reduce job-stress — goal setting.

Mentally check off each tip that is an activity you do now. "Unchecked" items are your new goals.

PREPARATION (At home)

- Sleep about seven hours nightly.
- Use a "friendly" alarm clock (No cannons!).
- Eat a good breakfast (Low blood sugar causes stress).
- Make optimism your breakfast of champions.
- Exercise three times weekly vigorously (e.g., walk) with a responsible "motivated" partner.
- Limit daily caffeine to two cups of coffee or two cans of soda.
- Maintain normal weight.
- Manage your time and budget.
- Do something fun (hobby) you have complete control over.
- Express affection with "loved ones"/socialize with friends/enjoy your pets.
- Hold a brief, informal family meeting weekly to discuss plans, victories, etc.
- Vent problems/complaints with focus on solutions.
- Get outside daily (Sunlight puts people in better moods). Allow as much sun in the house as possible.
- Home "work" should "contrast" job "work" (e.g., yard work vs. sedentary mental work).
- Take warm baths/get massaged.
- Prepare for work the night before (clothes, keys, breakfast).
- Use *Assertive Discipline for Parents* (Canter) if children's behavior is a stressor.
- Celebrate life's "little pleasures."

CONTACT (!) (At work)

- Arrive early.
- Do the most difficult tasks first(if possible).
- Reduce "brainstrain" by writing things down.
- Focus on doing one thing well at a time.
- Smile/laugh when you can. (Laughter releases the brain's natural tranquilizer.)
- Challenge yourself to continually improve your job skills, job relations and assertiveness skills (if needed).

REWARD and RECORD

- Keep your eyes on the prize (tangible rewards with specific dates for meeting goals).
- Take one day at a time.
- Keep track of tips you don't currently do. Practice one new one per week.
- Reward yourself daily.
- Maximize your physical comfort within company policy (comfortable shoes, ties, extra seat support if needed).
- Stretch for ten seconds every two hours. Focus your eyes at far distance hourly.
- Manage time, clutter and difficult people before they manage you.
- Make your work area "homey" (pictures, trophies, music).
- Practice one-minute breather.
- Develop trusted friends.
- Change what you can, accept what you need to, but know the difference.
- At day's end, write down tomorrow's priority plan; next day, follow the plan.
- Take breaks with positive people.
- Walk (outside) at lunch if you can.
- REMEMBER TGIE (Thank goodness I'm employed). Job hunting is very stressful.
- Listen to positive motivational tapes while driving or at home.

"STRESS BAGGAGE" — DO LEAVE HOME WITHOUT IT!

---

5. Dealing with Mondays: Hardly a fun day but …

Mondays are rough on the nerves because you are using your "right brain at the wrong time." Consider your left brain to be "forward" gear on your car and your right brain to be "reverse." We need both left and right brain functions to navigate through life, just as the best car must have reverse gear to be of any use.

During the workweek your left brain takes care of business, dealing with time, money, numbers and words. Your left brain strives to be positive, detailed, prepared and controlled from 8 to 5 — five days a week.

Shifting to the right brain

Nearing the weekend we start "downshifting" to a more relaxed right brain gear. Your right brain enjoys spending the leisure time and money your left brain has earned. Your right brain likes doing what you want when you want.

Mondays: The right brain at the wrong time

Before we know it, Monday morning is here, and we are daydreaming on the way to work about what we did or didn't do on the weekend. Still in this "right brain daydream" mode, we arrive at work on semi-conscious "automatic pilot." We approach our workstation looking like a dazed deer on a dark road blinded by car lights. We put on the brakes on daydreaming, and try to shift to our "left brain business" gear. Realizing we are really back at work, we again use our left brain to deal with deadlines, projects, following a team plan and controlling emotional impulses. This sudden shifting on mental gears is physically stressful.

Justifiably, we celebrate weekends with recreational dining and snacking. We may have extra coffees, sodas or treats at our leisure. On Mondays at work, we drastically change what and how we eat and drink. Withdrawing from leisurely weekend eating habits can be taxing.

An interesting case in point is the "standing room only" cafe. A major metropolitan city caters to those "eating on the run." The "standing room only" cafe has waist-high, small, red, round tables, with no chairs in sight. The customers, seemingly stuck in fast forward, feel they must stand to eat, so there is no need for seating. Without a doubt, these urgent diners go through weekend withdrawal in terms of how they eat on Monday.

Mondays can also be hard on your heart. Monday is the most frequent workday for heart problems. Since the major cause of Monday stress is "brain shifting," a partial solution may be learning how to ease from right brain to left brain behavior and thinking. Sunday may be a good time to start shifting rather than putting all the shift stress on Monday morning.

The command to rest: 3,500 years ago a command to rest every seven days was "carved into stone." The Commandment, "Remember the Sabbath," recognizes the deep human need for devoting ourselves to something beyond work.

Take time weekly to focus on the "wide-angle" landscape view of your life rather than on the "zoom close-up" of daily details. Constant fixation on details without considering personal meaning can make you near-sighted, narrow and inflexible. Scientists call this obsessive-compulsive thinking. You can become a robotic, colorless achiever without even knowing it.

Make Sunday a special day. Below are some tips to help you enjoy Sunday more, think about Monday less and even sleep better.

- Take a walk or exercise.
- No caffeine after lunch.
- Eat a light Sunday evening meal.
- Take a warm bath before bed.

- Don't turn your bedroom into a boardroom by talking about business.
- Set out your keys, clothes, etc., the night before.

Monday is a fun day — Hardly! You can make it easier by trying these "foods that soothe" to counteract "weekend treat withdrawal."

- A banana with Monday morning breakfast (It lowers blood pressure).
- Carbohydrate/protein rich cereal (commercially-available cereals) with milk.
- Fruit juice or vegetable drink mixture.
- Extra fluids while at work.
- Writing your Monday "To-Do" list on Friday so you can forget about work and you don't fumble around confused on Monday.
- Taking a shower before you leave for work.
- Leaving home five minutes earlier.
- While commuting to work, sharpen your left brain focus by doing 10 to 1 countdowns (silently) by ones, then by two's (10, 8, 6, 4, 2, 0). This is like saying, "Check, check" to make certain a microphone works before the big show. Math calculation is simply a "left brain check" to see if all (or at least enough) cells are working for you to work. Recall simple multiplication table facts (3x7 = ?). Make a game of it.
- Break your day into manageable chunks and take your breaks.
- Plan and enjoy some type of "Monday-night delight," a ball game, etc. for holding it together on Monday.

SUMMARY

Five basic tools for your on the job tool kit were provided in this chapter: 1) Don't complain — train, 2) The 20/20 rule, 3) Preventing "job rust-out," 4) Reducing job-stress, and 5) Dealing with Mondays. Highlighted in this chapter is how to push your own "reset button" (instead of the panic button) which is a fast, simple and effective way to calm down. It was suggested that before the next stress storm you learn by heart, "Reset when upset." The next chapters will deal with a simple but effective method for managing job-stress — the ABC's of job-stress management.

FOR FURTHER READING

Waitely, D., & Reni, L.W., (1985). *Joy of working, the 30 day system to success, wealth & happiness on the job.* New York, NY: Dodd Mead.

6

"POWER" ATTITUDES

"A man's mind, stretched by a new idea, can never go back to its original dimensions." - *Oliver Wendell Holmes, Jr.*

In this chapter you will learn the method (not mystery) of having a positive attitude. You will also learn that you are your own major stumbling block, having about three-hundred negative thoughts a day that you have to counteract. The eight key points of this chapter will address:

- Harvard Medical School's 2002 scientific breakthrough: Positive thinking proven to promote physical health and healing.
- Advice from the world's "smartest" person on the power of attitudes.
- "Small thoughts vaccine" for negative thinking on the job.
- Assessing chinks in your "attitude armor."
- "Hold that thought" — bringing about an attitude adjustment in a 75% negative world. Negative thinking changes your brain chemistry.
- Professional "attitude adjustment": Center for Creative Leadership.
- Don't wait for perfect timing.
- America undergoes a dramatic "faith lift": After 40 years, the dramatic return to the power of faith to help move a mountain (World Trade Center, 80 ft. of rubble from 110 stories).

Negative attitudes are energy vampires draining enthusiasm out of you.

Wearing his typically sour face, Bob entered his supervisor's office. "You're a bad apple, and insubordinate," said his supervisor. "You complain about me to others and spend more time whining than working. Tattoo this on your brain: 'When you pout you're out.' There are ten people willing to fill your shoes at this job." Only getting a verbal warning, Bob, although shaken, vowed he would be more positive, or at least less negative. His boss thought, "Only time will tell."

1. Harvard Medical School's scientific breakthrough 2002: Positive thinking proven to promote physical health and healing.

At the top of the "Best of" list is the Harvard Medical School's study (April,

2002), "The mind and the immune system." See "For Further Reading" for the complete reference.

Harvard Medical School reveals that positive thinking is proven to promote physical health and healing. The boss's bottom line for this mental-physical health link: You can take this to the bank — it's less expensive to be more positive because of less sick-(of)-work days by employees.

Also revealed in this study is that emotional counseling improves physical health, so employee assistance programs are definitely worth the investment. The stressed are four times more likely to get colds, or the flu. The stressed actually take longer to recover from surgery. Even for the hard of heart, the message of this landmark 2002, Harvard study is loud and clear: Miserable employees are actually physically sick more.

Sick people are less productive. So . . . being positive has a "bottom line benefit" of indirectly improving productivity. Like it or not, being nice is a better business practice.

Stress and sudden death at work

It is now common science that stress affects how long you live. It is common sense that we all die sooner or later. Stress makes our deaths sooner rather than later. Monday is the leading cardiac death day at work. If you can, lighten your Monday workload, somehow.

Office optimism — a refresher course

For the best of how-to materials for being positive at work, see Anne White's ***Twelve Commandments** for People who Work with People,* and Scott Ventrella's *The Power of Positive Thinking in Business: the 10 Traits for Maximum Results,* in this chapter's "For Further Reading" section.

"Positive thinking" movement turns seventy, making it an institution, not just a fad

As far back as 1932, the great power of positive thoughts was recognized, as expressed in Emmet Fox's pioneering book, *Power Through Constructive Thinking.* His "Fifteen Points" (p. 272 of his book) predate most positive thinking movements and exemplifies one of the best minds of the 19th century (Fox was born in 1886). Dr. Norman Vincent Peale, considered one of the ten most popular men in the world in the 1990's, carried the "positive thinking" torch to light the darkness with his best-selling classic, *The Power of Positive Thinking,* published about 20 years after Fox's groundbreaking book on positive thinking.

---

2. Advice from the world's "smartest" person on the power of attitude.

Marilyn vos Savant, who has the highest-measured IQ (230) in the world, believes that "…thoughts generate emotions. You may not necessarily choose your emotions, but you control the thoughts that produce them."

In essence, attitude is everything in terms of stress management. The old joke, mind over matter (if I don't mind, it doesn't matter) contains a kernel of truth. Your stress begins and ends with strong attitudes. Perceptions are real, whether they are really right or not.

If you work at it, you can maintain positive attitudes 90 to 95% of the time.

---

3. "Small thoughts vaccine" for negative thinking on the job.

"SMALL THOUGHTS VACCINE"

(Prescription — take seven times per "small thoughts" attack)

Dr. Ron Rubenzer © 2003

1. *This job is a drag; there is too much change; these computers are driving me nuts!* Work is fun, change is good: A poor workman argues with his tools, so get back in the loop of the 21st century program!
2. *I have to.* I want to. If I do what I have to now, I can do what I really want to do later.
3. *I think I can't (change).* I think I can.
4. *You are told: You will never have a perfect "score" (grade).* No monument was ever built to honor a critic. What are my LFT's, "Look forward to's"?
5. *This job is too stressful. I can't take the stress of these computer courses.* Job-stress is better than jobless stress. Choose to convert temporary stress into long-term satisfaction (e.g., taking those computer courses now for a better job life later).
6. *The only person who likes change is a wet baby.* Change is the only sure thing in life. You couldn't even eat if food didn't change form.
7. *Why am I in this job (course, etc.)?* What are my LFT's, "Look forward to's"?
8. *She is impossible to get along with.* I'll try the JLU, "Just like us" approach, by finding something in common with her (dress, food, hobbies, interests).
9. *I give up.* "It is better to light a candle than to curse the darkness." (Dedicated to E. Roosevelt by Adlai Stevenson upon Roosevelt's death in 1962.)
10. *I can't take this pressure anymore.* The glass is both half empty and half full. There is some balance between good and evil.

When stuck between a rock and a hard place, become a diamond. (Use the pressure to become the world's most-brilliant and strongest element, just slow the pressure down.)

THE ONLY THING YOU CAN CONTROL ABOUT THE PAST IS YOUR ATTITUDE. YOUR ATTITUDES ARE AN INDESTRUCTIBLE SOURCE OF STRENGTH.

World-famous psychiatrist, Dr. Victor Frankl, successfully survived the ravages of a Nazi concentration camp by sheer "will of attitude." Although his chances of staying alive at Auschwitz and Dachau were about 3%, he coped by developing the foundations of and using what would become Logo-Therapy. Most basically, he said if we have meaning in life we can survive anything. Three ways to find meaning in life are by doing a worthwhile deed or completing a work; encountering someone or experiencing something (love, truth, beauty, etc.); and managing our attitude toward unavoidable suffering. Dr. Frankl's secret to survival also included a sense of humor, even a grim sense of humor, toward one's own situation.

Victor Hugo once said, "Winter is on my head, but eternal spring is in my soul."

Using grim humor to cope with chronic illness

Bob's friend, Ed, was undergoing treatment for a nonfatal, degenerative disease requiring antibiotics for life. Dealing with the nausea caused by the medication was getting on Ed's "last nerve" which was aggravated by the need to perform a medical procedure every few hours, for life. After about a month of this routine of medication and procedures, it dawned on Ed that he would just have to get used to this new lifesaving "lifestyle." He was told that the medical procedure would be easier if he relaxed while doing it. He discovered that having a sense of humor about this medical challenge, in general, actually helped him to relax.

Seeing his friend Bob, he quipped, "I am on so many antibiotics, I could live in a leper colony, unscathed . . . . After a nuclear blast I would be the only thing to survive, along with the cockroaches . . . . I have been to the doctor's office so many times the nurse jokingly said, "You either have to go on payroll or we'll have to start charging you rent."

Ed should not quit his daytime job to become a comic, but being able to make fun of his own situation actually made it bearable, easier and medically more effective.

---

4. Assessing chinks in your "attitude armor."

Dr. James Loehr developed a mental toughness test measuring your "attitude reflexes" and key wellness practices. This self-test provides a most valuable "benchmark" on how world-class achievers react successfully to situations. This 60 item self-report, MENTALLY TOUGH TEST, is featured in Dr. Loehr's book, *Stress for Success,* in which he offers tips on developing healthy, productive work attitudes.

Sample true or false questions from Dr. Loehr's MENTALLY TOUGH TEST include:

- I can create the state of fun almost anytime at work.
- People would agree that I look confident, energized, relaxed and positive most of the time.
- I can perform at high levels on demand regardless of circumstances.
- My job helps fulfill important needs for me.
- I bounce back emotionally from bad news very quickly.
- I can laugh easily at myself.
- I can make myself change from a bad mood to a good one very quickly.
- I can leave the problems of work at the office. I don't take them home.
- I've learned to trace negative emotions to their source.
- I can summon and sustain the emotions that bring out the best in me during work.

Review this checklist weekly to see if you are "on course." The more "yes'es," the more mentally tough you are.

To truly gauge your mental toughness, take the complete MENTALLY TOUGH TEST, available from LGE Performance Systems, Inc. Corporate Training Programs. The advantage of taking this true-false test is that it will help you pinpoint your strengths and areas for personal growth.

Through his Mentally Tough corporate training program, Dr. James Loehr has taught Olympic athletes, such as gold medallist, Dan Jansen, and executives to summon emotions necessary for top performance at will. His "full engagement" training enables individuals to alternate between high stress and deep recovery, which is the key to peak performance. That is, they peak when they need to for best performance.

---

5. "Hold that thought" — bringing about an attitude adjustment in a 75% negative world. Negative thinking changes your brain chemistry in just two weeks.

People spend at least 75% of their time being negative, according to renowned stress consultant, Loretta LaRoche, of the Humor Potential. Positive people are going up the down stairwell crowded with angry, frustrated people. Without becoming preachy, it is important to give yourself a fighting chance at being positive by having reminders (carrying cards, etc.) and surrounding yourself with positive people (the other 25%). The average person has a negative thought every two and one half minutes, or about three-hundred negative thoughts a day, according to the Midwest Center for Stress and Anxiety, Inc.

The best book to help you learn and practice positive thinking is by Lucinda Bassett, founder of the Midwest Center for Stress and Anxiety, Inc. Her book, *Life Without Limits,* provides practical proven ways to change your mind to change your life.

Consider this: If you are not in control of your thoughts and actions, who or what else is?

Synchronize your mind with your watch

Get in real time, not lost in the false memories of the past or the future imaginings of things that may never be. Be "present" in the present. Living in the past breeds regret, living in the future breeds fear. Try to keep in the "here and now" making a "pleasant present" when possible. Surround yourself with the good and positive when you can. Try to keep in the "here and now" for just one minute, not letting your mind drift off into the past, future or someplace else. Taking ten deep breaths will take you about a minute. Feel the cool air being drawn in your nose, and the warm air flowing out your mouth. Build your "here and now attention span" up to two minutes if you can. Brain research suggests that your attention span should be about 50 minutes, but if you can build your breathing attention span to 20 minutes, you will be peaceful in a hectic world.

Science has revealed that the brain will stop producing it's own natural pleasure antidepressant neurotransmitter within two weeks, if we do not think positively. Medication is then used to stimulate the production or delay the metabolizing of these hormones that naturally make us feel more optimistic. It should be cautioned that there are many other causes of nonproduction of serotonin and endorphins, so always see you doctor to pinpoint the problem. A depletion of some chemicals is age related, for example, melatonin, which helps you sleep.

Try one or two of these dozen tips that best fit your situation. Even Albert Einstein allegedly stated that he could only really concentrate on one thought at a time. To "hold that thought," displace a negative thought with one powerful positive thought, through repetition and sheer force of will. These 12 tips, with examples, may help:

- Talk yourself into positive attitudes. Even a "writer's mantra" is featured.
- Continually build your own emotional trust fund (savings account).
- Avoid crossing your "fault line."
- "Fly swat" negative attitudes as you would swat an irritating fly or mosquito. You average about three-hundred negative thoughts a day.
- Carve out a ten-minute block for relaxed renewal daily to recharge your batteries.
- Have a theme song (e.g., "I did it my way").

- Use clip-notes to become a "card-carrying" optimist.
- Routinely resist "choral whining." Those who gossip to you, gossip about you.
- Exercise your mental flexibility to avoid arthritis of the attitudes.
- To keep your sense of balance, practice your sense of humor.
- Downward compare only when you are really "down and out."
- Don't become a bad news-junkie.

These twelve keys to an attitude adjustment are fleshed out below:

Talk yourself into positive attitudes

The key to turning your attitudes around is simply, "practice until you believe." It has been estimated that negative attitudes are several times stronger than positive attitudes. To excel in terms of stamping in positive attitudes, remember, practice makes permanent. Just as your office has dress codes, you follow different attitude codes at work. Helpful attitude codes follow:

- Easy always does it.
- Pain is unavoidable, suffering is optional.
- TGIE (Thank God I'm employed).
- "Line by line, things are fine; page by page, I've got it made," is the "writer's mantra," useful for any type of writing.
- Your enemies will become your stepping-stones if you are patient. (Janet Harrell).
- There is no danger.
- There is enough time.
- This too, shall pass. Everything is temporary.
- Don't give up.
- Don't take it personally. Do not be like the "princess and the pea" overreacting to the smallest pet peeve. "Jerks at work" are probably not aiming to hurt you personally, but only trying to help themselves.
- Divide and conquer your problems. Divide your problems into steps that can be dealt with one at a time.
- Live your life in daytight compartments. Like the rising sun, your energy will rise for the day if you let go of yesterday and concentrate on doing well today.
- Relax. You are not the center of the universe but you are central to the universe. We are actually centered in the universe, midway in size between stars and atoms. Our true life cycle is from "stardust to stardust." We are composed of stars and we will return to stars.

- Instead of saying, "I hate....," say, "I pity...." Instead of saying, "I dread doing ...," say to yourself, "I dislike doing...."
- "It takes confidence to win, and it takes winning to have confidence," according to a statement credited to Andre Agassi, world-class tennis player.

On the humorous side, if writing brings you to your knees seek divine intervention (silently). St. Francis de Sales is the patron saint of writers. It can't hurt to ask for help from beyond yourself, because, when you quiet your mind, you'll be giving your left brain, the writing side, a break and activating the right side's creative, inspirational part. It beats cursing, which is the dark side of the right brain's potential. Writers have been seeking inspiration from the muses for centuries. Many writers have pictures/books of long deceased heroes for inspiration. Many people still have St. Christopher medals or even statues in their cars. In childhood many of us said the prayer, "Now I lay me down to sleep," which comforted us. Millions of grateful adults still say grace before eating. Some coaches in private schools even have a team prayer before games. But again, keep your prayers to yourself.

Continually build your own emotional trust fund

Really think about whom you can trust, (loved ones, friends, colleagues, sources and causes beyond yourself). Encourage trust in others by keeping promises, caring, loving and consoling when needed. If you work in an anti-trust job where no one is trusted, it is even more important to build your trust fund with those you can confide in.

Avoid crossing your "fault line"

"Being conscientious "to a fault" can keep you sleepless at night with worry. You can be "generous to a fault" with your free time, by over-volunteering in activities that take you away from your family. The constant, continual improvement is called Kaizen in Japanese, a worthwhile goal. But living Kaizen to a fault could be distorted into the "pointless pursuit of perfection." Sometimes miscalled obsessive-compulsive disorder, one must repeat a ritual (e.g., washing hands, "quadruple" checking to make sure the iron is turned off). On the job the almost fanatical spirit of Kaizen is a good thing, while at home it'll land you in the doghouse or divorce court.

Quickly "fly swat" negative attitudes as you would swat an irritating fly or mosquito

It may be there but you do not have to let it land on you and bite you. You may not be able to control every thought you have, but you can control whether you entertain (feed and encourage) those thoughts. As stated above, research shows that you have about three-hundred negative thoughts a day which works out to about one negative thought every two and one half minutes. Chances are, you are even denying that fact you may have this many negative thoughts as you say to yourself, "I am not a negative thinker", which is a negative thought in itself.

Carve out a ten-minute block for renewal daily, to recharge your batteries

You can learn to attain a state of relaxed readiness, which will boost your performance.

Have a theme song

Sports and political rallies have theme songs because they motivate. Play (perhaps mentally) a personally meaningful song. At the right times whistling or humming that chosen song to yourself can be calming to help you concentrate. Some people march to the beat of "I did it my way," by Mr. Frank Sinatra. The song, "Somewhere over the rainbow," by Ms. Judy Garland is supposedly one of the most played songs of the 20th century. The fight song to the movie, "Rocky," may pick up your spirits. Another blast from the past century is, "You've got to be strong," by Desiree on her hit 1994 CD, "I ain't movin," from Sony Music Entertainment. From the dawn of the 21st century comes the best-selling song by LeeAnn Womack, "I hope you dance," under the MCA label, Nashville, Tennessee, 2000.

Use clip-notes to become a card-carrying optimist

Write down your personally uplifting attitudes on three by five index cards and clip them to a clipboard. Carry a card with you or place it where you can review it for several days. There are also commercially-available calendars and books that feature tried and true "attitudes." Use the "blue dot" special technique of putting a blue dot on your calendar as a cue to remember to try to be positive. Carry pictures of your "pride and joy," to remind you of why you are working.

Routinely resist "choral whining"

Whine-o-holics (whining addicts) love company and always have something negative to talk about. December 26 has actually been set aside as National Whiner's Day. Peer pressure increases pressure about neutral or already negative situations. Remember, those who gossip to you will gossip about you, perhaps as soon as you leave. Avoid "pity parties" when possible. Instead seek out positive, even humorous individuals in your situation who have learned to thrive rather than just survive. Do not contribute to "global whining" by being positive.

Exercise your mental flexibility (use it or lose it) before you get hardened attitudes. Life is "negotiated compromise" between our "ideal" and the "real." Being flexible closes the gap between what we want and what we get. A full range of flexibility includes the ability to wisely: control, accept, rest, or enjoy.

Your situation may demand using one "gear" often, but you should still be able to use "reverse" occasionally. For example, accept rather than control. As you read in Chapter 5, the finest car without a reverse gear is not marketable.

Use your sense of humor for your sense of balance

Well-used, humor can "defrost" and lighten up a situation. You may want to keep a "humor first-aid kit" file of your all-time favorites. Routinely reading the "funnies" in the newspaper can counterbalance the heaviness of the daily news. If you must read the obituaries, rejoice in not having found yourself featured. Calendars featuring daily comics are also available.

Downward compare only when you are really "down and out"

If you drift into feeling sorry for yourself, volunteer to do Hospice work, visit a nursing home, cemetery, or hospital. Remember those who have had things worse than you do, and still prevailed. Consider Christopher Reeve of Superman fame; Dr. Victor Frankl, Nazi concentration camp survivor and author of Logo-Therapy; Helen Keller, famous deaf, mute and blind author; and Dr. Stephen Hawking, quadriplegic, famous astronomer, and author. Remember, jobless stress is usually worse than job-stress. It is usual to contrast and compare your situation with folks who, not just in their own minds, are really "down and out."

Homeless — the really "down and out" A sad but true story

John Doe became homeless almost over night. As a machinist who lost his job, he went from making two-hundred-dollars per week to being homeless and jobless literally overnight. He had suddenly joined the ranks of the poor (poverty level = just under $9,000 per year). On April 6, 2002, he along with four other young homeless sitting outdoors in a makeshift tent, fought off freezing temperatures and biting wind by maintaining a fire in a big barrel. Another homeless person, who had a campsite within view, had managed to find water for bathing and drinking to bring to John Doe.

The "whining wall"

John Doe's story above was typical of the three-hundred known homeless in the area.

If and when you feel sorry for yourself, log on to your local newspaper and just search for homeless. Print up the story, then post it on a wall. This is your "whining wall" which you should go to and review as soon as you feel sorry for yourself. As a practical matter, you may want to mount articles about the homeless on the inside of a closet door, so you can inconspicuously view them when you feel like whining. When you feel you are really "down and out," make sure you fit the real federally defined description, you make just under $9,000 per year, which is the poverty level, as of April, 2002.

Don't become a bad news-junkie

"If it bleeds, it leads" is the motto of most news services. There are TV, movie, book and tabloid storylines which make anyone's life seem wonderful by "downward comparison." These items are littered with once in a lifetime traumas impossibly compressed into every character's daily life. Continual viewing of the horrific World Trade Center suicidal bombings resulted in some individuals developing serious emotional difficulties (acute-stress disorder). Unchecked, this acute-stress disorder can become a post-traumatic stress disorder (PTSD).

Distilling every tragedy experienced by six-billion people into one half hour may present a distracting, interesting, but highly warped, cynical, and hopeless view of life, especially for the young who can't use judgment in what they watch. As stated above if you are going to downward compare to get perspective on your life situation, stick to your own neighborhood which is more representative of real life. Stress experts state it's better to get "bad news on your doorstep" through reading once in the newspaper than viewing through a broken record technique of other media.

Dr. Denis Waitely, in his book, *Joy of Working*, suggests that you can be happier at work if you have a positive attitude, expect the best from others and yourself, and practice flexibility in terms of accepting change.

ATTITUDES IN ACTION: Emmy award-winning Hugh Downs, co-host of an acclaimed TV program, *"20/20,"* points to three key positive attitudes for success and satisfaction in life: a positive attitude toward productive activity; a fearless attitude about survivable failures; and an attitude of being totally in the "here and now."

---

6. Professional "attitude adjustment": Center for Creative Leadership.

The world-renowned Center for Creative Leadership provides individualized, objective and practical assessment of attitudes and behaviors related to successful leadership. This several day diagnostic-prescriptive assessment is custom-tailored to each business's corporate culture, goals and each individual's strengths and weaknesses. The outcome of this assessment is a detailed plan for success that fits the individual and his/her company. The CCL (Center for Creative Leadership) faculty is composed of seasoned, successful business leaders and top echelon leadership researchers. Fortune 500 companies regularly send employees to CCL as part of their corporate leadership grooming experience. The main headquarters and training facility for CCL is in Greensboro, North Carolina, with other training facilities in San Diego, Colorado Springs and Europe. For program information, call (336) 545-2810 or visit their website at <http://www.ccl.org/search>.

Positive thinking on the job

Scott Ventrella, in his 2001 book, lists ten do-able positive thinking steps for the job. Of course, calmness, patience and persistence are key factors. Faith in one's self to have a positive outcome, even when times are tough, tops his list of things you can do on the job for effectiveness and success.

A very useful and visually appealing list of "**Twelve Commandments** for People Who Work With People" is offered by Ann White. Her corporation can be contacted at (864) 463-6709, or <www.annwhite.com>.

---

7. Don't wait for perfect timing.

"When I graduate I'll . . . ; when the kids stop fighting I'll improve my. . .; I'll finish that report when my desk is cleared, all my papers are filed AND all my pencils are sharpened . . . ; I'll go to Tahiti when I can afford it . . . ; I'll improve my romance life when I lose more weight; We'll leave for vacation when the house is spotless and could pass "the Martha Stewart" inspection.

---

8. America undergoes a dramatic "faith lift" adjustment.

After 40 years, there is a dramatic return to the "power of faith" to help "move a mountain" (World Trade Center, 80 ft. of rubble remaining from 110 stories). The results of a 2001 Gallup Poll that was conducted the week after the terrorists' attacks reported that more people in the United States had attended a worship service over the previous weekend than any other time dating back to the early 1950's. As secular as our society is, one prayer on everyone's lips or heart was "God Bless America."

SUMMARY

The headline for this chapter could read major scientific breakthrough: Harvard Medical School reveals that positive thinking is proven to promote physical health and healing. The Boss's Bottom Line for this mental-physical health link: You can take this to the bank — it's less expensive to be more positive because of less sick-(of)-work days by employees. Also revealed by this Harvard Medical study: Emotional counseling improves physical health, so employee assistance programs are definitely worth the investment. The stressed are four times more likely to get colds or the flu. The stressed actually take longer to recover from surgery. The hard of heart, sick and miserable employees are not productive employees.

In this chapter you learned that we can control our thoughts although we can't always control our emotions. You were provided with a "small thoughts vaccine" to immunize you from ten contagious negative attitudes. You were provided with the eye-opening fact that you have about three-hundred negative thoughts a day, or about one negative thought every two and one-half minutes. No wonder thinking positively can be an uphill battle, but worth winning. You were provided with a self-assessment tool to see how mentally tough you were and you were given 12 tips on attaining and maintaining a positive attitude. The dramatic "faith lift" (return to church) after 9/11 is discussed. The next chapter focuses on relaxation breathing, to provide you with the concentration and oxygen needed for keeping calm on the job.

For Further Reading

Brown, L. (2002, April 7). The rural homeless: Nowhere to go. (Greensboro, NC. *News & Record*), A-2.

Center for Creative Leadership, Greensboro, NC, with other training facilities in San Diego, Colorado Springs and Europe. For program information, call (336) 545-2810. CCL's head office is located at 1 Leadership Pl. Greensboro, NC 27410. Visit their website at <http://www.ccl.org/search>.

Frankl, V. (1984). *Man's search for meaning.* New York, Simon and Schuster.

Fox, E. (1932). *Power through constructive thinking.* New York: HarperCollins Publishers).

Klein, A. (1991). *Quotations to cheer you up when the world is getting you down.* New York: Wings Books. Offers 750 quotes as spirit lifters. Many of the quotes are humorous, all of them are uplifting.

The mind and the immune system - Part I (2002, April). *Harvard Mental Health Letter 18,* pp. 1-4. <www.health.harvard.edu>.

Potter, A. (2001). *The positive thinker's 10 commandments.* New York: Berkley Publishing Group.

Sports Legends on Success. 5 North Main Street, Natick, MA 01760. Phone 1-800-585-1300, Website: <WWW.SUCCESS.ORG> American Success Institute, Inc., or e-mail: <info@success.org>. Author.

Ventrella, S. (2001). *The power of positive thinking in business: the 10 traits for maximum results.* Free Press.

White, A. (2001). ***Twelve commandments** for people who work with people.* (Laugh and Learn with Ann White). For ordering information call (864) 463-6709, or <www.annwhite.com>.

7

Breathing Easier

The Key to Stress Management is Right Under Your Nose!

Breathing relieves pain, relaxes and enhances concentration and athletic performance.

The Coach's Corner: The newspaper sports page read, "Focusing on breathing is key to runner's success."

This high school senior blocks out all distractions to focus on her running. Her secret is to breathe in and breathe out. As soon as she "mindfully breathes" from one to ten, every muscle in her body relaxes. Her routine is also to inhale then exhale while reciting a Bible verse. This outstanding athlete is then able to get into her starting block, and stares down the track with laser-like focus. She is not even aware of the other competitors or the rest of the world. This concentrated breathing has earned her the best time in the entire state with 11.67 seconds for the hundred-yard dash. Her hero is Marion Jones. In her upcoming meets there will be scouts, hoping that she will attend their college on scholarships.

What is this super athlete's response to this pressure? Focus on her breathing, while closing her eyes to meditate. She asserts that concentrating under these conditions is always the hardest part for her. She reported that at state competition she used to hold her breath for the entire race, causing her to pass out twice on the track last year. This "passing out" lost her for junior season. A coach in Virginia helped her work on her breathing routine, with top award-winning results in her senior year. The lesson to be gained is that to be at the top of your game, relaxation breathing should be part of your training routine.

Believe it or not, people under stress forget to breathe. Lack of oxygen to your brain will naturally make you feel tense, confuse your thinking and even make you pass out. A simple and highly-effective way to bring yourself into the "here and now" (which is always manageable) is by concentrating on your breathing. Seven major topics we will address in this chapter are:

- If controlled breathing calms during childbirth, it will work on the job.
- Excellent sensory perception through deep breathing.
- "Fill in the blank" of boredom with breathing.

- Breathing instructions: Easier done than said!
- Learn from the experts and get group support.
- Relaxation breathing is now standard preoperative procedure for hospitals.
- Harvard Medical School recommends relaxation breathing even after 9/11.

---

1. If controlled breathing calms during childbirth, it will work on the job. (Unless your job is worse than childbirth).

Why does deep breathing work?

According to the National Institute of Mental Health, "People who are anxious often hypervéntilate, taking rapid shallow breaths that can trigger rapid heartbeat, lightheadedness, and other symptoms." Slow deep breathing stops unpleasant anxiety symptoms.

Your brain is very "high maintenance" in terms of its need for oxygen. It needs ten times more oxygen for its body weight compared to other parts of your body. Breathing deeply and slowly will automatically provide energy to your brain, which is the first defense against stress.

Relaxation breathing calms

Dr. Andrew Weil, M.D., Harvard-trained physician and best-selling author, strongly advocates concentrating on your breathing for five minutes per day to lower stress and blood pressure. In fact, he states that relaxation breathing is the single best treatment for anxiety disorders. Deep breathing actually improves your ability to think quickly and speak more effectively because filling the bottom part of your lungs delivers more oxygen to your brain.

Although highly controversial, it has been suggested that one of the calming methods behind smoking is the long deep inhalations taken when drawing on a cigarette. One commercially-available smoking withdrawal technique actually has the consumer sucking air through a hollow, small white tube to help simulate the deep inhalation action of smoking. Perhaps deep breathing may help smoking withdrawal, however only as a support to standard, medically supervised smoking-cessation programs.

Just three minutes of deep breathing can help you reduce job-stress. Dr. Jon Kabat-Zinn, director of a nationally-acclaimed stress-reduction program, has trained thousands to calm themselves under traumatically stressful conditions. The key to his method is to focus on the gentle rising and falling of your breathing. Insurance companies reimburse for this "breathing training" because of the highly-successful results in reducing stress.

Dr. Fernand Lamaze found that those faithfully practicing relaxation, muscle control and breathing benefited by reduced pain during childbirth. Rare would be the job that would equal the labor of childbirth.

The World Health Organization or WHO (not the band!), has approved relaxation response as part of the treatment for high blood pressure. Relaxation exercises, however, are no substitute for medication and diet. The prestigious and conservative Sloan Kettering Hospital in New York employs deep breathing to ease the distress and pain of terminally-ill cancer patients. Relaxation even helps in the performance of very painful techniques that must be done in a conscious state by a patient. Many of these self-administered procedures must be conducted for the life of the patient (e.g., self-catheterization, insulin injections, etc.). Relaxation may not reduce the pain, but it does reduce the suffering. Suffering dangerously raises your blood-pressure, causing even more problems. Relaxation breathing can reduce your experience of pain.

---

2. Excellent sensory perception through deep breathing.

Relaxed breathing focuses you on the "here and now" by actually bringing you to your senses. Relaxation breathing improves your ability to smell both the coffee and the roses. How many times have people and things around us gone unnoticed because our minds were not focused on the "here and now", the only reality? We spend most of our time living in an imaginary future or a faded, often incorrect memory of the past. Relaxation breathing helps you get into the "pleasant present" moment.

Concentrating on the "here and now" is the best way to improve memory, performance and relationships. Have you ever felt annoyed when you are talking to someone and they are looking at their watch? The phrase, "You just don't listen to me," has probably echoed through millions of dysfunctional homes.

Try this exercise to see how excellent your sensory perception is. From memory simply sketch out in the smallest detail the dashboard and steering wheel part of your car. Spend about fifteen minutes. Picture your dashboard as activated (all systems on as if you were driving normally). Try to picture the exact mileage on your odometer, etc. When convenient, go to your car, turn on your ignition (if you need to) to activate your dashboard. Take your sketchpad, and as you carefully observe what your dashboard really looks like, just check off the exact matches between what is actually on your dashboard and what you sketched. You will be amazed that our sensory perception is probably about C+ even when we are concentrating on our surroundings while driving. Do this sensory perception exercise where appropriate in other environments. We often look but don't see.

"This one thing I do"; both Einstein and Michelangelo advised concentrating on one thing at a time. Your attending physician, surgeon, airline pilots and tax accountants all focus on one thing at a time....

Training your attention to "stay put" in the "here and now" is like trying to train a puppy to "come here-now" and "stay put" without a leash. At first this is almost impossible, but with lots of tender loving care, your attention will "stay put" in the "here and now," just as your puppy, with training, will eventually "stay here-now" by your side without a leash.

3. "Fill in the blank" of boredom with breathing.

During those no-brainer activities, (being stuck in traffic, listening to senseless chatter, waiting in a line at the store), do some deep breathing. It is mental housecleaning. Even a few minutes will help you combat feeling bored (or baffled) and it will help you get your breathing practice in.

4. Breathing instructions: Easier done than said!

Obviously if you are reading this page, you are breathing and do not really need breathing instructions. In fact, relaxation breathing, is actually easier done than said, because it is second nature. Every time you sigh, you are relaxation breathing. Just try breathing a little easier, slower and deeper. Begin your breath with your stomach first.

Try the following RELAXATION BREATHING exercise lying down.

Notice the rising of your stomach, then your chest as you slowly inhale. Your goal is belly breathing in which the belly fills with air before the upper lungs do. Notice your chest falling and then your stomach flattening as you slowly exhale. Putting your hand on your stomach will help you feel whether you are belly breathing. Practice this belly breathing when you go to bed for a few days until it is a habit.

The best commercially-available tape for relaxation breathing is offered by The Midwest Center for Stress and Anxiety, Inc. The tape, one of a dozen tapes in the kit, incorporates the best of breathing, deep muscle relaxation, visualization and positive self-talk techniques. It is less than fifteen minutes long. This would be an ideal tool for an adult counseling department or for the self-study of anxiety management. The Midwest Center for Stress and Anxiety, Inc. has provided very effective self-help stress-management materials to over a half-million people over fourteen years. Call 1-800-944-9428 for more information. Their excellent materials would be very useful in starting a large scale program for a school or business requiring funding of known, proven materials. One could adapt and adopt such materials to custom design a local program.

BREATHING BY THE NUMBERS

Breathe in on odd numbers, breathe out on even numbers up to the count of ten. For example, breathe in on the count of one, breathe out on the count of two, breathe in on the count of three, breathe out on the count of four. Five in, six out, seven in, eight out, nine in, ten out. The numbers give you something to think about while you are feeling your breathing. Practice "breathing by the numbers" several times a day until you can breathe to the count of ten some of the time without thoughts interrupting.

BREATHING TO THE COUNT OF TEN

Duke University anger research proves that if you can delay overreacting to an "incoming" stressor for 20 seconds you are more likely to think rather than get upset. Breathing by the numbers (inhale on odd numbers, exhale on even) to the count of ten will give you a 20-second stress buffer. Breathing to the count of ten prior to a stressful situation will take the sting out of the stressor. Start small with little irritations to build your stress tolerance. For example, breath-count before you make a stressful phone call, talk with a difficult person, or open bills.

BREATHE WITH "MEANING"

Once you can breath-count to ten, substitute a single word or short phrase for the numbers. For example, say silently to yourself on your inhalation, "In relaxation," then as you exhale say, "Out tension." (In relaxation [as you inhale] — Out tension [as you exhale]). Or try, "I am — relaxed." You may want to try saying to yourself more (on the inhalation) relaxed (on the exhalation). To review, some self-calmers are "I am [inhale] — relaxed [exhale]," "Just for now — I'll relax," or if you are religious, "This too — shall pass." "The peace that passes all understanding." It is most useful to select and practice your single favorite self-calmer. Change in itself is stressful. Stick with your best single calmer word or phrase for at least three weeks. Then try another for three weeks. Think of your top self-calmer, sleep on it, and start grooving it into your memory tomorrow.

To build habit strength, it is important that you pick one single phrase to practice with for at least three weeks. The phrase should be short and peaceful, not "More — money or work — faster."

If you are trying to doze off to sleep, say as you inhale, "Deep," and as you exhale, "Sleep."

5. Learn from the experts and get group support.

Contact your local hospital's cardiac rehab or wellness center to locate an expert in relaxation techniques. Carefully select someone who is certified, trained and proven to be effective. Certification in biofeedback relaxation training is a stamp of approval for legitimate practitioners. Also, licensing as a practicing psychologist or counselor would guarantee a high level of professionalism. Simply see your Yellow Pages.

A quality checklist for selecting a practitioner consists of the following:

- If the person you contact seems relaxed.
- If he or she demonstrates techniques, step-by-step, so you can take notes.
- Gives you homework (daily exercises at home and a way to track your progress).
- Provides support (through newsletters and testimonials from people you can contact).
- Has regular booster sessions.
- Has you keep records of your progress.
- Does not promise you the world. (No one becomes a gold medallist with one practice.)
- Contact a licensed psychologist or counselor in your area for advice.
- Ask whether he or she is trained in biofeedback and other legitimate relaxation and therapeutic techniques. At first consider getting outside help in relaxed breathing, like using training wheels on a bicycle. You should be able to get it on your own after a while, and like riding a bike, you will never forget.

A top professional, having helped more than a thousand clients over twenty years, is Dr. Richard Pinneau of Winston-Salem, North Carolina. He provides face-to-face breathing relaxation training, weekly booster sessions and follow-up through a weekly newsletter that is part of his Center for Life Enrichment (<CLEOffice@aol.com> or 336-768-0558).

6. Relaxation breathing is now part of standard preoperative procedure for hospitals.

Realizing the calming, oxygen enhancing and lung clearing benefits of relaxation breathing, hospitals now have included deep, relaxation breathing as part of preoperative preparation for surgery. Deep breathing has now become part of mainstream medical treatment.

7. Harvard Medical School recommends relaxation breathing even after witnessing 9/11.

The January, 2002 issue of the *Harvard Mental Health Letter* clearly states that in addition to physical activity and distractions, . . . "breathing exercises may help even dealing with the unbelievable devastation of the WTC and Pentagon."

SUMMARY

Relaxation breathing is actually easier done that said. In this chapter we looked at how deep breathing can work even on the job (It works for childbirth). Real-life benefits of better breathing are presented, such as excellent sensory perception, and overcoming being bored or baffled. A few tips on breathing instructions were provided. Some tips for selecting an expert in "breathing training" were provided. Deep breathing has now become part of mainstream medical treatment. Armed with the power of positive attitudes and relaxation breathing, you will now be able to take on the work world by using your Freedom of Choices, which the next chapter addresses.

FOR FURTHER READING

Carlton, J. (2001). "Focus on breathing helps Parker inhale competition, exhale records." Greensboro, NC. *News and Record,* 5-18. Section C.

Lamaze, F. in: Tanzer, D., & Block, J. L. (1972). *Why natural childbirth?* Garden City, New York: Doubleday & Company.

Noble, E. (1983). *Childbirth with insight.* Boston: Houghton Mifflin Company.

Pinneau, R. Winston-Salem, NC. Center for Life Enrichment (<CLEOffice@aol.com> or (336) 768-0558).

Zinn-Kabat, J. (1990). *Full catastrophe living: using the wisdom of the body and mind to face stress and pain-illness.* (Program Stress Reduction Clinic, University of Mass. Medical Center). New York: Delacorte Press Bantam Doubleday Dell.

8

WIN/LOSE – YOU CHOOSE:

YOUR FREEDOM TO CHOOSE

No statue was ever erected to honor a critic.

Choice is the C in the ABC's of Industrial-Strength Stress Control formula. Within reason, we have freedom of choice in how we handle problems. Consciously choosing how we handle hassles frees us from the involuntary stranglehold of job-stressors. Four proven choices for taking C.A.R.E. of business are:

C ONTROLLING,
A CCEPTING,
R ESTING,
E NJOYING.

This chapter deals only with the choice of Control in the C.A.R.E. package. Controlling the four C's of job-stress will be presented.

The four C's of job-stress are struggles with:

CONTROL (p. 90),
CHANGE (p. 96),
CONFLICT (p. 97),
COMPLAINING (p. 100).

Two other concerns directly related to the job environment are:

JLU, "Just like us," principle, the key to getting and keeping a job (p. 98);

Diversity and harassment on the job (p. 102).

The male equivalent of labor pain? Bob's experience

"Are you still with us, Bob?", asked the nurse as she inserted another tube in a place where Bob didn't know a tube could go. The doctor said, "Relax, relax, it will go easier on you." The attending doctor and nurse were worried that Bob was slipping away from consciousness, and unfortunately they needed his cooperation to complete the tests. He was told to "breathe deeply so we can finish this now."

Bob, mustering all his energy to fake a smile, thought of the Lamaze classes he had taught, and how the research proved that deep breathing helped relax and reduced pain. All this knowledge was not helping Bob now. So he started breathing deeply, and much to his amazement things started going better in the medical tests. He was later told, by the female nurse, that this procedure was the male pain-equivalent of childbirth. He thought to himself, it's a miracle that any woman would have more than one child if it hurts this much.

Take time to fill your tank, check your oil, check your tires and pack carefully. It's a long trip — your life on the job.

You will spend the equivalent of at least 15 full years (24-7) of your life on the job. Although it is important to use both your "head" and "heart" at work, you need to emphasize "head skills" in the work force because you are paid to deal with problems and people you would probably not deal with on your own. Employee assistance programs are routinely provided as part of an employee package because about one in ten employees will need to get help in coping with stress. On a positive note, it has been found that overall, working may be therapeutic if you have a reasonable sense of control and satisfaction on the job.

Industrial-strength stress control will be yours through building your force of habit in habitually making choices known to reduce stress. "What-to-do-tomorrow" tips are offered for you.

Tossing and turning, Bob mumbled in his sleep, "Abandon all hope, ye who enter here." In the most vivid dream he had ever had, he saw these hopeless words carved deeply into the cold granite over the door of the factory he worked in. Still dreaming, he entered the hot, furnace-like factory, turned around and again read the statement with one modification, "Abandon all hope, ye who enter here, NOT." He remembered the "No fear" license plate he had just put on his car. Waking from his disturbed sleep, he remembered he had just been promoted to floor chief. He now had a choice of using hope or despair (fear) to lead his crew. Being young and optimistic he vowed he would use hope to motivate and lead. Time will tell if he stays true to this "compass heading" of hope.

Again, using Choice as the C in the ABC's of industrial-strength stress management, we will offer tips on how to choose to rule over the four C's of work: control, change, conflict and complaining. Select one of these C's that is a roadblock to your success and satisfaction on the job. Get control over it (it may take weeks) and watch your job-stress decrease.

GAINING CONTROL OVER THE NUMBER ONE REASON FOR YOUR JOB-STRESS (The first C in the four C's of work) CONTROL

Three key ways to get control over your work are:

1. *Increase your knowledge. Find a need and feed it.*
2. *Play by the company rules.*
3. *Plan and pace yourself with time management. Use computerized "brain extenders."*

A large portion of this chapter will be devoted to time management because it is central to getting control over your job. Time management will help you from feeling overwhelmed while making you successful at the same time.

The specifics of these three key points to gaining control over your job are now detailed.

---

1. Increase your knowledge.

Knowledge is power, more than ever. The world's most financially-powerful person is the "knowledge baron," Bill Gates, developer of Microsoft computer software.

Find out what the company needs by finding out what people are rewarded for producing or providing. Who gets the "employee of the month" awards and why? Who gets mentioned in the company newsletters as examples? Look at others' success and make their success yours. It may require extra effort, taking courses, dealing with difficult people or problems, staying late, coming in early, etc. Again, it may be one of those like-it-or-not situations. What you like to do may not be what is valued in the company. So get a hobby, and do what you like to do when "off the clock."

The good news is that sometimes there is an actual marriage between what people like to do and what they get paid for. These are called trophy jobs for obvious reasons.

A good resource for getting, keeping and succeeding at a trophy job is a book by Joyce Richman, *Roads, Routes & Ruts, A Guidebook for Career Success.* Richman an internationally-recognized speaker and career coach, can be contacted at <JERichman@aol.com>.

A NOTE ON WORKING SMART. To work smart you have to be sharp. Paul Rosch, M.D., President of the American Institute of Stress, lists six practices to sharpen your concentration, memory and decision-making. These practices are: getting enough exercise and sleep, lowering your stress, controlling caffeine, avoiding prescription drugs, and eating a balanced diet for good blood sugar.

---

2. Play by the company rules.

Listen and watch for what the boss expects, don't be too perfectionistic, do more than the minimum, try to solve your own problems, accept your mistakes, use common sense, do not complain, and be on time.

---

3. Plan and pace yourself with time management. Use computerized "brain extenders."

One hour of planning saves you three to four hours later and achieves better results.

It is now the 21st century. Electronic markers have replaced paper and pencil. Try to use your left brain extenders — computers. Excellent time-management programs are available. Hand-held electronic calendars actually relieve you of cumbersome paper and pencil.

I've fallen behind, and I can't catch up

This is the theme song of the time-management impaired.

Hint: Corporations develop their master plan using computer calendars and planners. To give you a sense of control, get with the program, the computer program. Just as you weren't born knowing how to write long hand, you can learn to use computers.

Time management is considered one of the best job-stress managers for Type A's and for adults diagnosed as ADHD. Type A's tend to be constantly urgent individuals. Some Type A's tend to be impatient and easily agitated and angered. The angry Type A's triple their risks of heart attacks. ADHD is a medical designation that stands for attention-deficit disorder with hyperactivity. This is from the American Psychiatric Association's *Diagnostic Statistical Manual IV* that is a guideline for classification of mental-emotional maladies. ADHD adults are plagued with problems with attention, impulsivity and hyperactivity. ADHD symptoms usually occur by seven years of age.

The key to time management for Type A's and ADHD individuals is to pace oneself to work on one thing at a time. The inability to focus on one thing at a time is like a racecar with no steering wheel; when things speed up you will spin out of control. The Conners' Adult ADHD Rating Scales is a valid tool for measuring possible ADHD traits in adults.

The plane left without me! Why time management is so important.

Delia and Bob were rushing out the door for the airport when the phone rang. Delia had a feeling she should pick it up. It was her friend Lucille, who was supposed to be arriving within a half-hour at Bob and Delia's airport. With tears in her voice, Lucille said, "The plane left without me." All's well that ends well. She took a later flight and Bob and Delia met her at the airport.

The story came out that while waiting to board her flight, Lucille had started talking with her friend, Ethel, whom she unexpectedly met at the airport. Lucille was enjoying catching up with Ethel so much, that she just plain missed her flight. Lucille explained that she heard the last call to board the plane and thought she had time to catch it since she could see the boarding gate for her flight just down the hall. Lucille said, "Just because the plane was taxiing, they would not let me on."

To this day Lucille struggles with time management, hates being rushed, but is loved by all.

Work is especially difficult when you are required to do something complex, quickly. Develop or use already proven systems to handle your work. Simplify your work whenever you can. Develop good work habits by doing something correctly and consistently for about three weeks. Force of habit will take over after time, making the task easier.

For a good time: Use time management

- A Quick Quiz — How to know if you really need time management.
- How are time management and stress management connected? Improving your quality of life on the job and at home.
- What to do on Monday? Basic steps in time management. A Time-Capsule is provided in the Appendix.

Time is relative.

How long a minute seems depends on which side of the restroom door you are on when "nature calls urgently."

---

1. A Quick Quiz.

You really need time management IF:

1. *You are continually apologizing for showing up late.* For a month, start earlier for work, enjoy conversation or a warm drink with your spare time.
2. *You just "have to" do everything yourself because nobody else gets it quite right.* Take baby-steps in assigning tasks to others, enjoy trusting others.
3. *You are always misplacing your door keys, glasses, handbag or briefcase.* Always put your keys on your key rack at home.
4. *You have piles of unread newspapers and magazines.* Sit with each day's deliveries, and sort into trash, A-1 important, and bottom of bird cage when finished reading.
5. *You always need to search even for those kitchen items you use all the time.* Take one junk drawer at a time [15 minutes daily], organize it, and even label it until everyone gets the hang of the new system.
6. *You often feel exhausted because there seems to be so much to do and no time for you.* For one month, have a daily "To-Do" list or system, to reach weekly activities that reflect longer-term goals, go to a movie at week's end.

If some of these statements sound just like you, you are only human. You are not born with time-management skills any more than you are born knowing how to deal with money. Our notion of time is a made-up (but important) convenience. Even Einstein, in 1932, said: "For us . . . the distinction between the past, present and future is only an illusion, albeit a stubborn one."

Time is a convenient way for us to agree to meet (or not to meet) at the same place at the same time with the proper materials. Imagine if you will, even a simple four-way intersection, with stoplights that were not properly timed . . . ouch! Time is not only money, it is the way we measure life.

Plan to plan, today!

---

2. How are time management and stress management connected? Improving your quality of life on the job and at home, giving you a sense of control and predictability.

As said before, a high-energy person without control is like a racecar with no steering wheel. Both will crash and burn.

Time management gives you a sense of control and predictability, reducing your anxiety. It is considered one of the top ways to manage job-stress. Time management is a most critical key factor in helping Type A's, Type T's (thrill-seekers) and ADHD or ADD individuals gain control of their environment. Well-disciplined Type A's, Type T's (thrill-seekers), ADHD or ADD adults are simply called "go-getters, movers and shakers." In business, these high-energy, highly-paid executives are like thoroughbred racehorses. They leave the gate running and never seem to get tired. As mentioned earlier, the Conners' Adult ADHD Rating Scales (CAARS) is a quick (20 minute) accurate test for measuring possible ADHD traits in adults. See your human resources department for this test. Again, only physicians or clinical psychologists can confirm a diagnosis of ADHD.

If you are not a race horse type, but more of a turtle, you may need some "speeding up." Gaining a reputation of being on time or early will gain you respect, help you keep promises and accomplish your goals. A key "business winning strategy" is to under-promise and over-deliver. Translated this means, "I'll have the report to you by next Friday." If your client gets your report on the Tuesday before next Friday, you have made a good impression.

Fire—ready—aim

The opposite of managing your time well is captured by the uncomplimentary phrase of fire—ready—aim. You shoot for your target impulsively, without getting ready and then aiming. You may say or do things without taking the few seconds it takes to think first.

Don't wish for things to be over, because some day they will be — permanently.

If you don't know where you are going, any road will get you there.

Bob's very successful, top-executive friend relayed this true story that really captures the spirit of the saying, "If you don't know where you are going, any road will get you there."

He missed the job by five-hundred miles.

Jimmy-Bob had received the letter that he was to be interviewed for a fast-track-to-the-top job in the Fortune 500 Company he had applied for months ago. Not taking the time to read the letter carefully, (a good example of fire, ready, aim), he called the booking staff in his office suite and said, "Book me a flight to Trenton, near New York." The secretary, who was a seasoned traveler and a real company pro, said, "But Jimmy-Bob, are you sure this is where you want to go?" Jimmy-Bob said, "Well, our corporate center is paying for this, so just don't send me to Trenton but send me first class. Book it for a Monday morning flight, April 1st. My job interview isn't until four P.M." Again, the secretary tried to intervene and said, "But Jimmy-Bob, don't you think it would be a good idea to check out the corporate center the night before in Trenton?" Jimmy-Bob, in his typical Type A style, rudely clipped the secretary mid-sentence saying, "My son has a soccer game that Sunday. I'll expect to have an e-airline ticket by tomorrow morning."

Then came the big day, April 1st. Jimmy-Bob even put on a fresh tie, and with his e-ticket confirmed, boarded the plane for Trenton near New York. He arrived at 11:00 A.M. at LaGuardia airport, a half hour from Trenton. Hailing a cab, he was confident that if he went over the notes he had thrown together, he would ace the interview. On his departure from the plane in Trenton, however, he suddenly noticed no one from Corporate Office was there to meet him. No one was waiting in Trenton (near New York) with a Jimmy-Bob sign to provide him a ride.

Sadly, but true, a corporate executive was waiting at the Trenton (near Cleveland) airport for the Jimmy-Bob who had missed the entire interview by five-hundred miles. At the same time, in Trenton near New York, Jimmy-Bob carefully read the letter from Corporate Center. His first clue that he was in the wrong place but the right time, was the corporate letterhead, which clearly originated from a Trenton, but not the one Jimmy-Bob was in.

Needless to say, Jimmy-Bob did not even make the first cut for this scheduled interview, and eventually was cut from his job.

The author is tempted to end the story by saying, "He now works for a map making company", but since this is a true story, the author confesses he doesn't know whatever happened to Jimmy-Bob after he missed the interview by five-hundred miles.

---

3. What to do on Monday? Basic steps in time management.

Keeping time "the old-fashioned way," the "To-Do" list.

Time management is simple, but not easy. Keeping up your SINGLE daily

"To-Do" list is the heart of effective time management. Take advantage of the already constructed time-management (calendar) program in your computer, which does everything for you except make judgments of what items should come in which order. They even gently remind you of undone tasks without nagging. You have the great option of putting the reminder "to sleep" so it doesn't bother you.

Make fun of time by getting a humorous calendar, such as Page-A-Day distributed by Workman Publishing Company, Inc. in New York. Each day is provided with a helpful, often humorous tip on how to reduce stress. You may contact them on line at <www.workman.com>.

The basic steps to time management are simple, but not easy (requiring discipline). Again, daily use of a "To-Do" list is the heart of time management. Carry this habit for one-hundred days, and then it will carry you.

Time-Capsule

To save you time, an expanded version of the tips below can be found in the Time-Capsule (Appendix B).

Sweeping the crumbs out of your pantry may be a level C goal in September, but will quickly become an A-1 goal when mice start munching on those crumbs in October.

In the human race, you will simply spin out of control without time management.

GAINING CONTROL OVER CHANGE: (The second C in the four C's of work)

The only person who really looks forward to change is a baby in wet diapers.

How to handle changes on the job.

1. Stretch for flexibility. Train yourself to do your best, like it or not. You are paid for the "or not" part.

Honestly take stock of your job by making two columns with "like it" on the top of one column, and "or not" on the other. List the "like it's" and then the "or not's" under these columns. Try to enjoy the "like it" aspects of your job more, and just accept the "or not's." You might try doing the unpleasant "or nots" the first thing or on a regular schedule. Break down the tasks into small fifteen-minute "chunks" over several days if you need to. Use the if-then reward system, if I do such and such, then I will see a movie or do some other enjoyable activity.

As previously stated, "nimble" is the key word to survival in today's business. If you have a hard time changing your routine, just put the word "nimble" on an index card and carry it with you. Then say the "nimble-jingle" you learned as a child (Jack be nimble, etc.) to yourself.

2. Deal with love/hate at work. Many people have a love/hate relationship with their jobs, they love their jobs but hate the details of their work. There is some middle ground between love and hate. You may not be happy with a job, but that does not make you automatically unhappy.

GAINING CONTROL OVER CONFLICT: (The third C in the four C's of work)

Why should you try to control conflict? Conflict actually makes a worker dread coming to work.

Gaining respect from your boss protects you from "burnout." "Boss respect" is more powerful in protecting you from "burnout" than salary is. Tough bosses demand consistent, high-quality work, whereas brutal bosses will humiliate you in public. Try to fight for and earn respect from your boss rather than fighting with your boss.

Fighting with your supervisor is unhealthy as well as unwise

One out of five workers has a very difficult supervisor. Conflict with your supervisor can dangerously increase your blood pressure. For this and other reasons, learning to play on the team is a competency that must be acquired.

The hand that feeds you: working with your boss.

Points to consider when working with your supervisor:

1. *Try the JLU, "Just like us," principle. Try to fit in whenever possible.*
2. *Reducing the stress of your boss reduces yours because stress flows downhill!*
3. *It's their dime, so it's their time. You are paid to play on a team.*
4. *Accept criticism as a "need statement" from your boss.*
5. *Save up six months' pay to reduce your "what if" fears.*
6. *Talk with the "employee of the month" to find out what has made him or her successful.*
7. *Remember the success formula: Time on Tasks = Tasks on Time (TOT squared).*
8. *Be stress-intelligent.*
9. *Be civil: Your boss is under pressures you may not be aware of.*
10. *List and review positive things your boss has done and would do for you. Plan to ask for reasonable favors and needed advice to help increase your sense of positive control.*

We now provide a more detailed explanation of these tips to deal with conflict on the job.

Try the JLU technique. It may be like trying to find a needle in a haystack, but make every effort on a job (especially those first critical 100 days), to find common ground with your boss and co-workers. Your colleagues are a great support system and can provide you with very important "off-the-record" information to help you do your job better. Sometimes humor is a good bridge. The four magic words or phrases, sincerely said, that may pave the way when trying to fit in are: "Please, thank you, you're right, I am sorry."

"Just like us"

The well-groomed senior physician and CEO of the medical clinic stood at the head of a long mahogany table surrounded by richly leathered swivel chairs occupied by well tanned, healthy-looking doctors in lab coats. The CEO, Dr. Xavier Ray, smiling at the 12 medical practice colleagues and the computer specialist sitting around the table, began to speak. "After interviewing 35 applicants, we have found our best candidate for the job — Dr. Rentkin. You all know that four of us interviewed him, and found he was the strongest candidate by far to join our practice. The key point in our making the decision to hire Dr. Rentkin is that after all was said and done he is "just like us." The enormous success of this clinic is based on the hard-earned wisdom that people who are "just like us" fit in as team members. He even plays golf with the same handicap I have." One of the doctors at the table added, "Dr. Renktin knew all about the Beatles and the Kennedy assassination. We have had applicants who didn't have a clue about who the Beatles were." All his colleagues laughed, with good reason, because the clinic had made a record profit that year, and they were expanding their clinic because of the national service award they had just won.

Dr. Rentkin then entered the room, feeling he had made a good decision to "join" this practice.

The "just like us" key to success: About as many people are hired (and fired) because of their human relations skills as because of their technical skills. In fact, leadership-training courses suggest using a dual approach in selecting those to be promoted or demoted. Each employee is rated on a scale of one to nine on how well he gets along with other staff members and how sharp his technical skills are, again on a scale of one to nine. Those achieving a score of 9/9 (top score for human relations, top score for technical skills) are the first to be promoted and the first to get raises. The least preferred co-workers or LPC's (usually lowest in relationships and skills) are the first to be cut. With equally credentialed employees, many companies are actually giving the ability to get along more value than technical skills because technical skills change so fast and many of the technical skills are being taken over by computers. Also, credentialing levels the technical skills playing field.

Other tips in dealing with conflict

1. *Don't be paranoid. Get the facts about unfriendly competitors and then take action.*
2. *Know your enemies.*
3. *Have a good offense.*
4. *Disarm your enemies.*
5. *Face backstabbers. Confront backstabbers about what they have said and ask them to spell out their accusations to you face to face.*
6. *Deal with difficult people: Major tip — Turn up the AC (agree and comfort).*
7. *Use the "sandwich approach" (compliment-request-compliment), if you must get cooperation from these whiners.*

Ways to implement these tips are now provided.

Turning up the AC (agree and comfort) to cool down hotheads.

Sincerely agreeing with a distressed person may help cool him down. Carefully listen to the person, and rephrase what they are saying and feeling. For example, "I understand you are upset because the check (that is in the mail) did not get to you in time. I would be upset too." You might comfort this person by saying something like, "This won't happen again; How can I help you in this situation?" Pulling out your calendar or planner, to write down their concern, may help convince the person of your sincerity to help. Even writing down a date when you will follow through may be useful. Remember, you can't get inside the other person's head, so you are not responsible for how they react. Give yourself credit for doing the right thing even if things do not turn out right.

Be realistic in realizing that you can't change another person's behavior. Avoid the difficult person, or change your responses to that person. You can change your responses to a difficult person by applying the ABC's. Control your Attitude, Breathing, and Choices you make in responding to the difficult person. You are responsible and in control of your attitudes and choices you make. Breathing slowly and deeply for a few times, will quiet down your alarm reaction and help you think more clearly. Appreciate your own effort to relax under fire, whether you get the desired outcome or not.

Don't be a "reactionary." Don't be surprised every time a difficult person acts "difficult." Research on moral development, by Dr. Lawrence Kohlberg of Harvard, stated that only 10% of people reach the highest "Universal Principle" level, doing the right thing just because it is morally right. The golden rule, "Do unto others as you would have them do unto you," only works with some who play by these rules. Expect the best from yourself in how you respond, but say to yourself, "It's no surprise (INS) that ____ acted this way." Telling yourself INS let's you get the jump on controlling your response rather than "gut reacting" every time this person aggravates or irritates you. Planning ahead on how you are going to respond keeps you from being an emotional "reactionary."

Marcus Aurelius, one of the "good" Roman emperors (121-180 A.D.) and a philosopher quipped, "It is foolish to expect bad men to be good." He had spent decades on battlefields, but still maintained his moral "compass heading" through the brutality of war.

Be part of the solution, not part of the problem. You may be a "jerk-at-work" to others. Stress is contagious and people don't like to catch it from you. Smiling, while using calm gestures and a pleasing voice, can go far in reducing defensive, difficult behaviors in others. Don't be loud and annoying.

CONTROLLING COMPLAINERS: (The fourth C in the four C's of work)

Why control complainers?

Complainers feel better at your expense. Complaining does relieve stress for the complainer, while increasing it for the recipient. Complainers seek out those who will lend a sympathetic ear. Complainers become irritated if you disagree or do not respond the way they wish.

Treating complainers

Remember that complaining is like sneezing in public. It makes the sneezer feel better, but if you get too close you get sprayed and may even become infected yourself. The best advice for repelling complainers is do not be receptive, without being rude. Try to humor the person before they start on the "whine-o-thon." Have them put their complaints on a "whine-list", then have them rank the number one complaint they have. See if you can "problem solve" with them (if that is what they really want). Often whine-o-holics are addicted to whining and will always find something to whine about, not really caring about solutions.

Don't ration your compassion, but do avoid martyrdom. There are those who are the working wounded — wounded by life, but still needing to work. So before you ration your compassion, find out if the person is whining or wounded.

NATIONAL WHINER'S DAY — **It takes serious time to unwhine —** DECEMBER 26 (Fortunately most of the whiners are not at work on this day).

You may want to remind yourself that there is actually a National Whiner's Day. Whining for some may be a form of recreation. They get a lot of attention for it, and they have no intention of giving it up. A humorous approach to National Whiner's Day would be to generally challenge whiners to stop whining for 24 hours on National Whiner's Day. This "Whine-Off" would be the equivalent of a smoker's "Smoke-Off" day that occurs once a year. Tell these whiner's that they will be on their honor not to complain, because chances are they will be on a holiday break on National Whiner's Day.

How not to become a lightning rod for complainers? Complainers are always negatively charged up, just looking for a place to strike. Seven tips on how not to attract their thunderbolts include:

1. Don't ask how things are, if a person is a whine-o-holic. Be polite but don't invite complaints by asking, "How are you feeling?"

2. Avoid storms: If you step into a whinery (a room full of complainers), you are bound to get struck by complaints.

3. Be well-grounded to dissipate critical strikes. Put things in perspective when thunderbolts are thrown at you. Is there a kernel of truth? Does this person have a personality problem? Place the criticism on a scale of one to ten, with 1, 2, 3 being irritating but not dangerous. Most complaints will fall in this area.

4. Give yourself credit: To put criticism in its proper place, take and give yourself credit when due. If needed, keep a log of your key successes to give weight to your credit/criticism balance. (Share this list only if requested.) Reviewing your "credit balance" privately will give you confidence in your skills to persist in improving and growing from criticism.

5. Employ the "In one ear out the other" which you used with your parents and many authority figures as a child.

6. Try the phrase, "How can I make you happy? Or what can I do to make you happy?" (Retired corporate executive, Woody Mansir).

7. If you have to administer these whiners, try the "sandwich approach" (compliment-request-compliment). Find something you can compliment them on, sincerely, then make the request, then compliment again, with reassurance that you wouldn't ask them to do this thing if you didn't think they could. This technique came from the "heartless-land" of America, where people just want to be in control, even if they have to be nice. Again, remember, compliment, request, compliment. The compliments are the outside pieces of bread, covering the real meat, the request. It's easy to recognize this approach to manipulation, but at least the person is trying to make you swallow their request with some ease.

There's no pleasing her, so please, please yourself

By way of summary, this chapter looked at the C of the ABC's of Job-Stress Control-Choices. Reasonable choices can be summed up in a C.A.R.E. package. This chapter presented the most important choice, gaining Control over time/skills, change, conflict and complainers. The other three Choices in the C.A.R.E. package will be addressed in following chapters. (The other three choices are Accepting, Resting and Enjoying.) If you spend 80% of your effort to gain control over your work, you will greatly reduce your job-stress and maybe even experience job satisfaction.

You have freedom of Choices to gain control over the four C's at work:
CONTROL over job skills (including time management),
CHANGE,
CONFLICT,
COMPLAINING.

Dealing with diversity/harassment: Make sure the impact and intent of the message match

When in doubt, cut it out in terms of saying something you may regret later. What we may consider friendly could be taken the wrong way, by the wrong person. It is very important that you make every effort, in a sensitive situation, to be sure that the impact and intent of your message match up. The impact of your statement about someone's appearance may be much different than your intent. Feeling genuinely sorry for Bill, a co-worker, because you know he's been ill you say, "You look awful. You look tired and worn out." Now Bill slumps even further into his chair. If he did not feel bad before, he does now, after the impact of these words hits. The intent of what you said was compassion; the impact of what you said was discouragement to Bill.

An even more-sensitive dilemma occurs when someone asks you how she looks with a new hairdo, or dress. "Does this outfit make me look thinner?" The basic principle still applies; will the impact of what you say match the intent of what you are trying to say? An excellent resource by comedian Jim Dale is *Rules for husbands* and his companion work, *Rules for wives*. This 2001 publication gives men some clue as to how to navigate the sometimes treacherous verbal-seas they find themselves in. For six specific rules to get along better with the opposite sex, see the "Rules for the sexes" in the upcoming Chapter 19.

In the more serious arena of diversity/harassment, before you say anything that may be offensive, try to see how it sounds from the other person's point of view. Make sure the impact and intent of your message match. If you are "blessed" with a good sense of humor, this may be a good time not to use it if you have any doubts. Don't provide grist for the rumor mill. As said previously, those who gossip to you, will gossip about you as soon as you're gone.

Treat co-workers as if they were truly your sisters or brothers. In sensitive situations, perhaps in dealing with angered people, you may even want to script out what you are going to say to them. Wait a day, go over the script again, make any changes and practice a relaxation reset exercise, and then deliver the message. Drill into your mind the impact/intent principle.

SUMMARY

The C, standing for Choice, in the ABC's (Attitude, Breathing and Choices) of job-stress management, was featured in this chapter. Making better choices in dealing with the four C's of job-stress will go far in reducing job tension and even gaining job satisfaction. The four C's we can choose to deal with at work are Control (over job skills, time management), Change, Conflict and Complaining. The golden key to choosing to gain control over your job is to find a need and feed it.

A good resource for getting, keeping and succeeding at a trophy job is a book by Joyce Richman, *Roads, Routes & Ruts, A Guidebook for Career Success.*

We also briefly looked at the JLU, "Just like us," principle, which is key to getting and keeping a job. The opposite of the JLU principle is the LPC, least preferred co-worker. LPC's are usually targeted for "extinction" as soon as possible. We looked at the ever-growing and sensitive issues of diversity and harassment on the job. It was also discussed that when dealing with diversity/ harassment, make sure the impact and intent of your message match. *Rules for husbands* by comedian Jim Dale, and his companion work, *Rules for wives* were highlighted as good "word-maps" to avoid saying the wrong thing that could be considered harassment. Using the "sandwich approach" (compliment-request-compliment) to gain cooperation from whiners was discussed.

The next chapter deals with what could be considered the fifth C, Computers. Since more than 50% of adults avoid using computers, the need for CyberStress management in the computer age is obvious. Since many professional licensing/certification exams are now being given by computers, it would behoove professionals to overcome their computer phobia, if they plan to climb career ladders. At the other extreme of emotional-computer attachment is the new CSA, Computer-separation-anxiety, which will also receive attention in the next chapter.

FOR FURTHER READING

Barkley, R. (1998). *Attention-deficit hyperactivity disorder, a handbook for diagnosis and treatment.* New York: Guildford.

Long, G. (1909). *Meditations.* (New York, NY: P.F. Collier & Son).

Richman, J. *Roads, routes & ruts, a guidebook for career success.* Ms. Richman an internationally-recognized speaker and career coach, can be contacted at <JERichman@aol.com>.

Stokes Publishing Company, (1292 Reamwood Ave., Sunnyvale, California, 94089), offers a calculator-sized countdown timer that can be projected as a very large image, by a transparency projector. 2001 Price, $52.31 including tax and shipping. Ask for Teach-Timer (item 2-5850-007-412-000-621-00).

9

2001: A CyberStress Odyssey

COMPUTER ANXIETY

Your PC contains more programming capacity than the computer on the first manned space flight.

Too much technology causes rage

Too much technology combined with too little time are the root causes of rage in America today, according to C. Leslie Charles, author of *"Why is Everyone So Cranky?"*. Desk rage is probably caused by CyberStress, which results in people's maliciously planting viruses, or going on shooting sprees.

This chapter will focus on the why's and how-to's of dealing with CyberStress.

The **why's** of dealing with CyberStress discussed are:

- Half of adults avoid computers.
- Watch your language (your computer's language, that is). Is fatal really fatal? How illegal is an "illegal operation?"
- CyberStress is highly prevalent, yet America's largest online service cures it.
- Excessive computer use leads to depression or computer-separation-anxiety.
- Existence of web widows.
- Why should you try to like computers? So you can take your credentialing exam.
- Why is my VCR still unprogrammed?
- When your computer has a lobotomy or why computers may be stressful.

Eleven **how-to's** of managing CyberStress are provided with additional tips on how to deal with CyberStress depression. You may even experience separation anxiety from having to give up your computer, since over 55-million computers will become obsolete by the end of 2003. A tip from two-time Emmy award-winner is provided.

---

1. Half of adults avoid computers.

Over fifty percent of adults in America do not have access to the Internet and have no interest in connecting with the World Wide Web according to a 2000 study by a Pew Internet & American Life project. In fact the survey revealed that these individuals "liked" not being connected. Women were more likely to avoid computers (57%) compared to men (43%). Almost 60% of adults 60 and older were not interested in going online. Since this is the dawning of the information age, helping the other half feel comfortable with computers is essential to their success and satisfaction.

2. Watch your language (your computer's language, that is). Is fatal really fatal?

Fatal, schmatle — no one has ever died from a FATAL ERROR message from his or her computer. Watch your computer's language. Sometimes you have the option of disarming the fatal time bomb messages you will see on your screen. These skull and crossbones messages really just mean "get help from somebody who knows what they are doing."

If you perform an "illegal operation," can you get a computer lawyer to keep your program from shutting itself down? I don't think so.

Bob was confident when he sat down at the huge main frame at the Ivy University computer center. It was the early 1980's even before PC's. He had just taken a course in FPL, First Programming Language, which supposedly prepared him for writing software. His final assignment in the FPL class was to write a simple program to calculate the batting averages of a certain number of players. Each Ivy University student was allotted an hour a week on the mainframe, so time was important. After receiving about ten fatal error messages on the computer, his frustration was growing as his precious computer time was down to ten minutes.

Being a doctoral student in his late twenties, he was too proud to ask the 16-year-old whiz kid next to him in the computer lab to help him out. Finally, Bob broke down and politely asked the boy for help. The boy said, rolling his eyes, "I was wondering when you were going to ask for help." Making matters worse, there was an impatient woman from his FPL class standing right behind Bob, waiting for her turn. With wizard-like precision and speed the 16-year-old unlocked Bob's screen, eventually allowing Bob to finish the program. Bob could have gotten the answer faster by counting on his fingers, but it was the dawn of the computer generation. Although Bob has taught and taken numerous computer courses since, his level of CyberStress has remained the same, because every time he feels, "I've got it," a new form of hardware or software is introduced.

---

3. CyberStress is highly prevalent, yet America's largest online service cures it.

CyberStress, or computer stress, is as real and as common as the common cold. Out of the 40-million computer users, up to 8-million workers are at risk for computer stress. The easily-treatable CyberStress includes: eye strain; headaches; pains in the neck, shoulders, arms and legs; and a negative attitude about computers.

What the Internet giveth, the Internet taketh away: America's top ISP speaks out.

The largest Internet service provider offered an excellent feature on "Job got you down?" as presented on January 15, 2002, on this ISP. This computer-based article dealt with how to deal with job-stress. So what the computer creates in half its users, stress, can be managed by using a computer.

---

4. Excessive computer use leads to depression or CSA, Computer-separation-anxiety.

Fifty percent of high-tech workers in Finland report sleep disorders and physical pain resulting from stress. High-tech workers are at particular risk for anxiety disorders and clinical depression because they often sacrifice human relations to stay on the cutting edge. People in high-tech jobs often feel frustrated because they will always be behind the technological advances. New research reveals that people actually suffer from depression from computer information overload.

Computer-separation-anxiety

On the other hand, some people can get so attached to their computers that they go through separation anxiety when their PC's bite the dust. It is a fact that 55.4-million computers were retired and needed to be replaced before the year 2002. Placing your retired computer in landfill is not a good idea for environmental reasons, such as the batteries. It is strongly recommended you erase your hard-drive <www.comtechnologies.com> before you donate your computer. At this point, the author speculates that Goodwill Industries may be able to reuse your old computer. Also, "Get a life." Do you have emotional attachments to your lawnmower, rake, dishwasher, or other labor saving device? Why get upset when you have to "junk" your computer?

---

5. Existence of web widows.

Obsession with computers is probably as unhealthy as an unreasonable fear of computers. Many partners complain that they are computer widows, having lost their spouses to the web. If you spend more time with the computer than you do with your family and friends, you may want to consider withdrawing yourself somewhat before you become too taken with the computer.

6. Why should you try to like computers? So you can take your credentialing exam and other reasons.

Computers, testing us? Definitely.

Almost no technological advance has so revolutionized the work world in such a brief time as the computer. The 21st century exam has even been computerized. Licensing exams are now being given on computers instead of the respondent's filling in a paper and pencil exam. The financial world has embraced computerized testing, so it is quite likely that if you desire to be promoted through licensing or credentialing, you will have to try to like computers. In only twenty years, the personal computer is now used by 40-million workers in the U.S. alone.

Computers explosively increase our "collective wisdom" by linking up "electronic brain cells" (computers) throughout the world. The benefits for medicine, engineering, education, other sciences and entertainment are greater than ever. Never before has such problem solving and communication power been at our fingertips. Many workers do not have to leave the comfort of their homes to do their work. Students have access to the greatest libraries in the world at the press of a few buttons.

7. Why is my VCR still unprogrammed?

Regardless of time zones, millions of VCR's are all flashing 12:00 in unison in the U.S. because of our hesitancy to tackle those VCR manuals written in computerese. Although a VCR is a very simple computer, most people are gripped by a mild case of computer phobia and avoid attempting to program, even for fun, under no pressure.

8. When your computer has a lobotomy (hard-drive failure) or why computers may be stressful.

Hal 2001, revisited — Bob's stressed-out computer needed a lobotomy

When your computer suffers from IOS, "Information overload stress," from its stressed-out operator, your computer may need a computer lobotomy. This author overstressed his computer with too much information at once. To make a long story short, his computer needed a lobotomy, that is, its whole brain was wiped out and replaced with a new one. This was enormously stressful for him.

Now we will explore four major reasons why computers can be stressful.

Reason one: discomfort of "letting go" of paper/pencil and books

Computers represent the biggest change since books in how we store and use information. For over a thousand years, books were the primary means of storing and passing on knowledge. Most people today still remember when the accepted way information was recorded was through books or writing. This book tradition goes back 45 generations! The personal computer tradition goes back only twenty years.

Books are hands-on, requiring no special equipment to read; to read a disk requires a machine. The trust level in computers may have been further weakened when people were seemingly replaced by computers. Only the youngest in our society grew up along with computers, so they comfortably trust and even like computers.

Many adults do not share this comfort level with computers. So if you feel uncomfortable with computers, relax, you are in the "normal majority." If you are among the lucky few with the natural inclination toward computers, congratulations. This is your time to shine!

Computers are the 21st century equivalent to the technical leap made when printed books were first mass-produced in 1456, with the introduction of the *Gutenberg Bible*. To help dismantle computer phobia, it is helpful to understand why computers may be stressful. Ironically, computers themselves have been used to pinpoint causes and cures for computer stress. Computers can be both physically and emotionally taxing.

Reason two: trying to "muscle" computers

Using advanced "muscle movement measuring devices," it was found that computing workers have a tendency to tighten and hold muscle tension in the neck, shoulders, and arms. Users tend to tighten and hold muscle tension in areas not used for data entry, including the back and legs, and tend to hold muscle tension even when not entering data.

Reason three: getting emotional about data

It was found that entering data arouses a "startle response" which some individuals perceive as unpleasant and emotionally draining. This "startle response" can also be interpreted as excitement, depending on one's attitude, actually giving data entry workers a "power surge."

Reason four: not watching your language

As mentioned above, those menacing skull and crossbones messages on your screen really just mean, "Get help from somebody who knows what they are doing." One computer system even features a bomb with a fuse that is burning down. Your insurance is to save your information every couple of minutes.

Some programs already have this feature built in. Another wise thing to do is make sure you don't use someone else's computer unless they have taken you through the proper boot-up and power-down procedure.

Other Reasons: why computers may stress you out

Rule shifting: The more rules a situation has, the more stress is generated. Computers are now designing computers. But with advances such as WYSIWYG (What you see is what you get), the rules may be less mystifying in the future.

Lack of control: computer "gridlock" happens, or information "disappears"

Keyboarding: Letting your fingers do the talking is easier said than done. Until computers are voice driven, some people may feel as if they are trying to type with boxing gloves on, simply lacking typing skills.

Mind-numbing: Working at a computer all day can be like watching movie credits on a TV screen for eight hours. Unless the credits contain the name of a relative or friend, you get numb. However, working at the computer, you may still have to pay attention even though the material has no meaningful information for you.

CYBERSTRESS CURES

Adopt a humorous sense of perspective.

Remember, you can always pull the plug, after the recommended shut-down procedure is followed. The information processor in the box is only the servant to your personal "thought processor," your brain. Display your sense of humor with cartoons taped on your computer or workstation area.

Eleven tips follow:

1. Read the Consumer Reports *article, "This @!*# Computer. How to Handle Ten Common Gripes." (March, 2001, p. 65).*

"This article clearly addresses ten of the most stressful computer problems faced by common users. These problems include why crashes happen, how come startups and shutdowns can take so long, what about rebooting, do you really need an upgrade. If you are not too frustrated try the Consumer Report's email address <ideas@techlife.consumer.org>.

2. Scientifically learn muscle tension awareness/relaxation.

Employee assistance programs can provide this over a few weeks. Progressive relaxation, combined with muscle tension biofeedback, is the easiest and best way to recognize and relax muscle tension. Muscle tension is responsible for most headaches, some back problems and grinding of teeth at night (bruxism).

The best of biofeedback appears to be *Freeze-Framer™ emotional management enhancer.* This state-of-the-art, biofeedback stress-management system provides colorful, entertaining stress-reduction training using heart-rate self-regulation to consistently bring about deep states of relaxation. This enjoyable, but highly accurate and effective biofeedback product makes relaxation training fun and fast in almost any setting (business, school, stress-control coaching setting or home.)

Freeze-Framer™ emotional management enhancer is so effective it was commissioned in April of 2002 to help heal toxically-high levels of stress, inflicting about 200,000 of New York City's one-million school children. The *Freeze-Framer™* and Heartmath professionals were called in for emotional rescue work on Staten Island according to Mr. Jeff Goelitz. HeartMath immediately came to the mind as one of the leading institutions specifically geared to help with traumatized children and adults. The ingenious *Freeze-Framer™* works with PC's to redirect and focus one's attention to inner states of relaxation in a safe, pleasing manner.

It is very unlikely that any organization has been as traumatized as this 9/11 ground-zero school system. It would behoove any school system or business under the siege of stress to give the professionals at HeartMath a call.

On February 7, 2001, CNN, with an audience of 22 million, recognized the *Freeze-Framer™ program* by HEARTMATH as so effective it significantly reduces stress in teachers, students, and even policemen. Call Heartmath, 1-800-372-3100 or email: <info@heartmath.com>.

3. Rest your hands on your desktop or in your lap whenever possible.

Keeping your hands on the keyboard for longer than a few minutes strains your arms, shoulders and neck muscles according to computer-user muscle-tension research.

4. Blink. Also a tip from an Emmy award-winner to reduce eyestrain.

Staring at a screen can dry your eyes. Also, enlarge the font whenever convenient.

It's better to light a candle than to..., a tip from a two-time Emmy award-winner. Rex Best spends 60 to 70 hours per week writing at his computer. The quality of his performance is gauged by the Nielson ratings for his segments of the TV show. Best's tip is to light a candle to soften your environment. Gaze at the candle periodically to regain your focus. An aromatherapy candle would be even better. But of course, use caution, because computer workspaces are usually littered with paper and cords everywhere. Be sure to blow out the candle before you turn off your computer or whenever you leave the room. Of course use normal caution with candles if children are present.

5. Look away whenever you can.

Fix your gaze at a pleasant "target" across the room or outside.

6. Take a mini (minute) break every 15 to 30 minutes.

Unfreeze your muscles momentarily. Check your posture.

7. Breathe slowly and deeply for a few breaths as you sit down in front of your computer to counteract the involuntary "startle" response which occurs for some computer operators. Make certain you are not holding your breath without knowing it.

8. Get an entertaining screen saver.

Data entry involves left brain processing. To prevent "left brain strain," animated "right brainer-entertainer" screen savers (flying fish, etc.) can give your left brain a break.

9. Consider learning computers to be like learning a foreign language.

Just do it. Take classes with friendly instructors.

10. Get a personal trainer.

Link up with a computer store or find an expert who makes you feel comfortable. Stephen Abondolo, president of Educational Technology Consultants, Inc., (336) 288-7768, is a valuable resource to help you demystify computer problems at work or home.

11. Make friends with a child who understands computers! Get back with your significant other if he or she has become a web widow.

Finally, when or maybe before all else fails, ask your child for help!

If you have made your spouse a web widow, get back to being friends with him or her. Although great, computers are just two-dimensional machines in a three-dimensional world of reality. You are missing a whole dimension of life if you are obsessed with your computer. Living in a two-dimensional world is like looking at a menu but never really eating (a three-dimensional reality).

OVERCOMING CYBERDEPRESSION

A final word about computer depression. Up to 50% of high-tech workers can suffer depression as the result of the isolation and "bottomless pit" aspects of computer information overload.

Tips in overcoming computer depression:

1. Set limits on the amount of time you spend each day learning how to use a new application or technology. Technology information flow out there is practically limitless, so there is no limit to the amount of time you could spend, so budget your time.

2. Concentrate on learning only what you really need to know about a new technology. Don't read the manual from cover to cover unless your job requires it. Sooner, rather than later, something is going to replace it.

3. In an office setting, remember that you are a team member. This will help you with a sense of commitment.

4. Avoid worshiping technology. It is not a purely good thing or a purely bad thing. Your computer is merely a tool, like a very smart typewriter.

SUMMARY

This chapter focused on attempting to control a relatively new but major source of stress, computers. It was revealed that over fifty percent of adults do not favor the use of computers, with women being more computer resistant than males, and older individuals (60 plus) being less receptive to computer technology than younger individuals. Watch your computer's language. A fatal message has never resulted in a fatality, yet. No one has been put in "computer jail" (to this writer's knowledge) for executing an "illegal operation" on a computer. The fact that excessive computer use can lead to depression was discussed. The existence of web widows was discussed, and eleven how-to's of managing CyberStress were presented. A tip from two-time Emmy award-winner, Rex Best, was also provided to relieve eyestrain and inspire the writer within you. The urgency of treating CSA, Computer-separation-anxiety, is highlighted with some tips on how to deal with this 21st century malady. CSA will inflict tens of millions of computer owners when their computers end up at yard sales — for parts.

Controlling the cause of stress is the best choice in relieving stress. The next chapter deals with other choices in the C.A.R.E. package, which are Accepting, Resting and Enjoying situations as coping strategies.

FOR FURTHER READING

Freeze-Framer™ emotional management enhancer. Call Heartmath, 1-800-372-3100 or email: <info@heartmath.com>.

Pew Internet & American Life Project: 2001: Survey: Women more likely to avoid computers (57% for women, 43% for men).

10

More Freedom Of Choices

In the C.A.R.E. Package

"God grant me the serenity to accept the things I cannot change, the courage to change the things I can, and the wisdom to know the difference." - Reinhold Niebuhr

We will now look at three other choices we have to manage stress: Accept, Rest and Enjoy. The previous two chapters looked at the C in our C.A.R.E. package, Control, where we should put most of our effort. A separate chapter was devoted to getting control over your computer, such is the influence of this data processor in most workers' lives.

Choice Two in the C.A.R.E. Package: ACCEPTING

Experts on peak performance and stress management agree that learning "to accept" is critical. A nationally-recognized sports psychologist states that to perform our best we have to "accept the bad, banish it from the mind and keep on plugging away." Dr. Paul Rosch, President of the American Institute of Stress, suggests adopting the prayer of acceptance quoted above.

Accepting limitations expands our boundaries

Marilyn vos Savant, measured to have the world's-highest IQ, advises that admitting to and accepting our mistakes is a true way to becoming smarter.

Blood pressure can be dangerously skyrocketed by overreacting to mistakes. People overreacting to mistakes had up to a 54-point blood pressure increase within only twenty minutes, according to a University of Western Ontario study.

Good driver/bad passenger syndrome: Most of us make better drivers than passengers because being in the driver's seat helps us control or at least predict what is going to happen. At work you are paid to be a team player and accept decisions and workloads. It helps if you know that you can control how you react to what happens to you. It's like being on a bus with a team, with someone else driving. You just hope the driver (your boss) knows where he's going and is a good driver. Your stress-management skills will act like a safety belt so you don't get knocked around emotionally when the ride gets rough.

ARE YOUR ATTITUDES HARDENING? Just as you can get hardening of the arteries from lack of exercise and poor diet, you can also get hardening of the attitudes, or intolerance of differences, from lack of stretching exercises. Are you easily upset by young people's dress, music or behavior? Are you annoyed by people who wear studs in every part of the body? Blackbeard and his sailors wore pierced everything. Do you feel as if your country is being invaded by foreigners? Do you think our institutions are becoming like the U.N., having to serve diverse populations? Fortunately our ancestors took the brunt of being the unwelcomed foreigners. Anyone who has arrived in North America after 1492 is a foreigner, so get a grip, foreigner.

HOW TO ACCEPT JOB-STRESSORS

- Prepare to accept occasional "down times/down people."
- Don't make "something out of nothing." A survival manual for dealing with "jerks at work" is presented (*Nasty People: How to Stop Being Hurt*). One out of a hundred wants to be a jerk.
- Know what you can control and what you need to accept.
- Be patient but not passive.
- Try to be tolerant of intolerance.
- Accept being bored or baffled occasionally.
- Accept challenges. When faced with what seems to be overwhelming work, look at it as a challenge, saying to yourself, I'll do a good job and show them how it's done.
- Replace your "I have-to's" with "I want to's."
- Accept waiting: Develop a waiting list of things to do while waiting.
- Remember: Acceptance does not mean agreement. You can learn to accept things you do not like.
- No one was ever fired or divorced for listening.

You may wish to apply some of these same principles in trying to accept events you cannot control at work.

Please take a number.

Bob and his wife, Delia, had enjoyed a day of backpacking in the beautiful Manzano Mountains near Albuquerque, New Mexico. Being famished by the exhilarating but exhausting 10-mile hike, they decided to go to town to get Chinese food for an early dinner. Entering the completely empty Chinese diner, Bob went up to the counter and asked for chicken chow mein. The restaurant owner behind the counter coldly said, "Please take a number." There was indeed a number ticket dispenser on the clean stainless steel top of the counter. There was also a sign that clearly asked customers to take a number and be seated. Bob reasoned that since they were the only people in the Chinese diner, they wouldn't need a number to be served. The kitchen had just opened and it was obvious Bob and Delia's food would be the first to be prepared that day.

Abandoning the idea that the customer is always right, Bob dutifully took a number tag from the dispenser, pulling off number one. They were still the only customers in the restaurant when the owner said to Bob and Delia, "Please be seated." The man then went to the large neon marquee mounted on the wall, turned it on, and pulled a chain that displayed the number 1 for all three to see. At the bottom of the marquee was the statement, "Now serving this number."

Starving, Bob and Delia sat on the hard bench. They could hear the clatter of pots and pans in the kitchen, and Bob clutched the ticket in his hand. After ten minutes, with Bob and Delia still being the only customers in the restaurant, the owner came out of the kitchen with the order, smiling. He then shouted, "Number one? Is number one here? Your food is ready." Amused with the absurdity of having to take a number and waiting in line while being the only customers in the store, Bob and Delia chuckled as they left the store. Then they headed for the New Mexico sunset to enjoy their Chinese food.

---

1. Prepare to accept occasional "down times/down people."

Criticism and conflict hurled at you are commonly stress-driven. Consider the source. Live in such a manner that no one believes unkind things said about you. Your work-life should be "mostly sunny with a 20% chance of rain." There is a 20% chance of emotional storms in the business world, according to Duke University research on anger, because one out of five people holds significant levels of anger.

You are not responsible for other people's irritable moods, no more than you are responsible for the weather. You are responsible for "getting in out of the rain" by controlling how you react to or even avoid storms created by "bad moods."

In fact Marcus Aurelius, the great Roman emperor, put it less delicately by saying that you are no more responsible for another's bad behavior, than you are for their bad breath. Just try not to get too close to them.

Don't take others' bad moods personally, for you may accidentally be in the path of a tornado "whipped up" before you came on the scene. Bad moods can come from too much or too little caffeine/sugar and sleep. As Benjamin Franklin is credited with saying, "Face the sun."

2. Don't make "something out of nothing."

Do not exaggerate the "cold shoulder," interruptions, obvious lack of interest (yawns) or even rudeness that comes your way. Tell yourself as often as you need, "No harm done."

If you must work with the emotionally-blind people, try applying the 1989 book, *Nasty People: How to Stop Being Hurt by Them Without Becoming One of Them,* by Jay Carter. In chapter four of Dr. Carter's book, entitled "What Do We Do About It?," he specifically lists activities to help you with the invalidator boss or spouse. He details conflict management or confrontation skills essential to maintaining your validation as a worthwhile human being. He gets inside the warped heads of nasty peoples' thinking, highlights warning signs of nasty bosses, husbands or wives and how to break the cycle of nastiness. It is even a self-help book for the nasty (what you should do if you think you are the nasty one). This book, is worth its weight in gold, and should be required reading for anyone dealing with people.

Basically, Dr. Carter says you need to know who the nasty people are. He states that about one percent of the population consists of conscious invalidators. That is, they consciously try to develop those traits in themselves to put others down. So in any group of folks, chances are there will be at least one to burst your bubble, and take pride in it. They never are remorseful about hurting others and never say they're sorry. Dr. Carter suggests a two-prong approach to dealing with invalidators: He advises to always try reason first (professional positive behavior) then cause and effect. He provides over 20 reasoning activities (do's and don'ts). Because many invalidators are unreasonable, he provides eight cause and effect strategies, or behavior modification (rat psychology) strategies to apply for those at the "rat learning" of moral development. Don't try this at home.

3. Know what you can control and what you need to accept.

Make two lists, one of those being things you can control, the other those things you need to accept. Decide the top things you need to control for now and the top things you need to accept. Your list will change over time.

4. Be patient but not passive.

You can temporarily accept something while patiently working on a solution to help you gain control over the situation or your attitude. Contact your professional organization if you need advice or someone you can trust.

5. Try to be tolerant of intolerance.

"Zero tolerance" for errors is an admirable but sometimes unattainable goal. Shoot for excellence over time, not instant perfection. Accept those who feel that it is either their way or the wrong way.

6. Accept being bored or baffled occasionally.

Being bored or baffled are stress extremes, ranging from understimulation to overstimulation. Remember, everything is temporary.

Workers on a cruise ship were asked what it was like to work at vacationing. Surprisingly they said, "It got old, and they could not wait to get home." Mind-numbing boredom can be overcome by putting personal meaning or self-challenge into the work.

Reward yourself for making "quotas," reaching "benchmarks," beating the clock, setting performance records, and so forth.

Three tips to conquer boredom: prioritizing daily work, doing the worst first, making your work a game with several small parts and short deadlines. Boredom is often thinly-disguised procrastination. Treat procrastination as you would boredom.

To help you put boredom in perspective, try repeating, "If it's their dime, it's their time." Your employers are paying for your time so they determine how you spend your time. Also remember, correctly setting up your paycheck is probably quite boring for your company's accountant. If your paycheck were late or short because the accountant was "bored," you would not be happy. Think of how doing your job well while being bored is just as important as the company's accountant doing your paycheck correctly. You would not accept boredom or procrastination for paycheck errors or delays. You certainly would not want your 747 pilot to doze off into boredom or your surgeon to quit in the middle of your procedure because he got tired of doing the "same old thing."

Chaos creates stress, but it can also create solutions. If your situation is chaotic try to learn from it. Learning something new may involve feeling overwhelmed or baffled for a while. "Relaxed exposure" to small pieces of what you need to learn will help you get used to the new. Try to make the learning curve less steep by taking small steps at first. Part of learning how to learn involves dealing with the mild frustration associated with learning something new. Remember, every problem has a solution.

7. Accept challenges.

When faced with what seems to be overwhelming work, look at it as a challenge, saying to yourself, I'll show them how it's done.

8. Replace your "I have to's" with "I want to's."

If your life is filled with all "have to's," try replacing some of them with "want to's" (I want to go to work because I want to have a nice house). It will increase your sense of control.

9. Accept waiting.

Develop a waiting list of things to do while waiting. Even deep breathing often works when you are stuck with nothing to do but wait. Look for pleasant or entertaining features in your environment to distract you when stuck in lines or traffic.

10. Remember: Acceptance does not mean agreement.

You can learn to accept things you do not like.

11. No one was ever fired or divorced for listening.

Sometimes it is better to silently listen and accept what is being said to you, especially if the other person needs to vent. Acceptance statements include: "I understand, I can accept that," "I see" or even, "How fascinating!"

Choice Three in the C.A.R.E. Package: RESTING

No one has ever been too tired to leave work and go home!

Have you ever gone into work in the morning to find someone asleep at their desk claiming they were "just too tired" to go home at the end of their shift? No, I haven't, either. People always seem to find enough energy, even after the worst day at work, to get themselves home. Rest is absolutely important, but some of the fatigue we feel at work is in our heads, and that is job-stress.

Why rest? A 20-minute power-nap recharges the most powerful man on earth, President Bush. Twenty minutes of rest will reset your brain back to optimal performance. If the President can carve out 20 minutes to power-nap daily, certainly you can. A 20-minute nap can improve your memory, sharpen your alertness and reduce fatigue.

Relaxation is the oil in your mental machinery. You may want to catch twenty winks after you get home and before you eat or exercise. Twenty minutes is also considered enough time to meditate for optimal benefit. Twenty minutes of breathing meditation gives you a mini-vacation. Saying on inhalation, "I am," and on exhalation, "at peace," can center you, improving your concentration and thinking. Sit up in a chair, and set a timer in a drawer, under a towel, to muffle the ticking sound, while allowing you to hear it go off after twenty minutes. You don't want to hear the timer ticking like the one on a popular TV show that features a stopwatch as its centerpiece for advertising. It could create more stress than it's worth.

Sometimes resting or retreating is needed for coping or growth to occur. A man went to his doctor for advice and said: "Doctor, every time I move my arm like this it hurts. What should I do?" The doctor said, "Stop moving your arm like that." This old joke makes an important point: Think about what you want, not what you don't want. If you want to feel more relaxed, think relaxing thoughts. Give your worries a rest.

Scientific research shows that merely thinking negative thoughts physically triggers your emotional "fight or flight" response, which can make you irritable, sick and tired. Bringing up the past in a negative way brings up the same stressful feelings all over again and prevents healing of old wounds. You spin your wheels while getting nowhere. Following are some tips for giving yourself a break or rest from negative thinking:

- Avoid thinking stressful thoughts. "Negative-thinking addictions" — how to recognize and overcome them.
- Avoid contagion.
- Does the shoe fit? Avoid job-stress extremes. You may need to retreat from a chronically stressful situation.
- Take your breaks.
- Take more or better vacations. Frequent/shorter vacations may be better. Try a virtual visit with a friend or relative.
- Remember, your job is not designed to be an endurance test or a "stress marathon." Become more sensitive to stress symptoms before it's too late.

---

1. Avoid thinking stressful thoughts.

Realize that negative thinking is a maladaptive habit that can be broken. A mental-health specialist may be helpful in establishing more rational, healthful thought patterns that reduce stress. Without knowing it, you may well be a victim of a "negative-thinking addiction," built-up and rewarded by a negative world.

"Negative-thinking addictions" — how to recognize and overcome them

Honestly ask yourself if you are addicted to negative thinking. If you always look for the downside, expect the worst, or find reasons why something won't work, you may be addicted to negative thinking. If you read the obituaries first (and are relieved if your name is not included), you are probably addicted to negativity. Like any addiction, a "negative-thinking addict" is constantly looking for their next fix. The fix is to look for trouble. If there is not enough trouble in your own backyard, you will borrow trouble from someone else through gossip or the media or borrow nonexistent problems from the future.

Overcome your "negative-thinking addiction" by blocking any negative thoughts for just half a day. An effective way to block negative thinking is to have a ready-made positive thought to substitute as soon as a negative thought invades your thinking. Keep trying to block all negative thinking for just one day until you are successful. Doing this on a weekend or vacation is best.

Anger research has found that the "chronically angered" bring up past, unrelated events to fuel their anger, setting themselves up to be more easily angered in the future.

2. Avoid contagion.

Emotional contagion research shows that stress can be involuntarily caught just by being in the presence of a stress carrier. Reduce or eliminate exposure to these people, or put on "attitude armor" if you have to deal with these individuals.

3. Does the shoe fit? Avoid job-stress extremes.

A major source of job-stress is a mismatch between worker skills and job demands. You may have to avoid or reduce exposure to jobs you cannot adjust to.

Popular personality "typing" research suggests there are at least sixteen personality types. Seven different types of intelligence have been identified. It may be that your personality/intelligence profile conflicts with job requirements. Police work would be very stressful to a shy writer. Being a research scientist would be a very stressful job for an outgoing social director.

Finally, you may need to retreat from a chronically stressful situation. Use your "head" and "heart" in making this decision, however. Plan ahead as much as possible. Get support (professional opinions) about your situation. Do not burn your bridges as you leave.

Avoid making gut-level decisions, because your gut level is at about a five-year-old developmental level. Your gut-level responses are almost completely right brained, and impulsive, survival oriented and about as delicate as a bull-dozer. As to every rule, there is an exception, even to the gut-level quitting rule. Bob, with all his "supposed wisdom" having taught human relations and leadership courses, was forced to make a literal gut-level decision to quit. The story follows below.

Bob, after nearly three decades of devotion to a job requiring lifting as much as the average mail carrier does daily, had to say, "It's time to say goodbye." Bob said, "Regrettably this is a gut-level decision I have no control over. My 'gut' just can't take it any more. This was Bob's poor sense-of-humor attempt at saying his new hernia would require him to quit his job." Bob truly held out from making a gut-level career move until his gut (hernia) made it for him. His workaholic motto was, "I would rather cave in than give in" to job-stress. He got his wish.

4. Take your breaks.

Try to take breaks around positive individuals. Walking can help relieve stress. For most adults, 50 minutes to an hour is about prime time to concentrate continuously on a project before it's time to take a break.

Concentration "errors" (daydreaming, looking around, losing one's place) start to mount the longer you delay taking a short break after this 50 minute prime time. If you use computers or do close work you need to refocus your gaze at some distant object periodically. Muscle tension headaches and overall stiffness set in after several hours in the same position. Stretch, even for a few seconds every hour.

---

5. Take more or better vacations.

Frequent, shorter vacations may be better. It may be more effective to take more frequent, three-day weekends than a three-week vacation only once per year. Firemen are often put on 72-hour breaks to help them relax and recharge so they can perform more effectively on the job. The old saying, "Out of sight out of mind," points us to the need to get away from work. It may take up to three days to really get work out of your mind, or to "unwhine."

How well rather than how long we spend our vacation time is important. You may not be able to control how long your vacation is, but you can control how well you enjoy it. Try to leave work at work, if you can. It is probably better to work a little longer on the job site than to drag work home with you.

On the weekends, try not to "work at fun" with long-term deadlines and never-completed projects. Break down weekend projects into small two to three hour blocks so you have a sense of completion and satisfaction even if your overall projects take several weekends. Writing each "goal block" on a three by five index card may give you visible proof that you got something done during the weekend.

Taking a "reverse cruise" to reverse stress

Being limited in time and money, Bob and Delia decided to try a cruise in reverse . . . that is, they watched ships cruise by as they "luxuriated" in their riverside hotel room in beautiful Savannah, Georgia.

Thinking it would be nice to share a get-away on the riverside, they booked a room at a hotel where huge cruise ships passed their room regularly. What was most enjoyable is that it did not matter if Bob and Delia were on the ships that were moving or watching the moving ships. The result was relaxation, as they watched the largest machines on earth float by at a leisurely pace.

It is important that you learn to disengage from work when the whistle blows. Your car may even be a good "decompression chamber," serving as a neutral zone of music and news between work and home, both with their complicated expectations. An excellent decompression audiotape is *"Handling stress with humor,"* by Loretta LaRoche.

When you get home, really look at the pleasant things about your house and yard, make eye contact with loved ones, play with a pet, and give yourself about 15 minutes to unwind after the trip home.

Change out of your work clothes. Taking a shower or a bath can recharge you and give you a second wind. Enjoy something daily that takes your undivided attention and that you feel successful at, such as getting through the newspaper sports or comic sections. Have relaxation rituals that work for you.

Try a virtual visit with a friend or relative

The marvels of modern computer technology now allow you to have video-phone conferences with friends and loved ones thousands of miles away. Once these video-phone programs are installed in your computer (check with major computer stores), you can have moving video images of your friends or relatives, at a cost lower than long-distance phone calls. There is no place like home, or family. Now you can have a virtual "live video" visit when both parties agree on a time. Anyone who is homesick or just missing loved ones can now just log on and visit with your significant others. This technology will only improve since the increased hesitancy to fly due to the 9/11 plane tragedies.

---

6. Your job is not designed to be an endurance test or a "stress marathon."

True quality work requires that your thinking equipment is fully charged, so learn to rest well whenever you can. In fact, in the excellent book, *Living at the Speed of Life*, the authors strongly suggest that we lower our stress tolerance. We do this by being more sensitive to stress, not less, because we may build our stress tolerance so high that we ignore dangerous stress symptoms until it's too late. We have strokes, heart attacks, irreversible high blood pressure, serious and permanent stomach disorders. In essence we need to learn to rest before it hurts.

Choice Four in the C.A.R.E. Package: ENJOY

"No pain — no gain" makes about as much sense as "Spare the rod — spoil the child." Both principles are wrong and abusive.

Pleasure-starved people are often irritable, inefficient and unfriendly. These people brighten the room by leaving it.

The inability to enjoy simple pleasures, called anhedonia, can actually be a warning sign of depression. Always see a mental-health professional regarding questions on mental-health issues.

Why enjoy life more? You may be suffering from a "fun-deficit." Enjoying life helps you enjoy health. A "fun-deficit" in your life will result in feelings of stress. You can correct a "fun-deficit" by paying attention to the last time you had fun, and planning for more fun. Furthermore, pleasure is important for health. You may not be able to avoid negative moods and nervousness at work, but you can cancel out the disease-promoting effects of bad events by being enthusiastic, positive and taking pride in what you do.

Fifty researchers in fourteen European countries concluded in a study that pleasure is healthy and lowers stress hormones in your blood. Commonly-enjoyed European pleasures included: music; eating out; drinking tea and coffee; eating cheese, cream, butter and red meat; eating chocolate; and shopping for pleasure. Other indulgences included watching TV, videos and sports, and engaging in romance. Feeling guilty about enjoying these pleasures cancels out the stress-reducing benefits of moderate indulgence in these pleasures.

Music cuts stress nearly in half

Listening to upbeat music has a strong impact on people's moods. It has been found that music reduces stress hormones by a full 41 percent according to Katherine Butler.

Chocoholics take heart: Scientists have proven that eating chocolate reduces stress and is good for you (within reason). It has been proven that chocolate is a mild antidepressant and the caffeine has a mild stimulating effect. It also may raise good cholesterol (HDL). The ingredients in chocolate are believed to stimulate endorphins. Why do you think we always give candy to "enhance romance?" It works to elevate moods. Every year the average American eats 12 pounds of chocolate.

Chocolate has a very healthy ingredient, called epicatechins, or in English, antioxidants. A study at the University of California at Davis revealed that after eating 80 grams of chocolate, antioxidant levels in the bloodstream increased 31%. Furthermore, the epicatechins levels in the blood increased by 12 fold in just two hours.

A note of warning however, chocoholism is a risk. Finnish researchers have found that chocoholics often have eating problems in general. To visit a place just for the chocoholics go to <www.cocoa.com>.

Whenever you are having fun, you are healing from the effects of stress, according to Dr. James Loehr. The young naturally know how to enjoy life. Simply reach back into your memory to relearn how to enjoy life. Eight tips on how to polish up your "fun skills" follow:

- Enjoy what you can, even your personal "golden oldies."
- Make and review a list of your "look forward to's."
- Try to humor yourself when you can.
- Keep your eyes on the prize. Look for and use any pleasant features in your situation as "pleasure islands" to calmly escape momentarily.

- Enjoy eye candy, something you look at which is pleasing to the eye. Read Diane Ackerman's, *Cultivating Delight: A Natural History of My Garden.*
- Practice your "eye-robics" by feasting your eyes on beauty in motion. Gaze upon a flock of geese in flight, rolling ocean waves, a hummingbird suspended in flight, a horse running in a pasture, clouds lazily drifting by in a crystal blue sky, even a jet plane leaving a chalk white trail in the sky. Follow the warm flickering glow of a candle or fireplace. Nothing is more enjoyable than watching a loved one enjoy himself.
- Conduct a "pleasure hunt" at work to look for the most pleasant elements of your job you can enjoy daily. Pride in what you do is a close relative of pleasure, so take honest pride in what you can.
- Remember "reward revenge" is also a way to get even with life's hassles. The phrase, "I deserve this _______ (dinner, movie, sports event, book, etc.)" will help you enjoy the hard-earned fruits of your labor. Enjoy your "creature comforts."

SUMMARY

No one can steal your free will from you, so you will always have freedom of choice with perhaps unexpected consequences that you can handle. Your Freedom of Choices includes but, of course, is not limited to what is called the C.A.R.E. package: Controlling, Accepting, Resting and Enjoying.

This chapter focuses on the other freedom of choices besides control: accepting, resting, and enjoying. Graciously accepting circumstances that we cannot change is a mark of emotional maturity and true understanding about how life works. A very useful survival tool, in case the "jerks at work" won't let you be, is discussed, entitled *Nasty People: How to Stop Being Hurt by Them Without Becoming One of Them.*

Under the Resting principle, it was also emphasized that no one has ever been so tired from work that they couldn't get the energy up to go home. This suggests that part of job fatigue is in your head, in the form of job-stress, which can be lethal. The possibility and benefits of virtual "live video" visits with friends or relatives at great distances using computers were discussed. Under the Enjoy principle, it was proposed that "No pain — no gain" is as outdated and wrong as "Spare the rod — spoil the child." Nature's plan for pain is to serve as an alarm to get out of the situation or stop what you are doing. You were introduced to "eye-robics" by feasting your eyes on beauty in motion. To motivate people it is better to use a carrot than a stick. When the punisher with the stick is not around, then the mice will play with a vengeance. The pleasant physiological change caused by music is examined. Scientific evidence for the common pleasure of chocolate is provided, to possibly counteract misplaced guilt when enjoying chocolate.

Technical skills are your "head" knowledge. You spend at least twelve years "schooling" your technical skills. Out of the 168 hours per week, you probably can devote at least a few hours working on your people or "heart" skills. To generate more power to you, you need to use both your "head" and "heart!"

The next chapter deals with generating the will power to do what you know in your heart will help you. The gap between doing what is in your "head" (the map) and what is in your "heart" (enthusiasm) is will power. By fine tuning your engine (your heart), you will have the will power to follow the ABC's discussed above. The next chapter will look at the REDS program, which will keep you from being run over on life's highway by those Type A's who believe, "You are either the steamroller or the pavement." You don't want to have a personal energy crisis in the middle of a traffic jam.

FOR FURTHER READING

Ackerman, D. (2001). *Cultivating delight: a natural history of my garden.* (HarperCollins).

Butler, Katherine. (2001, February 28). Stress Busters-Put on Some Music *Page-A-Day.* New York: Workman Publishing Company, Inc.

Carter, J. (1989). *Nasty people: how to stop being hurt by them without becoming one of them.* Chicago: Contemporary Books.

Carlson, R., & Bailey, J. (2001). *Living at the speed of life.* New York: Simon and Schuster.

Dement, W., & Vaughn, C. (1992). *The promise of sleep.* Stanford, CA: Stanford Alumni Association.

LaRoche, Loretta. "Handling stress with humor," Humor Potential, 15 Peter Road, Plymouth, MA 02360. Phone (508) 224-2280, Fax (508) 224-6457 E-mail: <stressed @tiac.com>.

11

Boosting Your Will Power

You are Either the Steamroller or the Pavement

Let's "get physical" about stress.

Why "get physical" about stress? Because what starts off in your mind is expressed through your body. Stress generated by your mind produces hormones (adrenaline, cortisol and also, testosterone for men). Your negative thoughts actually decrease the production of serotonin in the brain after about two weeks. Your thoughts become things (hormones), which are measurable and can't be thought away. Your body starts controlling your thoughts. Drinking ten cups of coffee (don't try this at home) will test your nerves, no matter how positive your attitude is. You will be a nervous wreck. Clinical studies show that if your body is made to feel nervous, your mind generates anxious thoughts to justify your jitters.

BODY-MIND — Divorce or dance? Placebo or "nocebo"?

A word about the body-mind relationship. Everyone knows about psychosomatic interactions, where your mind influences your body's health. (Psycho means mind, somatic means body). A placebo is the positive psychosomatic effect of your mind on your body (e.g., sugar pill cures). Marilyn vos Savant asserts that mind is created by the body. A strong mind requires a healthy body.

When your body divorces your mind

Try to at least make it a friendly divorce, where you are still talking to each other. When your body says, pay attention to me, then listen.

Sometimes our own mind "won't mind" us

For example, you've "made up your mind" to drop a habit, but your mind stubbornly resists (e.g., overeating, whining, etc.).

Making strong men faint: The power of negative thinking "nocebo" effect

The "nocebo" effect is just the opposite of the placebo effect, when your mind makes you sick physically or in some cases can actually kill you (e.g., Voodoo). Strong men fainting while waiting in line for an injection is an almost humorous example of the "nocebo" effect.

A new term you can impress people with at parties is "somatopsychic," where the body (soma) influences the mind (psychic). Dr. Richard Rahe, co-developer of the most popular stress scale ever used, said we often forget about the "somatopsychic" relationship of the body and mind. Your body directs your mind through exercise, caffeine, alcohol, nutrition, blood sugar, oxygen, sleep, fevers, insufficient oxygen, and of course, hormones. The body-mind relationship means that your body and mind are inseparably woven together, and can work together or in conflict. Without the body-over-mind interaction, medications would not work (e.g., anesthesia). The whole purpose of the REDS program is to get your body to work as an ally in the battle against stress. The REDS program will allow your body to dance cooperatively with your mind, instead of your body dueling with your mind. Ignoring your body while trying to manage stress is almost impossible, unless you are a long-time user of mind-over-body techniques (e.g., biofeedback, yoga, hypnosis, professional athletic training).

Lest we forget to respect when the body takes over

Since some folks are more "kinesthetic learners," who learn by doing, we offer a down-to-earth testimony of the body-over-mind relationship. This down-to-earth testimonial is based on an "indelicate but true life story," when Bob was driving from L.A. to Las Vegas. He had been the unsuspecting subject of a well-meaning herbal-purgative experiment. At the crack of dawn on the day of his L.A.-Las Vegas drive, his friend said, "Try this herbal-blast, it has natural action." Willingly, Bob swallowed a couple harmless-looking large green herbal capsules and jumped in his car, heading for Vegas. The rest of the story? Let's just say that the "Rest-stop-in-five miles" sign gained new meaning and appreciation for Bob, as he frantically visited every single rest stop from L.A. to Vegas. He had to "rest" so often because the herbal purgative was really purging as promised, even though Bob tried every "mind over matter" control technique he could think of. He even kept chanting to himself, "Attitude is everything, attitude is everything, attitude is everything," as he broke land speed records trying to get to each and every rest stop between L.A. and Vegas. All we can say is that Bob really appreciated seeing his tax-dollars at work, in the form of clean "rest stops" along that L.A.-Vegas interstate.

The point of this story is that fortunately the body has its own wisdom, and takes over when it needs to (e.g., when we are sleeping, etc.). Modern science has proven over and over again that it is not so much "mind over matter," it is more like "mind with matter" working together, in harmony, as shown in the "somatopsychic" relationship.

Closing the gap between knowing and doing what's right

The ABC's (Attitude, Breathing, Choices) map can direct you to inner peace. You may have the right compass setting but you still have to walk-the-talk.

Wanting and doing the right thing can be short-circuited by your feelings of fatigue and frustration. Using the simple REDS program described below will close the gap between knowing and doing what's right for you by increasing your will power. Using the REDS program works on the body-mind aspect of stress, producing anti-stress hormones (endorphins, enkephalins) to influence your mind.

Energy crisis: When you are too tired to get out of the way or play

Stress is energy. Each day you are allotted a full, but one day only, tank of this stress-energy. Since stress management is simply energy conservation, you can actually have an energy crisis if you waste your daily stress-energy supply by "burning rubber" ("hypering" around) in the morning. Just as you can get the most "miles to the gallon" by going a steady 55 mph, it is better to pace yourself in terms of the stress-energy you use. Most of us experience a real energy crisis around three o'clock in the afternoon at work. It is interesting to note that when we are on vacation we are charged with eustress (good stress), and we can get up to fish or shop at 5:30 A.M. and have all the energy we need till our heads hit the pillow. At work we are required to do screeching stops and jackrabbit starts which waste a lot of our fuel. The REDS program will both increase the size of your eustress (good stress) gas tank and improve the efficiency of your engine (your heart). Always see your doctor when you experience chronic fatigue, to rule out possible physical causes.

The REDS program is designed to tune-up your physical engine so you have the power to climb emotional hills in the work zone. Always consult your doctor before engaging in any type of exercise program. Being fit will help you feel somewhat more like "getting back to work," rather than getting back to bed. Guess which of these former mottos is held by those in charge? Remember the "Little Engine that Could?" Increase the size of your engine (heart) so you are the bigger engine that DID, not just thought it could.

Many executives already use something like the REDS program to keep themselves tuned up. Many Type A's truly enjoy and are financially rewarded for the attitude, "You are either the steamroller or the pavement." Which one would you rather be? REDS can help you choose not to become professional "road kill" so you are not steamrolled, overpowered by those with bigger engines. If you are in good shape, at least you can sidestep life's steamrollers.

Many wellness programs will actually pay you to use something like the REDS program. See your HR (human resources) personnel.

The four components of the REDS program and related issues are described below. You are probably already doing many of these.

- Relaxation: concept of "kindling" — "over-sensitization" to stress and relaxation-induced anxiety.
- Exercise: (Find out what the most friendly piece of exercise equipment is!).

- Diet: (including caffeine, alcohol and natural remedies).
- Sleep: When your engine won't stop with the ignition off.

THE REDS (RELAXATION, EXERCISE, DIET AND SLEEP) PROGRAM

BELOW REPRESENTS A GOOD ANTI-STRESS ROUTINE.

1. Relax — The R in the REDS program.

It is impossible to have relaxed muscles and feel nervous at the same time. Tapes are available to learn how to do "progressive deep muscle relaxation." The best relaxation tape available is offered by the Midwest Center for Stress and Anxiety, Inc. This tape combines that best of breathing, visualizing and positive self-talk in a very pleasing format delivered by a professional.

The concept of "kindling." (Increased chance of stress reactions)

It is important to be more sensitive to stress than less. In mental-health jargon, the term, "kindling," means that one traumatic event actually is "kindling" for your severe reaction to the next stressor. See *Harvard Mental Health Newsletter* of Fall 2001 for more details on "kindling." A real-life example of "kindling" would be your becoming nauseous at the mere mention of someone's name, even if that person's grim presence is not darkening the room and he's on vacation miles away. It is estimated that 5% of all sick days are mental-health days, because people are just "sick of work."

For the young, the mention of a pop quiz can raise any student's fear level, and make students anxious about any kind of future tests. This condition is called test anxiety. Stressful, numerous pop quizzes could eventually serve as "kindling," making students nervous even at the mere mention of a future test. The avoidance of tests because of test anxiety could seriously short-circuit a bright person's career, since all high-paying jobs require passing numerous, complex tests.

"Kindling" was exemplified by soldiers who were shell-shocked, falling to the ground at the sound of a car back firing in their own neighborhood, far from the battlefield. Many adults who are gun-shy about dating or relationships are victims of the "kindling" effect.

Bob and Delia go for a Sunday afternoon drive.

Bob was driving up Battleship Drive when suddenly, as if in a tornado, his wife and dog went flying in the car as the result of someone broadsiding them at forty-miles per hour. Although no major, permanent damage occurred, a decade later when Bob and Delia drive at that particular intersection of Battleship and Impact, they always feel anxious. This is a real live example of the "kindling" effect, where a previous real stressor, creates anticipatory anxiety about a possible future trauma.

Dampening the "kindling" effect, with specialized relaxation. (Systematic-desensitization [SD])

Again, using mental-health "jargon," systematic-desensitization (SD) used by a licensed mental-health professional could actually decrease the chances of the "kindling" effect. Contact your local American Psychological Association (APA) for more information on professionals qualified to provide systematic-desensitization (SD). As mentioned previously, by increasing your sensitivity to potential stressors you put yourself out of harm's way, or if you must deal with the stressor, you are prepared, especially if you use the REDS program.

It is strongly recommended that you see your doctor or a mental-health professional if you notice severe stress reactions at the mere mention of a specific situation or a person's name. Your fear was learned, so it can be "unlearned" in a few months.

EMT's — emotional detoxification is required

Even trauma-hardened EMT's, paramedics and first response personnel are required to undergo emotional detoxification immediately after dealing with unimaginable human tragedy. If you need help, again consult your APA (American Psychological Association) for guidance in selecting a mental-health professional.

Relaxation-induced anxiety (RIA)

As mentioned previously, some people are so uptight they become more anxious when trying to relax. This relaxation-induced anxiety (RIA) requires special treatment.

For the "garden variety" irritations and frustrations, excellent resources are offered by the Midwest Center for Stress and Anxiety, Inc.

2. Exercise — The E in the REDS program.

This is very important in stress management. Exercise changes your blood chemistry by metabolizing (neutralizing) stress hormones and introducing the brain's natural tranquilizers (enkephalins, endorphins). Just as you can't think away the jitters you would get from drinking ten cups of coffee, you can't just think away the build-up of stress hormones in your system.

Exercise also gets you away from your problems. Walking three times weekly (20 minutes) at a brisk pace is sufficient. You will be in "good" walking shape in about eight weeks. Change your routine to counteract boredom. The immediate feeling of relaxation will be with you for about six hours. Exercise no later than two hours before bedtime. Exercising Sunday evening will ease you back into work on Monday.

What is the friendliest piece of exercise equipment there is? According to renowned-fitness trainer, newspaper columnist, and president of PurEnergy Health and Wellness Services, Julie Luther, a dog is the best piece of exercise equipment a person can have. Walking your dog 20 minutes, three times weekly, will produce great results in terms of your cardiovascular system, psychological well-being. Also, if your dog is anything like this author's, a brisk walk will keep your dog from waking you up at the crack of dawn because she spent some of her energy on the previous day's walk.

Golfers take heart, it's good for your heart. According to Julie Luther, middle-aged men walking an 18 hole game of golf (without toting their bags) improved their aerobic fitness and also reduced their risk of diabetes and heart attack. Plus, because they enjoyed it so much they stuck with it more than any other previous form of exercise for cardiovascular fitness.

Wanting an effective stress-reduction program without exercise is just wishful thinking.

In her November 6, 2001 column, Ms. Luther asserts that if you are already feeling stressed out, exercise actually gets rid of excess cortisol in your body. As indicated before, cortisol is the main culprit in making you feel jittery, uncomfortable and edgy. Excess cortisol can lethally disrupt cortical (heart) functioning. Cortisol and cortical obviously have the same root, "cort", which means having to do with the heart. A heart-smart person would manage stress for heart-health. The connection between Type A (agitated, impatient) personality and heart problems is baseline knowledge discussed in high school health texts. A new theory proposed is that exercise greatly reduces heart attack risk (by as much as 73%) because adrenaline and cortisol, the stress hormones, are neutralized by exercise.

The excuse of boredom with exercise is just that, an excuse, not a reason for not exercising. According to the Surgeon General's 1996 report, there are at least 22 ways you can exercise (for three hours per week) that are effective. Tundra dwellers (those living in snow-zones) take heart. Shoveling snow for 15 minutes is only topped by stair climbing, in getting the most out of exercise. See "For Further Reading" on the Surgeon General's report. The bottom line is, if you want to live longer and better, exercise. If not, don't bother.

3. Diet — The D in the REDS program.

Mean without caffeine

Caffeine is medicine for some. They get mean without their caffeine. Excessive caffeine is a "stress amplifier." Excessive caffeine is six or more cups of coffee per day. About two cups/servings of caffeinated beverage will generally not contribute to feelings of stress. Three or more servings may result in a caffeine addiction and feelings of stress.

An April, 2002 study revealed that excessive caffeine, more than five cups per day, can cause heart attacks, hypertension and has been linked with low birth weight in pregnant women. The same study showed that drinking up to five cups per day improved cognition, including memory, especially for the elderly. In this study caffeine-fueled folks actually enjoyed an eight percent higher advantage on cognitive tests over the decaffeinated-coffee drinkers.

If caffeine were just discovered today, it would be a controlled substance, probably available by prescription only. Caffeine is America's drug of choice, being used in some form by nine out of ten adults, causing jitters in millions. If you are trying to cut back, taper off slowly. Don't cut back on the amount of liquid you are drinking, but on the amount of caffeine in the drinks. Making a half/half mixture (half-caffeinated, half-decaffeinated) might be useful.

Try tea

Besides water, tea is the most-consumed beverage in the U.S. Try green tea. Cup for cup, it only has about one third the caffeine of brewed coffee. Green tea also contains antioxidants that are heart-healthy. Polyphenols, which are the antioxidants in green tea, are more potent than antioxidants such as vitamin E and Vitamin C. Green tea may even help prevent or lessen the severity of arthritis.

Tea consumption even affects cholesterol build-up. A large-scale three year study in the Netherlands of 3,454 revealed that those who drank one to two cups of tea a day were 46% less likely to have severe cholesterol build-up (atherosclerosis). Atherosclerosis was 69% lower for those drinking four cups of tea a day. The cadillac of green teas is Lungching Tea, at $4.00/box for teabags.

Caffeine stays in your system about six hours. If you have difficulty sleeping you may want to skip caffeine at the evening meal. Of course, chocolate and many headache remedies contain caffeine.

Obsessed with weight loss after fifty: Get a grip

Unless you are a model, or dating one, you probably don't have to be stressed about being thin enough. If your doctor says your weight is appropriate for your age, you have to ask yourself, "When is my next modeling shoot?" If you don't see a big modeling agency date on your calendar, relax. (Major hormone shifts causing overweight can occur after forty.) Focus more on exercise and relaxation. Follow your doctor's advice about blood pressure, developing Type II diabetes, etc.

Fruit of the vine: No wine until it's time

A "tongue-in-cheek" look at any possible benefits of using alcohol to reduce stress follows. The adage, "It's better to have a bottle in front of me than a frontal lobotomy," reflects our society's hopeful view of the possible medicinal value of alcohol. These sentiments are echoed through the ages. About every other adult in our society drinks. The rule of two for alcohol (two drinks for men or one for women at most) appears to have some possible overall health benefits according to *Harvard Men's Health Watch* of November 2001. Low alcohol use (one drink per day) was associated with a 40% reduction in cardiac risk, (p. 2). Low alcohol use raises good (HDL) cholesterol, reducing heart attack risk. Low dosage alcohol use from any source (wine, beer or spirits) is about equal in its effects (as are the harmful effects). The article goes on to list 16 major health hazards of alcohol abuse (more than one drink daily for females, more than two daily for males). However, it is not recommended that you start drinking if you already do not, and it is recommended that you take a vacation from alcohol weekly. The use of alcohol is so prevalent because it seems to have worked in calming shattered nerves for millennia. (Sumerians were brewing beer about 5,000 years ago.)

The oldest form of medication? Alcohol (Paul Rosch, M.D., April 2002, p. 5).

Mad cow, drunk cow disease

You have heard of Mad-cow disease, but I'll bet you have not heard of drunk-cow disease. Even animals, eating certain naturally fermented grains, will go back to the bail, for just one more, to get intoxicated if possible. Rats will drink alcohol rather than water if they have a choice. Alcohol is a feel-good drug, even though too much is not good for you.

Alcohol as medication: To medicate or meditate, that is the question

Alcohol is classified as a minor central nervous system tranquilizer. As a minor tranquilizer it has withdrawal characteristics (hangovers) and addictive properties, that is, you may need more drinks to calm your nerves than when you were a "rookie" consumer.

Using common sense when drinking is even imbedded in our commercial pilots' corporate culture. "Twelve hours from bottle to throttle" is the mantra adhered to by commercial pilots. Twelve hours apparently is enough time for any alcoholic haze to lift so pilots are not in a mental fog when flying, and so they are able to pass the "surprise" urine tests they are all subject to (for which they get paid). It may be useful for anyone to take this "12-hour drinkfast" advice for activities demanding peak performance, such as your job or school.

It may help someone to make better decisions if we think of alcohol as potentially good medicine. If a laxative prescription contained only six pills in the bottle and read, "one a day and stay close to a restroom," most people would not take all six pills at once just because the doctor prescribed the laxative as a six pack. Think of alcohol as a "relaxative," having potentially good qualities for some, if not abused. This "relaxative," or alcoholic drink, is packaged as a six pack or in a bottle. Just because alcohol is dispensed as a six pack or bottle, does not mean you have to take the whole prescription (six pack or bottle) at once. Would you overdose on a laxative just because all six pills were there in one prescription bottle? After taking six laxatives, you would learn quickly that the mind-body link is not as strong as you thought.

One of the world's-largest beer distributors has been recently valued at five-billion dollars. This corporation has obviously found a need and is feeding it. This and other companies will spare no expense to remind us to "take our medication" in very-appealing drinking ads, where no one ever has a hanger-over or a "beer-belly." By comparison, we will hear a feeble voice, once in a while, advertise the virtues of meditation. So when it comes to the question, "Should I medicate or meditate," you could say both, just at the right time at the right place. If you tried to meditate at a lively pub, the owners would call for an ambulance because they thought something was wrong with you.

Natural remedies: "Not everything that is natural is good for you." (Janet Nicol, R.N.)

Snake venom is as natural as you can get, but lethal. There may be some calming benefit to the natural homeopathic remedies called kava and valerium. Always check with your physician for possible interactions with so-called natural remedies. Some natural remedies can do more harm than good. National Public Radio offers "The People's Pharmacy," which is a legitimate source of information on the use and abuse of natural remedies. Joe and Teresa Graedon are the resident experts on "The People's Pharmacy." They offer common sense answers to often-complex interactions of natural and/or manufactured medications. To contact "The People's Pharmacy," email <pharmacy@mindspring.com> or their website at <www.peoplespharmacy.com>.

Soothing foods

Oatmeal or yogurt for breakfast could start you off on the right foot. Pretzels for between meal snacks appear to lead the list for soothing foods. In general it appears that vegetables, fruits and lowfat foods are good at mealtime. Proper nutrition is so important because poor nutrition crimps the supply of oxygen to your brain. Milk contains a natural tranquilizer and has a calming effect on some people.

Brain foods — the best book

One of the top authorities on real brain food is M.I.T. scientist, Dr. Judith Wurtman. Her book, *Managing your Mind and Mood through Food*, shows how proteins and carbohydrates work together in the body to actually make the mind more alert or even relax and focus the mind.

4. Sleep — The S in the REDS program.

Insomnia: The car that wouldn't stop running

Bob, with dark circles under his eyes, said to his friend, "You know what it's like when you have an old car that keeps chugging on even after you have turned off the ignition? Well, my 'work engine' just won't stop, even when I go to bed. I just can't sleep because I worry so much about work conflicts." Bob's compassionate friend, Dr. Tom H. said, "Well, maybe like the car, you just need a tune-up."

Bob indeed needed a tune-up. He had celebrated many "anniversaries" of his 30th birthday, and his melatonin level, which helps you sleep, was pretty well used up. Also, even though he bought a thousand dollar treadmill, it was used more as a very expensive item to hang clothing on than to exercise. If you have trouble sleeping, you just may need a tune-up. But again, see your doctor first before trying any of these home-remedies.

You need sleep to live because it:

- Improves your mood;
- Improves athletic performance;
- Boosts your ability to remember;
- Sharpens your ability to understand what you learned during the day;
- Boosts the immune system, improving your chances of staying well;
- Restores energy.

Get about seven hours. Keep the bedroom "off limits" for business or other important matters. If you can't get a problem off your mind, get up; write a note about it, and go to another room to try to fall asleep. Using a relaxation tape right before bed will aid in sleeping. Take a warm bath prior to going to bed. Use a sound soother. Install room-darkening shades. Your body reacts to sunlight as a signal to wake up.

OTHER STRESS-REDUCING BEHAVIORS

- Stop smoking.
- Write an angry letter. Keep it to yourself, then destroy it.
- Spend quality time with loved ones.
- Get a pet. At the office, wet pets (fish) might be best.
- Get a massage from a professionally-qualified person. Contact your doctor for a referral.

SUMMARY

The key to closing the gap between knowing and doing what's right is will power. We talked about how your body and mind can dance together or divorce against yourself. The body-over-mind relationship is called "somatopsychic." The "Little Engine that Could" can become the little engine that DID by increasing the size of your physical engine (heart). Using the simple REDS program described above will close the gap between knowing and doing what's right for you by increasing your will power. Being fit will help you feel somewhat more like getting back to work, rather than getting back to bed. Many Type A's feel you are either the steamroller or the pavement. If you are in good shape, at least you can sidestep life's steamrollers.

The four components of the REDS program are described in this chapter. These are Relaxation, Exercise, Diet and Sleep. Relative to relaxation, the concept of "kindling" (i.e., being gun-shy, test-anxious) was introduced. In other words, you are more sensitive to stress in a specific situation because you are psychologically set up by a previous bad experience to overreact to future similar situations. A clinical method to deal with being overly sensitive to stress was also discussed. It was pointed out that wanting an effective stress-reduction program without exercise is just wishful thinking. It was also revealed that if caffeine were just discovered today, it would be a controlled substance, probably available by prescription only. One of the top scientists on brain food, Dr. Judith Wurtman of M.I.T., is discussed. Her book talks about how diet really affects attention and relaxation. The next chapter deals with how to refuse to lose your mind in the face of catastrophic events that you have no control over.

FOR FURTHER READING

Geleijnse, J. (1999). Drinking tea protects arteries from cholesterol buildup. *Archives of Internal Medicine,* 159: pp. 2170-2174.

Harvard Men's Health Watch. (2001). Good and evil: alcohol and health. President and Fellows of Harvard College. Boston. Vol. 6, No. 4, <www.Health.Harvard.edu>.

Harvard Men's Health Watch. (1996). No sweat: new guidelines for moderate exercise, physical activity and health: a report of the Surgeon General. U.S. Department of Health and Human Resources. Boston, President and Fellows of Harvard College. Boston. (December) pp. 1-4.

Licht, J. (2002, April 16). A good snooze goes a long way toward restoring the strength of the body and mind. Special to *The Washington Post.* (Greensboro, NC. *News and Record*, D6).

Luther, J. (2001, May 22). Group activities make exercising fun. Greensboro, NC. *News and Record.*

Rosch, P. (2002). Dietary supplements and related controversies. *Health and Stress. The Newsletter of the American Institute of Stress* 3. 1-8. (p. 2, the possible calming effects of kava).

Rosch, P. (2002). Health news: accurate or advertising hype? *Health and Stress. The Newsletter of the American Institute of Stress* 4. 1-8. (p. 4, the benefits/risks of caffeine, pp. 5-6, benefits and risks of alcohol).

Somer, E. (1995). *Food and mood: The complete guide to eating well and feeling your best.* New York: Henry Holt.

Tariq, H. (1999). Green tea antioxidants may fight arthritis. New York (Reuters Health): *Proceedings of the National Academy of Sciences* 96: pp. 4524-4529.

Willett, W. (2001). *Eat, drink and be healthy.* Boston: Harvard Medical School Publication.

Wurtman, J. (1986). *Managing your mind and mood through food.* (New York: Harper Row, [Perennial Library]).

12

Refuse to Lose Your Mind

Don't Let Stress Squelch Your Success

"That which doesn't destroy me makes me stronger."
- Arthur Schopenhauer (German philosopher; b. 1788, d. 1860)

Sooner or later everyone is "rocked" by a level 10 earthquake on the stress Richter Scale

Our nation quaked with grief in the fall of 2001. "9/11 Tuesday," September 11, 2001, was the worst attack on our country since 1812. In 1812, we declared war on Great Britain because of her assaults. By contrast, in this recent fateful attack by faceless terrorists, we had no "hard target" or distinct enemy to retaliate upon. Thousands of World Trade Center workers were cremated instantaneously as a suicide pilot slammed into the first Tower with a fully-fueled 757 jet. The first Tower acted as a super-heated, vertical oven fed by jet fuel. As the horrified observers in the second World Trade Center watched, another suicide pilot smashed into the second World Trade Tower, turning many of its occupants into dust from the extreme heat and instantaneous compression of over one-hundred stories to just eighteen feet of rubble.

The devastating bombings of the World Trade Center on September 11, 2001 resulted in an acute-stress disorder eruption for millions of people around the world. This is a fairly new type of stress disorder (DSM-IV) that can result from witnessing (even remotely) unimaginably horrific acts. It is like a level 10 shock wave on the stress Richter Scale. After 90 days, this disorder could solidify into a post-traumatic-stress disorder, a serious anxiety disorder that could even require medication.

What was once a source of pride for this author is now a source of pain. (I had worked at the World Trade Center while a doctoral student at Columbia University.) Five temporary "band-aid" measures to help you and your family cope with traumatic events are listed near the end of this chapter (pp. 146-147).

The main way to counteract great distress is with great eustress. Eustress is good stress, exemplified by patriotic or religious zeal, love and devotion to family and friends. This eustress can lift you above your present, unpleasant circumstances. Only great faith will neutralize great fear.

Job loss shook up almost a half-million workers during the first quarter of

2001. Another half-million workers have been laid off as the result of the World Trade Center and Pentagon attacks because of a real fear of flying. Out of 43 stressors that can lead to illness, job loss ranks number eight in all life's stressors, according to the gold standard measure of stress, the Holmes-Rahe Social Adjustment Scale. We grieve when we lose our job, which happened to about a million workers fired during 2001. When under extreme stress, try to remember that the quick cure is sometimes worse than the disease. Giving up, extreme overindulgence, revenge or withdrawal may be some of the cures that are worse than the disease (job loss, death of a loved one, divorce, etc.).

Don't let life un-nerve you

Resist the urge to apply a powerful and permanent cure to a bad but temporary situation. An example might be "going postal" with your words by really telling so-and-so off, falsely whistle blowing, or taking revenge. No matter how much it hurts, your true north emotional "compass heading" is something like Adlai Stevenson's comment, "It's better to light a candle than to curse the darkness." You have lost your direction if your main goal in life is to get even or get out of the race. Check your "compass heading" during these terrible storms when you can't see the light. Watch for your emotional lighthouses in loved ones and friends. Also, take advantage of professional therapy (counseling) that is usually offered by corporations. Eventually take advantage of outplacement services by your employer, whereby you will be provided with professional leads and job-interview advice. There is actually a website that tries to comfort the "newly displaced" called <pinkslip.com>.

If you are in a career slump, employ the services of a career coach. Joyce Richman (notice the uplifting name Rich-man) offers the seminar, "Yes . . . I can." These workshops are sponsored by Jan Star, a skills-training company, call (336) 294-8936 or fax (336) 299-0289. Preregistration is only $35.00, which is cheaper than a prescription for insomnia medication.

Taking the path of least resistance

In 1992, Bob's friend, JT, shouted over his fifth beer at the bar, "I know I am going to get fired, so why bother doing my best on the job? I am not attending these stupid workshops on how to do workshops. I hate this job, and if I am going down, I am taking some people with me." Sadly, JT was fired, mostly because of his negative attitude. He was replaced by someone with a younger, more vibrant and open-to-learning attitude.

At a picnic right after his dismissal from his job, JT was seething with anger. He shouted to Bob and Delia, "I am now teaching courses in New Jersey at a community college. My students love the war stories I can testify to about large corporations."

JT was following a bad shot (getting fired from his large corporation job) with even worse judgment (publicly putting down the corporation that had let him go). His attitude was so poisoned with anger that he even lost the community college teaching job. Corporation X was rehiring, but no one would touch JT because of the hatchet job he had done publicly through teaching and word-of-mouth. JT, previously healthy, suddenly died in his early fifties of a heart attack. Ironically, he had been a wellness trainer for the human resources department in the corporation and should have known stress-management practices.

HOW TO TURN FAILURE INTO SUCCESS — A DOZEN DO-ABLES

- Retreat rest, momentarily.
- Like President Clinton, be a "comeback kid" but with good judgment.
- Set reasonable goals that may be out of reach but not out of range.
- Have a plan B with tangible goals and progress markers.
- Confidently brace yourself for bumpy roads.
- Know yourself — realistically. Brainstorm resumé items.
- Read about heroic "successful failures."
- Truly believe in yourself (It is contagious).
- Keep your resumé up to date.
- Positive thinking on the job.
- Dealing with catastrophic events, until help arrives (e.g., 9/11 bombings).
- An invocation for strength.

1. Retreat — rest, momentarily.

Failure often triggers the urge to fight, flee or fume. If given the option, try to cool down for two or three days before taking decisive action. The bigger your "surprise" the more time you may need in your retreat. Plan activities that you enjoy and that get your attention.

If someone seems to be marching out of step, it may not be that he hears a different drummer. It may be that he is dodging bullets you can't even hear from your viewpoint.

2. **Like President Clinton — be a "comeback kid." See yourself succeeding in the future.**

An example of the power of attitude (even if misdirected) was President Clinton's almost supernatural ability to come back after public scandals that would destroy most people. On his last day in office, January 20, 2001, he said with a smile to the farewell crowd at a DC airport, "I am still here." This was his response to the reporter's pointed question, "Mr. President, will you remain politically active?"

This "comeback kid" saw himself succeeding, no matter what reality revealed. The point of this negative example is the power of an attitude to rise above circumstances.

Remember that failure is a temporary exception to the rule. Top athletes see themselves making the basket, sinking the putt, hitting the target. Court the friendship of those who support you. Provide yourself daily with small success experiences by doing things you know you can do.

3. **Set reasonable goals that may be out of reach, but not out of range of possibility.**

Employee assistance programs or career counselors can help generate plans of action to fit your skills and personality. Find a need and fill it. The more needs you fulfill in business, the more chances of success you have.

4. **Have a plan B with tangible goals and progress markers.**

Your plans should include markers to let you know whether you are being successful in your plan and whether your plan is truly successful in meeting your goal. For example, find out what a reasonable "yield" rate is for returns on "mailings" to prospective clients (e.g., 5 out of 100). If you are getting this yield rate within your timeline, proceed. If not, adjust plan A or proceed to plan B. Small business courses and counselors are available at most community colleges and universities to help you realistically build and adjust your plan. It may not hurt to give some thoughts to a plan C.

Your plan C is for what you didn't see coming.

5. **Confidently brace yourself for bumpy roads.**

Train yourself to relax when things do not go your way. Self-calming under pressure is a trademark of peak performers. Take a course in stress management. Besides appearing calmly confident, you will keep healthy and work-ready by achieving relaxed readiness.

Avoid the extremes of anger or anxiety and accept the fact that "overnight success" takes months and even years. There may be many "learning curves" in your road to success you did not plan on. Support groups exist to show that you can hold it together over the rough spots. "Professionals In Transition" is a support group to meet the need for emotional support.

---

6. Know yourself — realistically. Brainstorm resumé items.

Focus first on your strengths and then build up one key area for improvement. Take stock of your skills, and change your attitude and/or your skills. Make a list of your strengths, then ask someone you trust to add to this list. Post this list somewhere prominent in your house if necessary. Work on a resumé to be polished when you are thinking clearly. Step nine provides specifics and resources for this skill.

---

7. Read about heroic "successful failures."

Learn how successful failures such as Walt Disney, Henry Ford and Abraham Lincoln not only survived failure but succeeded because of their failures.

Distraction and distress have been initially isolated as causes of pilot/engineer error in experienced professionals, according to the National Transportation Safety Board. Training designed to calm down and improve concentration reduces the chances of "bad days," particularly for seasoned professionals. Fatigue and illness are also on-the-job factors that impair performance. To bring things into perspective, what if your medical doctor seemed tired, nervous and was constantly taking calls and looking at her watch while you sat there in one of those "breezy" hospital gowns?

---

8. Truly believe in yourself. It is contagious.

Being confident but not cocky will increase your chances of being successful. Take your opinion of yourself and give yourself a 10% ego boost. For example, Bob was told time and time again that his golf swing was adequate, but would never improve. Bob told himself, "I am not only adequate but I am good at golf even if only once in a blue moon." Having a positive attitude will instill others' belief in you and will help you persist so that your typical performance will some day be the same as your best performance. If you don't think professional athletes boost their own egos (by far more than 10%), just ask them. They have no difficulty accepting the fact that they make more money than the President. How would you feel if the surgeon about to operate on you said, "I feel I can do an adequate job on you today"?

"Do the thing and you will have the power" is what Thoreau is credited with saying. Basically he is saying, if you want to feel bravely, then believe and act as if you are brave. You will then become courageous. Our modern sage, Marilyn vos Savant, recently stated that when you feel fearful, act bravely, and you will become brave. If you can feel brave, you can relax. Her timely advice, after the WTC incidence, included having fun and taking a break (even putting together a colorful puzzle), and leaving a legacy by your brave behavior now. Engage in activities you can be proud of to relay to your progeny. She also suggested that is it less stressful to get your news from the newspaper than TV, because you only have to expose yourself once to the bad news in the newspaper whereas TV fills time with exacting and unnecessary replays. Even "professional sports" casts a suspicious eye on instant replays.

9. Keep your resumé up-to-date.

Love at first sight is the law which determines which resumés grab the attention of time-starved employers. First impressions of your resumé are formed within 20 seconds, according to Bill Holub, President of <eResume-Pros.com>. Your resumé should showcase your ability to problem solve on your own initiative (when appropriate). It is suggested you distill your resumé to one page, which should include at least your formal education, continuing education, certificates and even job-related workshops. You should spotlight the skills, accomplishments and honors you may have received. How many people are capable of reducing job highlights and unique skills into one page? Probably no one, unless you're in advertising. Seek help. A seven-step resumé model is offered by <www.7step-resumesampler.com>. An actual job-website is offered by <www.jobweb.com>. A good way to custom design a resumé is to analyze a "help wanted" ad, then mold your resumé to key into the main requirements of the job.

10. Positive thinking on the job.

Scott Ventrella, in his new book, *The Power of Positive Thinking in Business,* lists ten do-able positive thinking steps for the job. Of course, calmness, patience and persistence are key factors. Faith in one's self to have a positive outcome even when times are tough, tops his list of things you can do on-the-job for effectiveness and success.

11. Dealing with catastrophic events (e.g., World Trade Center bombings, anthrax anxiety).

Always consult with mental-health professionals, but some do-it-yourself measures, suggested by Lifeworks wellness consultants are as follows:

- Take care of yourself after a traumatic series of events, by eating properly, trying to sleep and giving yourself a "faith lift" if you are religious. In terms of exercise, doing a few jumping jacks will keep your blood from pooling where you don't need it (your seat or feet).
- Ease your family's fears and concerns and try to act calmly.
- Tell your children that is it normal to feel upset and worried when attacks and tragedies occur.
- Consider your various options regarding childcare if your child's school is closed.
- Call such an organization as LifeWorks at 1-800-635-0606 for more information.

The horror of 3,000 unfinished "To-Do" lists — a 21st century lesson in perspective

---

All your eggs in one basket:
The World Trade Center Tragedy, September 11, 2001

Dr. Bob, who had once worked at the World Trade Center as part of an internship, saw each of the two ivory towers for the country's best smashed into by 757 airplanes. Eventually, both of the twin towers pancaked, crashing one-hundred and ten stories into about ten feet of vertical rubble. Workaholism was the motto during Dr. Bob's tenure at the World Trade Center. He was being groomed for tireless leadership, and everyone drank at least ten cups of coffee a day. Windows on the World, at the top of the World Trade Center, is where Dr. Bob took Delia many years later. Dr. Bob was actually bursting with pride that he was selected to work at the Mecca of workaholics during his time as a graduate student. Many of the workers were obsessed with their "To-Do" lists, as Bob was. Most tragically, there are now thousands of "To-Do" lists left unfinished by the victims of the World Trade Center attack. The lesson to be learned: don't become check-list obsessed, for one day you won't be completing your "To-Do" list. It has been estimated that the average worker has about 40-60 hours of work left to do, when they are unexpectedly snatched from or snuffed out from their jobs.

Two other techniques that may be useful during a time of tragedy:

Ask yourself, "What possible good can come from this evil?" For example, the World Trade Center bombing put the nation in a "war zone" mentality, which actually lowers suicide rates. Why? Dr. Margaret Mead, a former Columbia University sociology professor, found that when there is a national cause of great importance, people find strength in a "call to arms" or a call to a national purpose. People become more selfless when a community is threatened.

Activities of daily living: ADL is a term used by medical personnel to help those maintain quality of life when there is a life-threatening illness. If you are ill, try to do those things which gave you pleasure before (within reason). If you are jobless — then "make a job" out of finding a new job. Network. Word-of-mouth advertising is the best way to get a new job. Get up, get dressed, have a "To-Do" list, enjoy whatever you are used to enjoying. Exercise. See your doctor while you still have medical insurance for suggestions on sleeplessness, irritable bowel syndrome, etc.

Harvard Medical School advice on the disaster and trauma of 9/11 can be summed up as follows:

You are only human if upset. New York City sleeping-pill prescriptions shot up 28% after 9/11, antidepressant medicine prescriptions climbed 17%.

Most extreme shock symptoms wear off in a couple of weeks. If not, get help if you are continuing to have problems such as headaches, concentrating, indigestion, nightmares, intrusive images, and fatigue. These were the symptoms of the bereaved, witnesses and relief workers in the 9/11 events.

As difficult as it may be, try to resume normal lives as soon as possible. (Adapted from the January, 2002 issue of the *Harvard Mental Health Letter*).

- Concentrate on the future, coming to grips with regret.
- Keeping faith in your own ability, but getting help if you need it.
- Seek solace at community meetings, religious services.
- Get physical activity, and try meditation, breathing exercises, and muscle relaxation, hugs and even massages (p. 1, p. 4).
- Seek out positive psychology. Positive attitude and good physical health are related.
- Stay engaged in pursuits that give you satisfaction, and have a sensible balance of realism and optimism (pp. 1-7).
- A major way you can tell if you have healed, is if you can be calm when you want to be, and only become vigilant when necessary (p. 4).

You can set your recovery "compass heading" on these principles. Harvard University is a world-leading authority on stress management. It is strongly recommended that you contact the "source" at <www.health.harvard.edu>.

---

12. An invocation for strength.

To conclude this chapter on how to keep your mind in the face of great challenges, we leave you with this:

"Let me not pray to be sheltered
from dangers
but to be fearless in facing them.
Let me not beg for the stilling of my pain
But for the heart to conquer it."
-Rabindranath Tagore

SUMMARY

In this chapter you learned how to refuse to lose your mind. The motto of this chapter is: "Don't let stress squelch your success." A dozen Do-Able tips are provided on surviving a level 10 earthquake on your stress Richter Scale. Former President Clinton is cited as an example of a "comeback kid" demonstrating the power of positive attitude, even if misdirected, to overcome circumstances that would destroy most people. The centerpiece of this chapter is how not to have life "un-nerve you." Marilyn vos Savant, our modern sage, offers tips to deal with life during catastrophic events, such as the World Trade Center bombings.

The role of how eustress, such as patriotic or religious zeal, love and devotion to family and friends is discussed. Resumé-building tips are provided for when you are ready to hit the pavement running. Five temporary measures to get through traumatic events until the "Calvary arrives" are provided.

Harvard Medical School offers a therapeutic "compass heading" to follow in the "doom and gloom" of tragedy. The highlights of these cornerstone articles on dealing with 9/11 (trauma and disaster) are listed as well as the benefits of positive psychology. The next chapter will explore how humor is your balance pole when you are walking on the tight wire of work.

FOR FURTHER READING

Kelleher, J.B. (2001, June 3). Employers shift from stock options to handing out pink slips. Greensboro, NC. *News and Record.* p. 4.

Miller, M.C., Disaster and trauma. The *Harvard Mental Health Letter.* Vol. 18. 7, 1-5.

Miller, M.C., (2002). The benefits of positive psychology. The *Harvard Mental Health Letter.* Vol. 18, 6-7.

Star, J., A skills-training company. Phone (336) 294-8936, or fax (336) 299-0289.

Vos Savant, M., (2001, December 2). You can nourish your mind during these uncertain times. *Parade.* p. 14.

13

MAKE FUN OF STRESS & SMILE

IT MAKES YOU *LOOK* SMARTER

A sense of humor makes people believe you are intelligent.
- Carolyn Dickman, Education Director, Midwest Center for Stress and Anxiety, Inc. (2001)

I took an IQ test and the results were negative.
As seen in *Interfax Daily,* used by permission.

This chapter will look at:

- Why it is important to have workplace humor.
- How humor lifts moods and improves relationships.
- How to inject humor into your life by knowing yourself.
- Going on a humor diet (e.g., *Interfax Daily*).
- Making fun of stress — Developing your sense of humor.
- Is there a place for grim humor?
- Watching the company you keep; locking it in.
- Remembering that your sense of humor is your sense of balance.
- Humor leads people to believe you have a higher IQ or "virtual intelligence," (Mark Lewis).
- How to introduce humor to your job.
- Getting in touch with the experts.

1. Why is it important to have workplace humor? It works.

He who laughs… lasts. Although leading a humorless life is not fatal, it can be unhealthy psychologically. Humor serves as a balance pole on the tightrope of life. Humor is a powerful force in releasing stress's stranglehold. In fact, humor is such a powerful antidote to stress that many corporations hire humor consultants to "lighten up" office environments.

What is the secret to dramatically improving the quality of your life? Increase your smiles per hour.

Laughter is a natural mood elevator, and according to a Cornell University study, it also increases creativity and flexibility of thought. Humor gives a more balanced sense of perspective. Appropriately timed humor has even been found to be useful in alleviating the pain of injections as well as post-operative pain. Hal Lancaster, of the *Wall Street Journal*, emphasizes three important benefits to humor at work. Humor can:

- Motivate,
- Strengthen bonds between workers,
- Reduce stress.

Humor can enhance your career up the ladder. One CEO says, "Competent people with a sense of humor are more likely to be promoted. People are more likely to want to work for someone who has a sense of humor."

Lancaster says that the key attribute of humor in the workplace is to motivate and create team spirit, without wasting time.

Humor should be used like a spice, to enhance your career. Overusing humor is like ruining a dish with too much flavoring. You should use the right amount of humor at the right time.

Humor works at the workplace

IBM executive, Karen Donnalley, attained a 30% increase in sales by injecting fun and humor into a very competitive, intense office. She is considered one of the top motivators for IBM. Some techniques she uses include having salespeople hit a gong for their first sale of the day, and then moving a race horse with their picture on it out of a starting gate.

---

2. How humor lifts moods/improves health and relationships.

The main mechanism of humor or laughter appears to be the release of endorphins or the brain's natural tranquilizer into the system. Laughing results in an "endorphin high." Furthermore, laughter stimulates internal organs making them work better through the increase of circulation that follows the vibrating massage that accompanies laughter and heightens resistive vitality against disease.

We smile because we are happy. Interestingly, it has been discovered that our smile also causes our feelings of happiness. The act of smiling elevates moods.

---

3. How to inject humor into your life.

Know yourself.

Find your "sore spots" and apply humor as you would a soothing salve. For example, if your daily encounter with a computer makes you sore, find cartoons that make fun of computers. (Whole books have been devoted to making light of irritations, such as *101 Uses for Your Discarded Computer*). You may want to put the cartoons in a file where you can pull them out.

4. Go on a humor diet.

Try *Interfax Daily*. Optimism is the breakfast of champions. Instead of waking up to "doom and gloom" news, listen to upbeat radio stations. Find a radio station that emphasizes humor. Calendars are available that feature a daily cartoon or joke. The nationally-syndicated radio station, WMAG, is a pleasing way to start the day. When reading the newspaper, focus on the "funnies" first before finding out all the negative things thousands of people have done lately. Watch movies, listen to tapes or read books that are humorous. Duke University Comprehensive Cancer Center offers a very extensive list of humorous books, audiocassettes, and videocassettes. There are cable channels that feature only "light" programs. Many TV networks offer comedy serials. These can be bright spots in your weekly routine.

The *Interfax Daily* is "America's original faxed newspaper since 1995." It is faxed daily from (336) 397-0000 at no charge, to well over ten-thousand offices daily, and then copied and distributed. A sample of their daily humor is, "What do you call a cow with no legs? Ground beef."*

*Used by permission, *Interfax Daily*, March 5, 2001, Vol. WZ1V7101.

5. Making fun of stress.

Develop your sense of humor. Humor is an art form that can be nurtured. Jeanne Swanner Robertson, a nationally-renowned speaker and author, offers the how-to's of honing your humor skills in her 1998 book, *Don't Let the Funny Stuff Get Away: Turn Everyday Experiences into Stories That Audiences Will Remember.*

Robertson suggests taking "humor breaks." Often people feel worse after listening to everyone's complaints during breaks, so choose to be around more uplifting people. The last chapter of her book details how to collect "humor cues." Organize a file of things that are humorous to you. Pull up these "humor cues" on a daily basis.

Children laugh at least 25 times more often per day than adults.

(Adults average only 15 laughs a day, children about 400 per day.)

6. Is there a place for grim humor?

Yes. The world-famous Viennese psychiatrist, Dr. Victor Frankl, who survived the atrocities of two Nazi concentration camps, recommended using a sense of humor to soften one's own harsh situations. Dr. Frankl felt that even having a "grim sense of humor" helps to protectively detach ourselves from unavoidable suffering. Of course, limit your use of grim humor to yourself.

Never give up. Even a blind pig finds an occasional acorn.

A sad song, but bounce back anyhow

With a tear in his voice, Billy-Bob whined, "My dog just died; my health, job and marriage have failed; and I just got a summons to appear in court for speeding." Billy-Bob took a breath and dramatically continued his sad song, "If I didn't have bad luck, I'd have no luck at all." Tired of Billy-Bob's constant whining, his friend, said, "Did you ever hear of Winston Churchill? Sir Churchill said, "I have cornered the market on Indian rubber, because I will always bounce back." Billy-Bob's friend continued saying, "Just like a superball, the harder you hit rock bottom, the higher you need to bounce back."

7. Watch the company you keep; locking it in.

Avoid "pity parties." Fly with eagles, don't flounder with turkeys. Seek out and be around people known for their uplifting jokes and/or sense of humor. "Pity parties" use sarcasm to vent complaints, but using negative humor can actually intensify negative feelings, especially if the unwilling target for sarcasm is not an exceptionally "good sport."

Stop crucifying yourself . . . someone else needs the wood for a picnic bench.

Treat yourself to a humor treatment on a regular basis. Don't let a day pass without some exposure to humor. Lock in your sense of humor by habit.

8. Remember: Your sense of humor is your sense of balance.

People who need humor the most, seek it the least. When you feel you no longer have the time or mood for humor, perhaps you should slow down, relax, and smile. If you can't smile outwardly due to the situation, imagine yourself smiling. Daydream about the most humorous memory you can (e.g., even a pet's antics can be funny). You may not feel like "jumping for joy," but the lift you get will empower you with an increased sense of control and a more balanced perspective.

9. Humor leads people to believe you have a higher IQ (or higher "virtual intelligence"© by Mark Lewis of Denmark).

According to Carolyn Dickman, Education Director, Midwest Center for Stress and Anxiety, Inc. (2001), an important relationship between our IQ and humor was found. She goes on to suggest if you want people to think you are smart, start smiling.

The esteemed Reverend Mark Lewis of Denmark talks of "virtual intelligence." VIQ (virtual IQ) is a simulated form of intelligence that seems very real. Again, having a sense of humor projects this "illusion of intelligence" called "virtual intelligence." It does not matter if you are really that smart or not. "Virtual intelligence" is a good thing to cultivate, because no one is intelligent in all 120 measured types of intelligence as discovered by IQ expert, Dr. J. P. Guilford. Sometimes you just have to fake it until you make it in an area you haven't mastered. The bottom line is that smiling persuades people to be believe you are "virtually intelligent" which is very important in any business or human relations setting. Anyone who works for a living on or with computers should make every effort to appear "virtually intelligent." When video-phones soon dominate communication, it would be great to have your stand-in dummy looking very "virtually intelligent" in your chair, until you can make it there yourself, smiling and secure. People take a mental personality "snapshot" within the first 20 seconds of meeting you, so smile for the camera.

It's just an act, and if people were as smart as they acted (a true measure of "virtual intelligence"), their brains would be so big they couldn't lift their heads from the floor. So explore your "virtual intelligence."

---

10. How to introduce humor to your job.

Hal Lancaster, of *The Wall Street Journal,* offers four tips for workplace humor:

1. Start with a little humor.

For example, put up jokes on a bulletin board to see reactions. Don't jeopardize your career in a totally humorless office by irritating humorless executives.

2. Meaningfully connect.

Squirt gun fights are probably pushing humor too far. To mix playfulness with productivity, try role reversal. Have an executive do your job for a day with you supervising. (Use caution with this approach.)

3. Renew the humor.

To keep humor from getting old, bring in new approaches.

4. Don't offend.

One approach that does not work is to have comedy skits about other departments that attack personally. Be certain not to question anyone's value or harm anyone with attempts at humor.

---

11. Get in touch with the experts.

For humorous props and workshops, contact the Humor Potential, a corporate training organization who specializes in injecting fun into the workplace. The "Joy of Stress" workshop by the Humor Potential was a nationally-televised, Emmy-nominated special, looking at the lighter side of stress.

The highly-popular "Dilbert" series takes the employee's side of stress at work. This cartoon series by Scott Adams is read by millions daily. It offers potential stress relief through downward comparison. In other words, compared to this cartoon strip, your job may not seem so stressful.

A positive motivational series is "Herbert," which specializes in producing large posters humorizing potentially tense situations. A classic film that pokes fun at stress is Mel Brooks', *High Anxiety.* It has some content that would be more appropriate for college students, but it is generally an entertaining, yet instructional tool to learn about anxiety.

Remember, "Humor is the spoonful of sugar that helps things go down easier."

SUMMARY

This chapter explores five major topics regarding humor: 1) Why it is important to have workplace humor; 2) How to inject humor into your daily life; 3) How humor makes you look smarter, (i.e., "virtual intelligence"); 4) Tips on how to inject humor into your work-life; 5) We also looked at how to get in touch with the experts. Your sense of humor is truly your sense of balance. The next chapter deals with the reported number one job-stressor — public speaking. We will attempt to humorously dismantle this fear by pointing out that public speaking just takes more "hot air" than private speaking. Tips from the American Society of Training and Development (ASTD) are provided to guarantee a successful, if not pleasant, speaking experience.

FOR FURTHER READING

Guilford, J.P. (1967). *The nature of human intelligence.* New York: McGraw-Hill.

Interfax Daily, March 2, 2001, Vol. WZ1V7951, Phone (336) 397-0000 for a Free-Daily humor fax. Baton Rouge, LA.

Robertson, J.S. (1998). *Don't let the funny stuff get away: turn everyday experiences into stories that audiences will remember.* Houston, TX: Rich Pub. Co.

14

Public Speaking: Public Enemy Number One

Private & Public Speaking are Basically the Same, You Just Need More "Wind" for the Latter

Call him Mr. Cologne, even though he's in Switzerland.

Bob was excited about his invitation to speak to some of the top people in the world at the Stress Conference in Montreux, Switzerland. Overlooking the heaven-on-earth view of Lake Geneva and the snowcapped French Alps, Bob was trying to practice what he preached, that is, trying to be calm. He was wearing his "lucky speaking suit." To ease his own stress, Bob told himself that half the people in the audience could not even understand English. He was faithfully practicing his deep breathing and went over his notes that he had carved into his brain through repetition for weeks.

What Bob did not count on was having to serve on the panel on job-stress at this world level conference, which included gold medallist scholars in the field. At lunch, right before his speech, he was surprised to find out that he would be speaking on this job-stress panel followed by an interview with the local newspaper. His prepared speech was scheduled for 2:00 P.M. His impromptu job-stress panel was scheduled for 2:30 P.M. and the newspaper interview was scheduled for 3:00 P.M. Bob, although trying to be cool, was nonetheless getting nervous as he paced in his richly-decorated hotel room facing the stunning view of the Swiss landscape.

Again, he told himself there was nothing to be nervous about, since half the people at the world conference did not speak English, plus his speech was already printed in the proceedings. However, this was like using a ping-pong ball to deflect a bowling ball's path. It worked a little.

It was 1:45 P.M. — only minutes before his world speaking "debut." His supportive wife was dressed at the level of elegance to match the ornate speaking room they were headed toward.

In an effort to at least have neat hair, Bob hurriedly ran into the bathroom one last time and grabbed what he thought was super-hold hair spray. After spraying his hair for about ten seconds, he noticed the smell of his wife's expensive spray cologne. In his hurry-worry frenzy, he had accidentally grabbed the spray cologne, applying it generously to his hair. Coming to his rescue, Delia grabbed her container of spray cologne, and without missing a beat, said to Bob, "Try this," handing him the hair spray which he sheepishly applied.

All's well that ends well. After the presentation, Bob stayed even closer to his wife than usual, so people would assume that sweet smell was emanating from her. The Swiss newspaper reporter, however, did comment on the sweet-smelling scent in the room where Bob's interview was held. Bob stated that his wife had just reinforced her dose of cologne before she left the room. He knew she wouldn't mind this "little story" told to the newspaper reporter to protect Bob's macho image.

The moral of this story: Public speaking can take its toll. By overpracticing his speech so it was automatic, however, he still "delivered" even though he did not remember what he said, which is probably a merciful form of amnesia. To his surprise, people, in addition to his loving wife, said he had done a good job on the speech.

In this chapter we will try to vanquish the number one job-stress enemy — public speaking. We will address the following aspects of public speaking:

- You just need more "wind" for public speaking.
- Mastering public speaking is an art.
- To disarm the number one stressor on the job, a step-by-step guide is provided:

    Doing a "Needs Assessment" *(p. 161).*

    Bells and Whistles. Eight tips to prevent you from boring or baffling your audience *(p. 162).*

    Content Development. Seven strategies to make sure you are on target, on topic, and getting audience attention *(p. 162).*

    Presenter Preparation. Tips to guarantee success including, Don't sweat, Attitude affirmation, and "Tattoo your speech on your brain" *(p. 163).*

- Pulling it all together with the step-by-step workshop checklist (p. 164).

---

1. You just need more "wind" for public speaking.

Most people will eventually overcome this stressor; public speaking. Probably the main reason public speaking is stressful is that we cut off our own air supply. We squeeze our own wind pipes. When we are not used to projecting our voices, we tend to breathe shallowly and quickly, almost hyperventilating. Of course, oxygen deprivation will set off all kinds of alarms in your brain, even leading to panic attacks. Seasoned actors know the importance of deep breathing to speak well and even feel well during performances. Take a deep belly breath, through your nose, breathe down to your belly, fill your chest with air, and hold for a few seconds, then breath out through your mouth. Repeat this twice, slowly. This whole "breathing exercise" takes about 30 seconds (Breathe in for two seconds, exhale for four seconds, three times). Do your homework and you will be fine. Start "smart breathing" about three weeks ahead of your event.

---

2. Mastering public speaking is an art.

How you react to the stress of public speaking is up to you. Many consider pre-speaking jitters as a sign of respect for your audience. As stated before, stress is simply energy, and stress management is simply energy conservation. Choose to use stress as an energy source. If you interpret the butterflies in your stomach as excitement, you are converting negative stress (distress) into positive stress (eustress).

To disarm the number one stressor on the job, a step-by-step guide has been provided below, based on information gleaned from the American Society of Training and Development.

The story of Mr. Green-Jacket: surprise, lights, action, camera

Bob and Delia had just returned from a great week at the beach. On the answering machine was a message from Dr. Lee Kinard, host and producer of the top Nielson-rated, longest-running local morning TV show in America. Dr. Kinard had asked Bob if he would do a week-long series on stress on the ***Good Morning Show****. Bob had taught a semester-long stress-management course at a local college for three years so he felt confident. The next morning Dr. Kinard called to say," Bob, bring down some notes to the station and we'll talk about setting up the series." The following day Bob typed out his presentation in kindergarten-letter-sized type, and Delia picked out attire for him that would make a fine impression. A bright, green sportcoat was what Bob was going to wear, because this was the color worn at the Golf Greater Open, held that week in town. Wearing the GGO color would impress Dr. Kinard, and perhaps land Bob the TV spot.*

Bob admired Dr. Kinard, voted the most-trusted public figure in an area covering one-million people. Dr. Kinard warmly shook Bob's hand, commented favorably on his bright green GGO sportcoat, and offered Bob a seat. Trying to look organized, Bob showed Dr. Kinard his notes. He said, "Bob, this series is not designed to cure anybody, but just give people some simple causes and cures of stress." We'll air the series each morning at 7:15. We'll make a copy of the series for you. Bob agreed and was already making plans on how he would schedule his rehearsals at home.

Reaching over, Dr. Kinard straightened up Bob's tie. He said, "We want you to look good for the folks." Getting out his calendar, Bob said, "When would you like to do the series?"

Dr. Kinard said, "Right now. We'll tape an hour with you talking, edit it, splice it in at 7:15 A.M. daily for the next week, and it will look like it's a live interview." Bob could feel beads of sweat form on his forehead, and could actually feel his blood pressure rising. "Now? I thought we were just going to talk about doing the series next week." Dr. Kinard smiled as the cameraman clipped the mike on Bob's bright green GGO jacket. He leaned over to Bob and said, "Bob, the best way to relax during this interview is just to concentrate on the questions I ask and don't worry about anything else."

Dr. Kinard's 40 years of TV experience were apparent when he took Bob's notes, looked them over briefly and pointed to the cameraman, saying "Roll 'em." He asked Bob well-formulated questions from his notes, and somehow Bob made it through the whole hour. Dr. Kinard's tip to just focus completely on one thing (his interview questions) actually did calm Bob down even under this high-intensity stress situation.

Leaving the ***Good Morning Show*** *TV stage, Bob asked if and when the series would be aired. "Next week, Bob. You did well. We'll edit out what we need to," Dr. Kinard said cheerfully.*

Bob learned from this experience that totally concentrating in terms of listening and speaking to the subject at hand will help you be successful even under the spotlight pressure of "surprise, lights, action and cameras."

Bob called his wife at work and told her the story. As always, she was comforting. Bob asked her to keep it "mum" until he could see what he came across like on TV. With masterful editing and artful interviewing, Dr. Kinard actually made Bob seem professional on the show. On Monday people at work congratulated him. By the Thursday installment of the series, people would smile when they saw Bob. By the end of the series, he found an envelope on his desk. It said, "office collection for a new sportcoat."

Because the show was taped in one hour, Bob wore the same bright green GGO sportcoat through the entire interview. People thought Bob had only one coat, having appeared five days in a row on TV with the same conspicuously bright coat. For better or for worse, that's what people commented on about the week-long interview. Bob took it in stride, smiled and had to laugh at himself when he viewed the video. Best of all, Bob landed a job from a prospective employer who had seen him on the week-long series, green sportcoat and all.

---

3. To disarm the number one stressor on the job, a step-by-step guide is now provided.

Lady luck favors the prepared

The smarter you prepare, the luckier you become. Usually it takes about three hours of preparation for one hour of speaking if you know the subject and have your materials. If you are starting from scratch (no information, no materials) it is about a ten-to-one ratio, ten hours of preparation for one hour of speaking. Effective public speaking truly requires the use of both your "head" and "heart." A listing and discussion of the heads-up skills and how to get to the heart of the matter are now provided. A single-page, workshop-worksheet checklist is provided to further demystify what goes into a good speech.

Heads-up skills

The four basic needs an audience wants to have met were presented by Dr. David Campbell, an award-winning speaker with the Center for Creative Leadership (Co-author of the Campbell Strong Interest Inventory). He emphasized the four basic components that successful workshop presenters need to have:

1. *Credentials/accomplishments of the presenters (Degrees, Associations, Publications).*
2. *Content: "What to do tomorrow" activities or information.*
3. *Entertainment: Relevant humor and "stories." Your presentation is competing with "popular media" as a baseline expectation. Use graphics, visual media when possible.*
4. *Resourcefulness of speaker to recover in case things go wrong (e.g., equipment failure).*

***Doing a "Needs Assessment"*: What is your training bull's eye?**

Ask training "needs assessment" questions. Are the training needs process or outcome based? Example of process goal: Train teachers about test-taking strategies and have students learn test-taking skills as part of the curriculum. Example of outcome goal: Test scores will improve.

Find out what results (goals) are most highly rewarded in the system. What goals/results receive recognition?

Spend 20% of the workshop finding out what the participants need. Write out workshop activities as they "connect" with the identified needs the workshop is to meet.

Single-factor emphasis: Most participants will only remember one simple fact one year after the workshop. Define, highlight and emphasize the most important thing to remember from the workshop.

Bells and Whistles

Here are eight tips to use in trying not to bore or baffle your audience. You are competing with sophisticated mass media (TV, radio). Learn from these media in terms of simplicity, colorfulness and appeal of your presentation.

- Use color where possible.
- Use music where possible.
- All overheads should be legible. (You should be able to read the material from a five-foot distance without projection.)
- Handouts should match overheads (where possible).
- Limit key points from five to seven maximum.
- Give people choice in participating in simulations.
- Use banners/props where appropriate.
- Provide snacks.

***Content Development*:** **Seven strategies to make sure you are on target**

1. *Incentive (Remember WII-FM — What's in it for me?) What will your participants gain personally and/or professionally from your talk?*
2. *E. F. Hutton statement ("Wow! I didn't know that" statements). Make bold and truthful statements.*
3. *Speak their language. Use the audience's language. People can only absorb five to seven new facts at a time. Know your audience.*
4. *Remember the 7-7 rule. Stick to seven major points; repeat the main points seven times (in different forms).*
5. *Take hourly breaks if possible. The average adult attention span is 45 minutes.*
6. *Did we hit the bull's eye? Or was there good R O I - Return on investment? For the investment (time/money), what measurable, positive change has been realized? Ask your participants what single change they will make as the result of the workshops. How will this change be documented? (It can be a process or outcome change.)*
7. *Attention-getter notes from the audience. Distribute two or three 3 x 5 index cards to each participant. Tell them ahead of time that you will randomly ask them to write down whatever they are thinking about at a particular moment during your talk. Have each participant do this individually, and anonymously. You may wish to delay telling them they don't have to put their names on the cards till right before they turn in their cards. This will increase their attention span. You are testing your attention-getting ability, not their listening skills.*

Have them pass in the cards (with no identification) right after you ask them to write down their predominant thought at that moment. Review these cards, and see how many bull's eyes you were hitting with your talk. Turn up the volume for points not getting through by reducing the number of points or increasing the interest level of your points.

Presenter Preparation: **Tips to guarantee success**

1. Don't sweat (while presenting).

Sweat while preparing. Ten to one ratio of preparation to presentation time is typical. (It takes ten hours of preparation for an hour of good presentation.) This includes needs assessment, product development and practice.

2. Attitude affirmation.

Repeat to yourself, "I know — that I know," to build your confidence. You will always know a little more than your audience (at least new jokes).

Smile and say to yourself and then to your audience, "I'm glad to be here," (whether you are or not, fake it till you make it). Smiling will make your audience think you're smart. Find one friendly face in the audience.

3. "Tattoo your speech on your brain."

Use the rule of 7. Go through your talk at least seven times. Practice once to a live audience (of one) sitting at the back of the room or tape record your speech. Make sure your practice audience feigns boredom and distraction so you are not upset when it happens in real life. Have your "guinea pig" audience sit at least twenty feet away from you so you learn to project your voice.

4. Double the amount of enthusiasm you speak with normally and slow down your pace.

5. Practice the main points of your speech right before you go to sleep. This will solidify it in your memory.

6. Drink a warm (decaffeinated) drink right before you talk.

It will relax you and your voice. Take three or four slow deep breaths, belly breathing if you can. Breathe in through your nose, exhale from your mouth.

7. Use cue cards and technology but don't depend on them entirely.

Have your major points memorized. TV personalities use kindergarten letter-sized type on their notes. Probably a twenty-point font size would be helpful. Also, you can even put breathing/pause marks in your notes so you don't talk too fast under stress. A breathing mark in your notes is simply a slash. Professional speakers use breathing marks in their notes.

Remember: Practice makes permanent.

Pulling It All Together with the Step-By-Step Workshop-Worksheet Checklist

(Check items as they apply. See text for explanation of each item)

NEEDS ASSESSMENT: WHAT IS YOUR TRAINING BULL'S EYE?

Four Basic Needs

- ■ Credentials of presenters.
- ■ Content "What to do tomorrow" based on knowledge.
- ■ Entertainment — Humor that is relevant.
- ■ Resourcefulness to recover (Plan B if Plan A doesn't work).

Other Considerations

- ■ Process or outcome (end point) goals of training defined.
- ■ Rewarded results identified and used as goals for training.
- ■ Twenty percent of workshop time used in "participant identification" of needs.
- ■ Workshop activities connect with identified goals/needs.
- ■ Single fact "to be remembered" is defined and highlighted.

BELLS AND WHISTLES

- ■ Color used where possible.
- ■ Music used where possible.
- ■ Overheads all legible.
- ■ Handouts match overheads (where appropriate).
- ■ Limit key points to five to seven items.
- ■ Give people choice in simulations.
- ■ Props, posters used.
- ■ Edibles.

CONTENT DEVELOPMENT

- ■ WII-FM (What's in it for me? Incentives for participants).
- ■ E.F. Hutton, truthful statements.
- ■ Speak their language (Know your audience).
- ■ 7 - 7 rule: (Limit to seven major points, repeat main points seven times).

- Hourly breaks (if possible).
- Was training bull's eye hit? Use an outcome measure (before/after quiz results on topic).
- Attention-getter notes. Randomly ask all participants to write down what they are thinking during the talk on three by five index cards given out earlier. No identification needed on cards submitted. Use feedback to improve your message and/or delivery.

PRESENTER PREPARATION

- Expect ten hours of preparation for one hour of initial presentation.
- Attitude affirmation to build self-confidence (I know that I know this material).
- Smile and say, "I'm glad to be here." Think of friends in audience.
- Go through talk seven times prior to speech.
- Double the amount of enthusiasm when you speak.
- Slow down your rate of speech.
- Practice speech night before with your warm-up audience "faking boredom."
- Drink warm decaffeinated drink right before talk. Take a few deep breaths.
- Use cue cards but memorize key points.

SUMMARY

This chapter looked at techniques to disarm the number one job-stressor — public speaking. Public speaking just requires a lot more hot air (in actually breathing and in amount of prepared material). Panic from cutting off our own air supply by shallow breathing may be the number one culprit in making public speaking stressful. Based on information obtained from the American Society of Training and Development, eight specific, proven skills are detailed to assure a productive and even pleasant speaking experience. You are provided with a one-sheet, point-by-point checklist of skills that will lead you to speaking as well publicly as you do privately. A trick of the trade to assure and assess audience attention is also provided.

Up till now we dealt with job-related problems and prescriptions. Even though we spend an equivalent of fifteen solid years at work, the majority of our life is still spent at home. Hopefully, you are working so you can live, not living so you can work. This next section talks about the great need for equipping today's children with the 21st century skills to manage stress at home and at school.

FOR FURTHER READING

Campbell, D., Center for Creative Leadership (Co-author of the Campbell Strong Interest Inventory, 1981).

15

CHILDREN: STRESS CURES AT HOME

LISTEN TO YOUR CHILD AND TAKE A REAL RECESS

I hope the old saying, "There's no place like home," is true for children. However, some children may not experience peace of mind at home. To help address the growing need for stress management for children, this chapter will examine the following eight topics:

- The epidemic need for stress management for children.
- Which children are at most risk for stress and substance abuse? You'd be surprised.
- Stress: a growing problem linked to increased drug abuse.
- Snapping under stress — the final act.
- Stress causes, warning signs of excessive stress and cures: The ABC's of stress management for children.
- The terrific or terrible teens; it is a choice.
- Seven tips for dealing with school stress.
- Getting off on the right foot; managing school mornings.

1. The epidemic need for stress management for children: A stress-status check.

- One-third of children in the U.S. have levels of stress ranging from moderate to extreme.
- Children may start having stress by age four (e.g., monsters under the bed) which is normal and treatable.
- Children have never been under more stress and this stress is predicted to mount. The reasons cited for this increased stress are the pressures youngsters are under to deal with academic demands and other tasks for which they are not developmentally ready.
- Almost no one is dealing with teaching children how to deal with stress, outside of a few school programs.
- Migraine Mondays are becoming a reality for many teenagers because of the stress they now experience. The flip side of the stress coin is that there are at least five key benefits to teaching children to manage stress.

Five benefits resulting from stress management in children include:

1. *Enjoying better physical health.*
2. *Increased resistance to negative peer pressure.*
3. *Less fighting.*
4. *Preventing and controlling emotional problems.*
5. *Opening lines of communication: Highly-anxious children may be afraid to displease their parents, and may even tend to hide problems. Unrelieved stress from a child's problems will eventually erupt.*

---

2. Which children are at most risk for stress and substance abuse? You'd be surprised.

According to a 2000 Yale University study, suburban teens were more prone to substance abuse and stress than low-socioeconomic counterparts.

---

3. Stress: a growing problem linked to increased drug abuse.

Drug abuse is on the rise for children. Sadly, drugs are used to alleviate unpleasant stress symptoms and/or to create pleasant stress (eustress-excitement). Adults, using the All-American drug cycle (caffeine, alcohol, nicotine), are perhaps unconsciously modeling behavior that says it's O.K. to self-medicate.

---

4. Snapping under stress — the final act.

The newspaper read, "Teen kills father, then self." R.C. was a quiet fourteen-year-old attending Pleasantville Junior High School in Europe. The day prior to the murder-suicide, his friends reported that he was upset about his grades, and he allegedly said, "I'll never get all A's." RC did not exhibit any warning signs of the tremendous self-imposed stress he was under. Everyone said, "He just snapped." The exaggerated fear of facing his father with another less-than-perfect report card was the "straw that broke the camel's back." He used a permanent solution to a temporary problem. A counselor at the school felt the story should be told to prevent this from ever happening again.

Snapping under stress is happening more than ever before. These five words (Teen kills father, then self) in the headlines provide more than enough justification for encouraging stress/anger management among our youth. Stress management for children is no longer a luxury, but sometimes a life-and-death necessity. Murder-suicides among children are supposed to be statistically rare (one in eighty thousand) but even once is too much. Always seek professional help if you have any doubts about your child's emotional status.

5. Stress causes, warning signs of excessive stress, and cures: The ABC's of stress management for children.

Today's children are particularly susceptible to stress and resultant "burnout" or "blowout." Some of these causes are listed below:

- Preschool competition, the media and family matters.
- Perfectionistic tendencies.
- Increased sensitivity to adult problems.
- Many children tend to be "info-maniacs" about what is going on in their environments, ranging from family problems to global issues.
- Developmental gaps.
- Peer pressure.
- There may well be a "tug of war" going on within a child between pleasing either parents or peers.
- Increased external pressures.
- Achievement anxiety: "Achieving to live" a satisfying, productive life is far better than "living to achieve."

TEN WARNING SIGNS OF EXCESSIVE STRESS

The more of these symptoms a child has, the more likely he or she may be suffering from excessive stress. (Physical complaints, overactivity and distractibility should always be investigated to determine or eliminate possible medical causes.)

1. *Sudden, dramatic increase or decrease in effort at school.*
2. *Major change in attitude/temperament (irritability, lack of enthusiasm, carelessness).*
3. *Withdrawal or outbursts.*
4. *Nervous tics, fidgeting, jumping from task to task, difficulty concentrating. Pulling eyebrows, twirling hair, bouncing knees, frequent unnecessary trips to the bathroom, can be forms of nervous energy overflow.*
5. *Complaints of fatigue and vague illnesses.*
6. *Difficulty sleeping.*
7. *Stomachaches, headaches.*
8. *Drug abuse.*
9. *Increase in allergic/asthmatic attacks.*
10. *Avoidance of school or testing situations by direct refusal or convenient illnesses. Frequent visits to the school nurse's office for no diagnosable cause.*

Mental-health professionals should always be consulted if one suspects a child is experiencing excessive stress. Stress is often an internal, quiet disorder, because highly-anxious children are overwilling to please and conform. Stress symptoms may be invisible unless you as a parent are sensitive to changes in the child's attitude, behavior or health.

CURES: The ABC's of Stress Management for Children

Stress does not go away; it is how one copes with it that changes. Successfully coping with stress should allow children to retain achievement attitudes of the "Type A" personality but exhibit "Type B" behaviors (relaxed, patient, well focused) that are conducive to high achievement and problem solving. The ABC's (Attitudes, Behaviors, and Circumstances) to promote relaxation are below. In no way are these suggestions a substitution for treatment provided by a mental-health professional.

Attitude

- Promote a positive, flexible, noncompetitive spirit.
- Encourage "one-thing-at-a-time" thinking.
- Get guidance when needed.

Behavior

- A key principle in stress management is that anxiety and deep muscle relaxation cannot coexist. By deeply relaxing muscles, anxiety states can be reduced.

Circumstances

- Watch out for excessive preschool competition, TV violence and family discord.
- Listen to the child.
- Get help with school work. Use Homework Hotline and WorldCat (a world-wide Research Engine). Combating being bored or baffled.
- Join the PTA.
- Tackle test anxiety.
- Have a real 20-minute recess with your child.
- Try not to "club your child" to stress with excessive clubs and after school activities.
- Encourage a stress-reducing diet.
- Use sports as a way to "blow-off" steam.
- Make certain your child gets enough rest.
- Provide a quiet environment.

- Pet your pet.
- Be tough minded but tenderhearted.
- MOST IMPORTANTLY: Be a "good example."

An expansion of these tips is provided below using the ABC of childhood stress management (focusing on Attitudes, Behavior, Circumstances).

Attitude

Promote a positive, flexible, noncompetitive spirit:

Overly competitive, impatient and angry attitudes dominate a highly-stressed child's profile. Encourage persistent, patient effort on the child's part. Teach the child to be firm but flexible when planning and working toward a goal. Encourage the child to have a "plan B" ready in case their first efforts are frustrated. You may want to ask the child how he/she feels about demands/pressures to gauge whether he/she is feeling overwhelmed and negative about their circumstances. Teach and show the child the value of trust in the trustworthy.

It is important to remember that the "dawn of reason" (knowing right and wrong) varies. Some say by age eight, others by age eleven. Most children are capable of reasoning by teenage hood, unless the hormone wars win.

Encourage "one-thing-at-a-time" thinking

Teach your child to concentrate on one thought or action at a time, at least on occasion. Constant chaos creates tension. Even imaging a pleasant scene for a few moments can be relaxing.

Get guidance when necessary

The 2002 pamphlet, *When Terrible Things Happen*, by Dr. Lewis Leavitt, helps parents and caretakers to respond to great trauma with age appropriate methods for each developmental stage, from preschool to twelve-years-old. (Please see "For Further Reading." American Academy of Pediatrics [April, 2002]). To access the on-line component related to helping children deal with trauma visit <www.jjpi.com>.

Behavior

A key principle in stress management is that anxiety and deep muscle relaxation cannot coexist. By deeply relaxing muscles, anxiety states can be reduced.

The physical strain from stress collects in the neck, head, shoulder, face and jaw muscles. To eliminate or prevent physical strain, one must learn the difference between muscle tension and relaxation. By tightening and relaxing their fists (at about 5-second intervals), children can feel the alternative states of relaxation in their forearms. Next have them try this tension-relaxing exercise in the shoulders, neck, and jaw muscle areas.

Finally, they should try to relax the whole body (without tensing), starting with the feet and progressing up to the jaws by major body sections: feet, ankles, legs, hips, stomach, chest, back, shoulders, neck, scalp, facial muscles and jaws.

In guiding your youngster with relaxation exercises, it is helpful to "suggest" the desirable behavior. For example: "Relax your feet (ankles, legs, etc.). Feel your muscles becoming loose, limp, heavy and warm." This should be done slowly with sufficient pauses after relaxing each major body section.

Circumstances: Treat the reasons

Treating the reasons rather than just the reactions to stressors is most important. Find out what the reasons are for the child's stress first. Watch out for excessive preschool competition, TV violence and family discord.

Just as you would not allow your child to stare at the sun during an eclipse just because he or she wanted to, exposure to excessive stressors at an early age should be limited also. Be alert for signs of excessive competition or criticism at school, even at the preschool level. A child may avoid going to school or even become sick if he feels too much pressure in school. TV violence should not be part of a child's diet during their mentally formative years when they often do not know the difference between fantasy and reality. Nightmares may suggest that a child should cut back on violent TV. Family feuds certainly do not need to be displayed in front of the child. He may even feel blame for family fights.

Listen to the children

According to Dr. Thomas Huberty of the National Association of School Psychologists, performance problems in school can often bring on anxiety. Listen with feeling to what your child says to you. Accept whatever your child tells you are heavy problems, and help the child solve the problems. For example, your child may feel terrified of the schoolyard bully, which most adults have forgotten about. Adjusting the child's reactions to these problems through attitude and behavior modification will provide the patience to work out the problems. (This may require professional help.)

An excellent resource to help you listen to your children is *Talking with Your Kids About Fear and Anxiety,* by Lisa O. Engelhardt and Dr. Lyn Sontag. This easy-to-read, succinct, illustrated manual looks at five activities to help you help your child with stress, starting at age four up to age twelve. (Call 1-800-325-2511 or write One Caring Place, Abbey Press, St. Meinrad, IN 47577.)

Other common reasons for childhood stress are: problems with being separated from home for the first time, time- and schoolwork-management, peer-sibling-family difficulties, self-concept, and competition in general.

Get help with school work: Being bored or baffled

Being baffled. As stated above, schoolwork is often a major stressor for children. Being bored or baffled in school are both stressful. If your child is having difficulty in school, have his/her learning abilities and interests assessed and look at the child's work habits. Often times children simply don't do their homework. Teaching and tracking time management for your child may be the most important thing you can do to relieve school stress. (Post the child's study schedule in plain view on a door so he or she can check off homework completion on a daily basis.) Rightfully so, more money is spent on educating children with learning differences who are having difficulty in school.

Also, make learning rewarding by celebrating project completions and showing your appreciation for the work done. Post awards and good grades on the refrigerator. You may have him "earn" allowance by making homework a part of her tasks. Have your child do his homework first and then have him enjoy privileges. Often children feel overwhelmed when they do not break down assignments into weekly or daily assignments. A child may panic when she realizes this semester's project is due tomorrow when actually she forgot about it. There are many good books on learning to do homework. Educational material stores offer many good time- and homework-management systems.

Obtain a tutor if necessary, take a closer look at the child's learning strengths/needs and help keep your child on a schedule for tests and assignments. Finally, reward your child on a weekly basis for sticking to a schedule until learning itself becomes rewarding.

An excellent reference for parents to help children with homework habits is *Homework Without Tears,* by Lee Canter and Lee Hausner. A useful how-to book for highschoolers is *Getting Smarter, Simple Strategies for Better Grades,* by Lawrence J. Greene and Leigh Jones-Bamman.

Join the PTA if you want to demonstrate to your child your support for his efforts in school. Of course, attend activities in which your child is involved.

Being bored. It is a reality that there are some second graders who already have academic skills at the eighth grade level. These children are our future scientists who will invent everything we use, enjoy and need (buildings, medicine, TV, computer games, airplanes). Obviously, if these children had not existed, we would still be living in caves with an average lifespan of 18 years. The downside of this ability is isolation and being teased because they don't fit in. Being bored is as stressful as being baffled. The common sense formula for personal happiness is "keep like minds in touch" but "keep in touch" with the world if you want anyone to listen to you. A feeling of loneliness can quickly lead to unbalance even if you are just one out of one-hundred.

If you had an IQ of 160 (top scientist level), you would be about 3 in 100,000. Imagine the isolation you'd feel sitting in a large athletic event center that could hold 100,000 fans. If only your "mental equals" were sitting in the audience area, there would only be two other people in the whole stadium, with 99,997 empty seats! Courses in common sense to learn how to relate to normal people are necessary and the opportunity to be with like minds is critical for healthy emotional development of highly gifted.

A great organization that parents and teachers can join is the Council for Exceptional Children, which embraces children with learning differences. Established at Columbia University-Teachers College 80 years ago, this well-defined organization provides support for parents and children with exceptional needs.

Tackle test anxiety

Test anxiety heads up the list of stressors for many students.

See the chapter, "Scoring Best on All Life's Tests." Something as simple as letting your child wear his/her favorite outfit to the test can help reduce anxiety. Treat your child to fruit (not candy) before a test. Set up a test-simulation with a timer so he/she learns how to budget time.

Dr. Thomas Huberty states that test anxiety is treatable by teaching your child: relaxation, realistic attitudes, positive self-talk, and practicing relaxation/positive self-talk/attitudes while thinking about or taking tests. The child should be rewarded frequently for positive attitudes and behaviors (studying according to a schedule) and should have a realistic attitude about test performance (it is not do-or-die).

Contact your local university or community college several months before important exams, such as the SAT, so that the child can start preparing before test anxiety has a chance to set in. Panic is unlikely if the child has practiced taking this type of test "a thousand times before."

Matt Oeschli of Greensboro, North Carolina is a national consultant who offers proven SAT preparation courses (Guilford College), and a book, *Mind Power for Students,* St. Martin's Paperbacks. His book provides methods that can raise SAT scores by 100 points, help students study better and take tests in general more effectively. The Matt Oeschli Institute can be contacted at (336) 273-6582.

Have a real 20-minute recess with your child

Authorities state that what is quality time for you may not be quality time for your child. A child may not enjoy a slow talk-while-you-walk event. Try to spend 20 minutes daily doing what your child wants, except perhaps watching

TV together. If the child likes playing catch, play catch. If the child likes to ride her bike, get a bike to ride along with her. Even go fly a kite with him if he asks you. You may want to talk to your child during this time, but focus on what is important to your child such as things he is looking forward to.

Try not to "club your child" to stress with excessive club activities, expecting him to join soccer club, French club and computer club. Your child may be trying to please you by taking up your every offer but wearing himself out doing so.

Encourage a stress-reducing diet

Caffeine and excessive sugar intake induce tension; therefore encourage children to limit, if not eliminate, consumption of food with these substances.

Use sports as a way to "blow-off" steam

Even a few jumping jacks will relieve pent-up stress. Jumping rope, playing ball games, swimming, soccer and other active sports can serve as a safety valve to relieve pressure. These activities can help a child sleep better and be less restless during periods requiring concentration. Do not counteract the benefits of exercise by overemphasizing competition.

Send your child out for errands on his/her bike when possible. Even having your child climb steps to the second story of your house will help vent some stress.

Make certain your child gets enough rest

Getting enough rest is one of the best ways to combat stress and boost a child's stress tolerance. Getting enough rest even determines how much a child will learn from the lessons taught that day, according to the latest brain research. Often individuals will have a difficult time sleeping the night before a big event. In this case, it would be best to make sure the child gets a good night's sleep two nights before the big event. The child can then tap in on energy reserves built up from the more relaxed sleep he had two nights before. Giving a child milk and cookies (or graham crackers) a couple of hours before retiring may help her relax. Taking a warm bath about an hour before bed may also be helpful. But playing competitive games, such as video games, may pump a child up too much right before bed, so have a cut-off time for games. Also, doing homework right before bed may be counterproductive and cause restlessness. Try to avoid touchy subjects (what the child has not been doing correctly) right before bed.

Provide a quiet environment

Silence is healing, in terms of repairing stressed-out nerves. Some quiet time will help a child relax, especially if combined with a simple relaxation exercise (like muscle relaxation) or pleasant thoughts.

Pet your pet

Research shows that caring for and enjoying a pet can help reduce stress. Even "wet pets" (fish) can help in focusing a child's attention onto caring for an animal.

Pet loss. Of course, the loss of a pet can be unexpectedly stressful, even on adults. The Argus Institute Foundation at Colorado State University suggests going to a vet who is known for their sensitivity about pet loss or joining a pet-loss support group. It is part of the normal grieving process to cry as you say goodbye to your pet. For more information on pet-loss support groups, contact your vet or a pet loss support group (Check your Yellow Pages under psychologists/psychiatrists or counselors). For reading materials and resources contact the University of California at Davis website <www.vetnet.ucdavis.edu/petloss/index.htm>. Unless you have experienced the sting of losing a favorite pet, you may be in for a very unpleasant reaction. (Buchalter, Gail. "When It's Time To Say Goodbye," *Parade*, June 3, 2001, pp. 8-9).

The best, most helpful and "to the point" pet-loss article this author has read is by Dr. Michael H. Andress, D.V.M., of Gate City Animal Hospital, in Greensboro, NC. The article, "Losing Your Beloved Companion," compassionately and sensitively deals with such topics as what to expect emotionally when we lose a pet, and tips on how to help your children, and even yourself get through this difficult period. (Dr. Andress' office can be reached at (336) 286-9500 or <www.gatecityvet.com>).

Just because you know the process of grieving, does not mean you are above feeling great distress when you lose a pet.

Be tough minded but tenderhearted

Children need structure within a caring framework. Constructive rules provide children with security because they know what will happen in the future. Rules will also teach the child the relationship between effort and results; cause and effect. This most often applies to studying for tests, doing homework, taking care of pets, keeping rooms clean, and getting along with siblings. Limit your rules to no more than five at time. Post the rules, state them positively and list many rewards for following the rules. Provide consequences (which you can follow through on) if sensible rules are not followed consistently after three weeks. Ask your school psychologist/counselor about good books on how to systematically enforce and/or discard rules. Of course, rules should have meaning. Explain the meaning of the rules when appropriate.

Be tenderhearted by giving your child "breathing room" about following the rules (expect eight out of ten times compliance unless for serious rules that involve safety). Do not bring up the child's past mistakes. Concentrate on the daily following of the rules. The Lee Canter series of books may be helpful in working with more difficult children. Refusal to follow simple rules may reflect other needs a child may have at the time. Seek professional counseling if it appears that he can't follow rules rather than that he just won't follow rules.

MOST IMPORTANT: Be a "good example"

Probably the most important thing to remember is to model the relaxed behaviors you are trying to cultivate in your youngster. Stress is very contagious. Your nonverbal behaviors (rushing, always seeming pressed for time, being impatient) will affect your child more than your reassuring, "Relax, don't worry." This is a clear case where "Actions speak louder than words."

---

6. The terrific or terrible teens; it is a choice.

Brain research shows that many children, having performed well up to about 11 or 12, can go through a learning slump in terms of academic performance in their preteens. On top of this brain-based learning slump, teenagers are going through hormone wars within and between themselves. Hormone-rage is probably more widespread than all road rage cases put together. Developmentally teens are testing their wings and testing your patience as they get ready to leave the nest. You suddenly start losing IQ points in their eyes as they get older (late teens) and wiser. This period of teenagehood has even been called the period of storm and stress.

Entire books have been written on dealing with teens. Basically it is better to be authoritative with tough love (not authoritarian with rigid rules). The apple doesn't fall far from the tree, in genetic terms, and they may be up to the same tricks that you or your mate once were since the expression of personality traits is based on genetics and environment. Perhaps things you were tempted to do, they are tempted to do earlier and with more opportunity. Teens undoubtedly are under terrific stress today. If your teen starts to display the stress symptoms listed above, it would be well to go to your family doctor first, and this professional could refer you to specialists, psychologists, or counselors.

Some tips to help avoid power struggles:

- Keep the peace. You can't give what you don't have. If you are mad, your child will "catch it" one way or the other. Once your child is defensive they turn a deaf ear to you.
- Have some "carved in stone" rules. You all remember the saying, "As long as you live under this roof, the house rules are to be followed." Don't make more than five serious commandments (You will always be home by 8:30 P.M., etc.). Be a broken record on these five rules (e.g., wearing a helmet on

a motorcycle, etc.). If you vary in your enforcement of important rules, the child will actually get a sense of excitement that gamblers get when they play the odds (Maybe I'll be lucky this time!).

- Prioritize your whining. Concentrate on a few rules that really do matter. Learn to compromise in setting your rules in stone. If your child is responsible enough, you should bid high (in expectations) so your child will feel that you're giving in a little. (e.g., Say, you are to be in by eight, then move it to 8:30 P.M.) Ask yourself, "How serious is this?", if Johnny wears certain clothes, or wants a certain hairstyle.
- Bring back the days of a benevolent dictatorship: Provide an environment where a child can make a mistake or two (85% compliance with any new rule is considered good in terms of behavioral management). Teach your child that they cause their own effects. In English this means there are rewards and consequences in the real world for behaviors.
- Give it a month. It takes about a month for a habit to "jell." Habits require a physical change in your brain. This takes time.

To help guide teens, it is well to start early. An excellent book is *Our Last Best Shot: Guiding our Children Through Early Adolescence,* by Laura Sessions Stepp, a *Washington Post* reporter. It provides realistic tips on how to help steer teenagers while they will still take direction. In the preteen years children are developing their lifelong behavioral maps and setting their compasses as they head out.

---

7. Seven tips for dealing with school stress.

School stress affects up to 10% of children to the point that they refuse to come to school. That can equal up to three children per class who are experiencing great, but treatable, anxiety. These children often end up in the principal's or nurse's office. They fake illnesses so they can stay home. They rarely mention what happens at school. They become visibly saddened or nervous when the subject of school is raised. Some of the reasons for their reactions to school follow, along with some remedies.

1. Achievement anxiety. Children with learning differences may constantly feel frustrated. It is not that "they won't learn, but that they can't learn" without additional help. To rule out physical causes for learning difficulties, have your child's vision/hearing checked out by a specialist. Also some children are hard-wired for hard-driving, perfectionistic tendencies. Don't wait until their "hard drive" crashes before you step in. (The next chapter deals with how to keep students cool at school.)

Children with learning disabilities may experience difficulty remembering what they hear. Since the majority of what is taught is often spoken by the teacher, this can be very frustrating for the child. Written expression is the most commonly required evidence for learning, so if a child has difficulty proving what he knows through writing, this can be stressful.

Learning differences can be identified and remedied by referring your child to a school psychologist or other learning specialists.

2. Personality clashes. Disciplinary/instructional styles used in the classroom may clash with your child's personality. Sensitive children may become highly anxious in a classroom strictly adhering to the "three strikes and you're out" approach. That is, the whole class may be disciplined for the misdeeds of a few students. An anxious child may take this personally. Also, witnessing disciplinary action directed at another child may create irrational fear in an innocent student. The child may fear, "I am next."

Having a heart-to-heart talk between the student and the teacher may relieve the child's fears. If the teacher's reputation for being a strict disciplinarian is true (which some children may actually benefit from), consider changing classrooms.

3. Bullies. If a child acts scared to attend school, she may be a target of a bully. Teach the child that there is "strength in numbers," and that he should hang out with his friends. He should avoid the bully's turf. Younger children may get help by talking directly to their teacher about the problem. Parents can appeal to the principal to reduce the child's contacts with the bully through schedule changes or different bus arrangements. The November, 2001 issue of The *Harvard Mental Health Letter* suggests the following steps on the school's part in their article, "Bullies and Their Victims." Involve the school by engaging bystanders, students more so than adults. The *Harvard Mental Health Letter* goes on to say that by age 11 or 12, if supported by adults, children will be able to at least report bullying. Bullying is inconsistent with most children's belief system (p. 5).

The best antidote to bullying is teaching empathy.

4. Fear of the unknown/Fear of failure.

If the child is nervous about entering a new school, make the child familiar with the new setting by having her meet the new teacher and learning her way around the new school.

Work at home to "disarm" the child's fears about "big assignments" by cutting the job down to size. At home, model positive thinking through such statements as, "You can do this," in place of the child's statement that, "I'm going to fail." You might want to place positive statements on index cards for the child to carry and review privately. Guide your child in the use of time management, in breaking big projects into smaller "do-able doses" which the child can handle on a daily or weekly basis.

5. Separation anxiety. Build your child's confidence and comfort level about leaving home by saying such things as, "I know you're going to have a great day; I'll see you after school." Do not fuel the child's insecurity by saying you will be there to rescue him if anything happens. Do not take off work in the anticipation that something might happen.

6. Rejection. Some children feel alone or friendless. They may even give away prized items to "buy friendship." Feeling rejected, a child may become conveniently sick to avoid field trips or class activities. To gain friends, emphasize or build a desired skill in your child. Developing athletic skills can improve the child's chances of being selected for a team. Nurturing musical talent can help your child feel successful and even part of a group (the band). Computer skills will win popularity. Even the ability to tell jokes can be an asset. Teach the child, "To have a friend you have to first be a friend." Have the child introduce himself with a smile and a handshake.

7. Be aware of the games your children play. Check out with the teacher claims your child makes. Try to pinpoint the true source of the child's stress. Almost every problem has a solution.

---

8. Getting off on the right foot; managing school mornings.

Organize the night before

Have your child select and lay out everything he is going to wear for the next day.

If inclement weather is in the forecast, know where the rain gear is. Find out whether the child has any special clothing requests at the beginning of the week. This may include clothes for gym or after-school sports.

Pack his/her bags

Place an envelope with his lunch money in his backpack, or pack her lunch with all utensils including desserts. Use obvious markings (different-colored lunch bags or boxes) to keep each child's lunch separate in the refrigerator. At the beginning of the week, find out if any special supplies are needed and on what day. The next day's school supplies, homework assignments, data disks, books and writing supplies need to be put in one carrying case or backpack. Put the completely packed tote bag by the door the night before. Some schools now require see-through tote bags or backpacks, so check with your school.

Wake-up calls

Use a clock radio and turn on the lights for wake-up calls. Have your child select his favorite radio station. Set the radio alarm to allow for at least nine hours sleep. The time the child's ride comes determines what time to set the alarm. Catching the bus at 7:00 A.M. means setting the alarm for 6:30 A.M. if your child can get ready in a half hour. Bedtime would then be 9:30 P.M. To make getting your child up on Mondays a little easier, try not to let them stay up too late on the weekends. Play "beat-the-clock." Set a kitchen timer to signal when your child needs to leave for the bus stop. If your child is out the door at the sound of the tone, he has then earned part of his allowance (or a TV or phone privilege) for that day. Playing this game for about three weeks will start a good habit of being on time. Drop back on the rewards at that time. Catching the bus on time, or getting in the car on time, will be reward enough.

Breakfast for champions

By the time breakfast is served, many children have not eaten for ten to twelve hours, so breakfast is critical. A quick, simple breakfast is best. The night before, have your child select from a "menu" which could include low-fat yogurt, bagels, cereal with skim milk and a banana, toast with jam. For meals on-the-run, graham crackers, dry cereal and a banana would do the trick.

SUMMARY

This chapter looks at the epidemic need for stress management for children. Upper-socioeconomic group children are actually at a higher risk for stress problems and drug use than their less privileged counterparts, according to a recent Yale study. Students under great stress are becoming a danger to self and others, because children under great strain are most likely to snap. Stress management among youth can be a matter of life and death in the 21st century.

Five benefits of stress management are listed, such as children fighting less if they are stress-intelligent. The ABC (Attitudes, Behaviors, Circumstances) approach to stress management for children is presented. (The ABC's are different for adults who have more control and greater wisdom than their children). Numerous tips are provided on how to help parents help their children deal with stress, using extensions of common sense activities. One new source however, is specifically designed to help parents and caretakers assist their children (from three to twelve years of age) in the face of traumatic events. This resource is offered by the American Academy of Pediatrics. How to deal with stress and future scientists of America is revealed. The number one antidote to bullying is revealed. How to keep the teenage years terrific, not terrible, is briefly addressed. Seven tips on how to deal with school stress are briefly presented leading into the next chapter dealing with the number one stressor for most children, school. **School is "job one" for most students, and they take school as seriously as adults take work.**

FOR FURTHER READING

American Academy of Pediatrics. (2002, April). *When terrible things happen.* (American Academy of Pediatrics, International Pediatric Association, Johnson & Johnson Pediatric Institute). Pamphlet on helping children aged 3-12, cope with trauma. On-line component at <www.jjpi.com>.

Andress, D.M.V., M. (1995). Death of a pet. *News-times.* (Burlington, NC).

Dr. Andress' Gate City Animal Hospital in Greensboro. NC can be reached at (336) 286-9500 or <www.gatecityvet.com>.

Anxiety Disorders of America. 6000 Executive Blvd., Suite 200, Rockville, MD 20852-3801, Phone (301) 231-9350.

Bramnick, L., & Simon, A. (1983). *The parents' solution book.* New York: Franklin Watts.

Buchalter, G. (2001, June 3). When it's time to say goodbye. *Parade.* p. 8-9.

The Center for Applied Psychology, PO Box 61586, King of Prussia, PA 19406. *Don't pop your cork on Mondays.* Children's anti-stress book. Stress Strategies, A game to help kids overcome stress, (2-4 players, ages 7-12).

Elkind, D. (1981). *The hurried child: growing up too fast too soon.* Reading, Mass: Addison-Wesley.

Engelhardt, L., & Lyn, S. *Talking with your kids about fear and anxiety,* Phone 1-800-325-2511 or write One-Caring Place, Abbey Press, St. Meinrad, IN 47577.

Huberty, T. (1999). National Association of School Psychologists Conference.

Luther, S. (2000, Summer). Professor Luther finds suburban teens prone to substance abuse and stress. NY. Columbia University's *TC Today,* p. 14.

Oeschli, M. (1996). *Mind power for students.* New York: St. Martin's Paperbacks.

Schor, E.L., (Ed.), (1995). *Caring for your school-age child.* New York: Bantam.

University of California at <www.vetnet.ucdavis.edu/petloss/index.htm>. (A resource for dealing with pet loss).

16

WHY KEEP COOL AT SCHOOL?

Nine-year-olds Taking College Entrance Exams!

School is "job one."

Let us now focus on job-stress management for children, that is, dealing with school stress in general. Children are learning more, faster and earlier, than ever before, which can be stressful. Children under ten are under increasingly intense pressure to score better and earlier on college entrance exams! With the suicide bombings of September 11, 2001, even schools are less safe, which makes stress management for children at school even more urgent.

The pressure is on. Nine-year-olds taking college entrance exams?

Children as young as nine-years-old are taking college entrance exams at a rate 20% percent higher than in 1996. Any parent who pays the $25.00 (April 2002 rate) can have their child take the SAT. It was reported that one parent was so excited about their elementary child taking his first college entrance exam that she videotaped the testing session. Some students have taken the SAT nine times before age eighteen. The reason that third grade children are being made to take the SAT and ACT is the belief that practice sessions will eventually result in better scores. Better SAT and ACT test scores at a younger age mean earlier entrance into the best programs.

Test anxiety for these young children is making them sick. But what is the test anxiety cost to our children? Potentially increased insecurity and test day accidents (e.g., losing one's "cookies, bathroom "leaks," nervous fidgeting).

Test anxiety: a half-century later, still a problem but now earlier

Even back in 1952, Professors Mandler and Sarason recognized the problem of test anxiety and how it makes children sick and unsuccessful. Dr. Sarason developed the Test-Anxiety-Scale for Children (TASC), which is a self-administered survey of test-anxiety symptoms. This instrument is a good starting point in identifying and treating test anxiety.

Test anxiety/poor test performance downward spiral

There is a real downward spiral effect between test anxiety and test performance. It doesn't matter which comes first. Test anxiety makes a child sick, which causes poor test performance. Poor test performance causes even greater test anxiety because of fear of failure, resulting in even poorer test performance. In the long run, a highly test-anxious child will avoid school at all costs. Avoiding school weakens skills, so when a child takes her next test, she will do even more poorly.

The lifetime cost of excess test anxiety? $100,000.00!

Test anxiety can make one underachieve at a whopping negative 15 percentile points. The more complex the tests, the worse test anxiety drags down performance. One may ask, so what? Underachieving on tests can make a difference of at least a $100,000.00 in lifetime earnings. How? Test anxiety drops one's performance from a successful college student level to a level where one may not be considered for college, even though the person has the ability. A college graduate is estimated to make about $100,000.00 more in lifetime earnings.

The dropout rate for college students is unusually high at the third year of college. And they quit for emotional reasons and not intellectual reasons. Why do these bright students drop out? Because these intellectually-capable college students "won't or can't" put up with the emotional stress of college. So even at the college level, stress management is extremely important.

The rat race at school

The rat race at school is more frantic than ever because children are smarter than we were at their age. We should start by saying that IQ's have been increasing greatly through the last several generations, according to Professor Robert Sternberg of Yale University.

More specifically we'll explore why males may well need school stress management more than females to keep schools safe.

Teachers play a key role in making your child's 30 hours per week, 12-year experience satisfying and successful. Some issues and tips for keeping children cool in school are provided below, though they are not designed to be a substitute for professional advice from your child's teachers and counselors. Always see your child's teacher and support staff if your child seems to be stressing out. Finally, we will hear from the President of the nation's best-teacher graduate school about lessons to be taught from 9/11 in the schools. He articulates what teachers might say about this tragic event to students.

In this chapter we will explore these ten key points.

- The Goldilocks key to school success.
- Misdiagnosing anxiety disorders for ADHD results in prescribing medications that worsen anxiety.
- How keeping an "even keel" can help teachers help ADHD children.
- Why focus on stress education for students? Another word for Character Cultivation (Education).

- Why males need stress management more.
- The incidence of school stress.
- The impact of school stress; including poor test-taking, unwanted teen weight gain, shooter's stress syndrome.
- Five benefits of student stress management.
- Cures: what teachers can do. What lessons should be learned from the 9/11 WTC bombings?
- The best of "biofeedback training" products.

---

1. The Goldilocks key to school success.

Too much stress in school results in a child's mentally dropping out at an early age by doing the least he can to get by, procrastinating and avoiding school. Too little stress breeds boredom, lack of motivation, procrastination and not preparing enough for life. The Goldilocks key to success under stress is simply to learn how to bring about just the right amount of stress at the right time. This key to success is one of the most important tools for school, home or work.

Teaching children to get into the key stress zone, will replace worry and test anxiety with constructive work habits and "test success." They will carry this mental habit into their adult lives and may even model it for their children.

Children now receive mixed messages about achievement in society. The tortoise and hare story tells them it is better to be slow and consistent, like the diligent tortoise who beats the aimless hare. The ant and the grasshopper story tells them to be vigorously and tirelessly working or you will starve like the grasshopper that rested and played. The Goldilocks story, in which the girl finds "just the right fit," is a better metaphor for achievement. Being able to have the right amount of stress at the right time is often the key to winning in the long run.

---

2. Misdiagnosing anxiety disorders for ADHD, results in prescribing medications that worsen anxiety.

Symptoms of ADHD can possibly overlap with a serious anxiety disorder called post-traumatic stress disorder or PTSD. Both ADHD (which is often treated with a stimulant medication) and the anxiety disorder PTSD can be characterized by problems with concentration, impulsivity, restlessness or irritability. The potentially harmful result of treating an anxiety disorder (like post-traumatic stress disorder) as ADHD is "increased levels of anxiety" as the result of adverse reactions to the stimulants used incorrectly according to Dr. Russell Barkley, a leader in ADHD studies and editor of the *ADHD Report* (October

2000). That is, if a child is misdiagnosed as ADHD only but actually has an anxiety disorder, the stimulant medication will make his anxiety worse.

It is critical that if your child has been described as being ADHD, the possibility of an anxiety disorder be considered. Anxiety disorders and ADHD can also coexist, concluded Dr. A.S. Blank. Because prescription treatment of ADHD is often long term, it is crucial that the possible existence of an anxiety disorder be properly diagnosed.

3. How keeping an "even keel" can help teachers help ADHD children.

According to an NEA publication, when a teacher calmly understands that a child's ADHD symptoms are caused by neureochemical imbalances beyond a student's control, the teacher is more likely to be tolerant and effective in working with ADHD children.

4. Why focus specifically on stress education for students?

Today's students need to be equipped with tools to control their stress. The incidence and impact of student stress spotlight the importance of "stress education" more than ever. Self-control is key to "Character Education."

5. Why males need stress management more.

Males under stress, aggress or will be hostile under stress. In school this means many more males will get into fights (verbal and physical) and will be more likely to damage property to get even. Why are males more at risk for the "fight or flight" response? Males are particularly prone to react to tension with hostility and aggression because their bodies are flushed with testosterone (aggression hormone). This testosterone flushing does not occur in females, who try to befriend potentially stress-producing people. Females only produce two major stress hormones, compared to males. Both sexes put out adrenaline and cortisol under stress, but males also put out testosterone, according to the April 2000, *Harvard Mental Health Letter*. The best form of socialized aggression for males is sports.

6. Incidence of school stress.

Today's students feel achievement stress

School is "job one" for most students. Students take school as seriously as adults take their jobs. School achievement surfaced as a top stressor for 60% of students, according to a survey of 135 ninth graders. Properly harnessed, this achievement stress can fuel determination to set and meet high expectations.

Student are under more stress

Nationally 10-15% of students are under chronic stress from various causes. Excess stress robs students of enthusiasm, enjoyment and achievement in school. Unrelieved stress explodes like a time bomb on occasion.

---

7. Impact of school stress; including poor test-taking, unwanted teen weight gain, shooter's stress syndrome.

Stress impairs performance

Ten-million elementary and secondary students suffer from test anxiety. Sixty-five years of research have proven that test anxiety lowers test performance.

Stress increases absenteeism

According to a survey conducted at East Carolina University, about one in six students missed an average of a week of school from stress-induced severe stomach pains. A 1993, *New England Journal of Medicine* study shows that the over-stressed are twice as likely to get the flu or colds, resulting in absences.

Stress leads to unhealthy "Type A" development

As early as three years of age, Type A habits are being crystallized. Untreated, these habits solidify into Type A personalities by fourth grade. Type A students are often inappropriately perfectionistic, competitive, urgent, overreactive and/or anger-prone. In fact, many students cannot relax by fourth grade. Tense, overly competitive, angry or urgent students often become emotionally fragile adults at great risk for health problems. The rate of teenage depression is higher than ever.

Stress causes obesity due to stress-relief eating

According to the March, 2001 issue of the *Harvard Health Letter,* stress is a leading cause of being overweight. Stress, along with food choices and eating habits, is something we can control. Genes play a significant role regarding the tendency for obesity (from 40% to 70%), but stress level plays a significant role in whether those genes produce obesity. Also, cortisol, a stress hormone, converts calories directly to fat. Sadly, when children are most sensitive about their appearance, the temptation to eat for stress relief is great. Obese children are a greater target of peer cruelty than handicapped children. This perpetuates the cycle of eating to relieve stress, gaining more weight, eating more to reduce the psychological pain, and then becoming an even bigger target for other children's slings and arrows. Getting involved in sports during this period may be the best way to keep weight down and gain respect for acquiring athletic skill.

Shooter's stress syndrome

Out of the over fifty-million students who attend our schools, even one violent death is too many. The deadly outcome of the Columbine shooting incidence at school focuses the spotlight on the extreme result of unrelieved stress. In other related events, all the school shooters were male. As stated above, males are more prone to violent acts when under extreme stress. In society in general, most, if not all "on the job" shooters have been male. This is why stress management is needed in general, and males may need stress management most of all.

---

8. Five benefits of student stress management:

"Taking off the edge" gives children "the edge" on tests

Fortunately, systematically reducing stress significantly improves test performance. Four decades of research solidly support the performance-boosting effects of stress control.

More teachable moments

Excess stress is a nonconductor of learning according to over a century of experience. Professionally-conducted relaxation training can improve concentration.

Curbing school violence

"To curb violence, it is essential to establish a relaxed, positive climate in school," says Cohn Greer, author of *"How Safe is Your Child's School?"*. Some schools have also instituted conflict-management centers.

Reducing drug abuse

The local D.A.R.E. (Drug Abuse Resistance Education) program points to stress as one reason people use drugs. Reducing stress reduces the risk of drug use for some.

Stress management as a lifesaver

According to the American Institute of Stress, "Teenage suicides have increased by twenty percent over the last decade." Increased suicides are primarily due to higher levels of student stress. These figures could be significantly improved by instituting proper educational programs in schools."

Coping with witnessing traumatic events like the World Trade Center bombing is the responsibility of older and wiser teachers. An excellent resource for dealing with childhood post-traumatic stress disorder is the book, *Disruption, Disaster, and Death: Helping Students Deal with Crisis*.

9. Cures: what teachers can do? What lessons should be learned from 9/11?

Model "grace under pressure"

Teachers are classroom climate controllers. Stress is contagious and students easily catch adult tension. Emotional contagion research shows it takes 30 minutes to calm down after being infected by a stress carrier. A stress carrier is one who brightens the room by leaving it. A positive, relaxed teacher can actually immunize students from stress contagion, helping them perform better during tests and other stressful events (public speaking, competition).

You can telegraph relaxation by smiling, talking and moving calmly but enthusiastically.

Try doing this during your personal high-demand teaching tasks.

Try the W.A.L.K.E.R. program

Students can exit the "stress express" through following the 6-step WALKER program. Encourage:

- **W**alking (briskly 20-minutes, three times weekly to burn-off stress).
- **A**ttitude (of positive organized persistence - POP).
- **L**aughter (Use a humor board for students' cartoons).
- **K**eeping up (with homework, studying, test preparation).
- **E**xpressing stress (through writing, art, music, sports, stress-control coaching).
- **R**ewarding (Teach students to keep their "eyes on the prize" — earn praise, privileges, pride, support cards along with report cards).

Offer specific skills training in test-taking, homework management and dealing with conflict/criticism

Your school psychologist and/or counselor can provide practical, proven tips on how to gain control over these major causes of stress (homework, and conflict/criticism). Test-anxiety management is the oil that permits a student to calmly apply knowledge and test-taking skills under pressure. Test-anxiety management provides students with confident self-control when faced with frustration, time pressure and uncertainty. Your school psychologist, counselor, or school testing coordinator can provide anxiety management information or you can contact Psychological Services for "test-taking tips." Test-taking skill mastery can make a test-score gain of 15% on standardized tests (from high average to gifted performance), at least one whole grade (from B honor roll to A honor roll).

Post up relaxation reminders

Motivation posters can serve as relaxation reminders and can help students remain calm during tests. Have students put stickers on their desks (just simple blue dot stickers) to remind them to relax.

The "perfect score" — just a "good day?"

A sixteen-year-old high school junior who obtained a "perfect score" of 1600 on the SAT humorously quipped that he must have had a good day that day. He also enjoys playing musical instruments and concentrates on taking courses he likes rather than being overly concerned about his GPA. Nationally less than 600 students a year get perfect SAT's.

Relaxation: the fourth "R" in education

Your classroom may be the only place where achievement-stressed students learn to identify and control stress. The turn-of-the-century curriculum needs to incorporate relaxation as the fourth "R" to maximize our students' success and satisfaction when challenges rise on the horizon.

What lessons should be learned from 9/11?

Dr. Arthur Levine, the President of Columbia University's top-rated Teachers College, talks about the lessons to be learned (and taught) from the 9/11 WTC bombings.

Key points from Dr. Levine's advice to educators on learning from the WTC follow:

- Teach more about the strength diversity has, and the importance of tolerance . . . "invite more foreign teachers and students to this country, even with the great pressure to do exactly the opposite."
- Improve civic participation.
- Match our deeds with our words.

Dr. Levine eloquently states many other extremely important lessons to be learned (and taught) from this history-changing event, in his *Alumni Letter,* which was published in its entirety one week following the World Trade Center bombings.

---

10. The best of "biofeedback training" products.

Biofeedback is considered to be the most effective way of stress-self-management in terms of how quickly and measurably relaxation is learned. An excellent way to work relaxation training into the curriculum would be through a unit in P.E., health, biology, psychology, or test-taking skills. A general principle is that once we can get "live" feedback on any of our systems, we can learn to control that system. How we can gain control over autonomic systems such as heart rate and skin perspiration, which are completely automatic, is not known yet. "Biofeedback training" provides "live feedback" on how relaxed or tense we are with a measurable record, so one can compare before and after results in a scientific manner. Actual classroom experiments can be developed to demonstrate the measurement and management of stress states. Biofeedback takes the guess work out of that slippery area of measuring emotions into a more scientific method of measuring physical states associated with emotions (stress, etc.).

The best biofeedback device appears to be the 2001, *Freeze-Framer™ emotional management enhancer* (See: COMPUTERS AS DESTRESSERS: *Freeze-Framer™ emotional management enhancer* reference in the "For Further Reading" section for details.) This state-of-the-art, biofeedback stress-management system provides colorful, entertaining stress-reduction exercises which are appealing to most children and adults. This program teaches the pupil or teacher to use heart-rate self-regulation to consistently bring about deep states of relaxation. Call Heartmath, 1-800-372-3100 or email: <info@heartmath.com>. This biofeedback product makes relaxation training fun and effective in almost any setting, (business, school, stress-control coaching setting or home.) This device was seen by twenty-two-million viewers when featured on the *ABC Nightly News* with Peter Jennings on February 7, 2001. The great effectiveness of the *Freeze-Framer™* made news when used in the classroom and even by police to remain calm under pressure. In May of 2001, CNN featured how using *Freeze-Framer™* actually helped students to concentrate better on testing. Dr. Jeff Goelitz of Heartmath was featured in the CNN report, and said that *Freeze-Framer™* can provide students with lifelong emotional-management skills.

A *Freeze-Framer™* team was called in to help New York's children and adults with the devastating emotional fallout from 9/11. Children on New York City's Staten Island were provided critical relief from the extreme stress levels that had not settled down after 9/11. Sadly, this truly 9/11 tragedy hit the country's single largest school system.

Tools and toys for "stress education"

Using these tools and toys of stress management may be useful in health/science units on the physical aspects of stress. Stress management should only be taught by qualified professionals. Two types of classroom biofeedback devices are listed below.

- "Biofeedback stress monitor:" This easy-to-use device allows you to listen to your physical stress converting your stress to sound. $13.99. Locally available. Radio Shack, Fort Worth, TX 76102.
- "Biodots;" adhesive, heat-sensitive 1/4 inch dots that convert your stress into differing colors. Includes a teacher lesson guide. Call 1-800-272-2340.

SUMMARY

School is "job one" for children. They take school as seriously as most adults take their jobs. Children as young as nine-years-old are now starting to take college entrance exams in hopes for early admission to special programs. Very early college entrance exam testing has increased alarmingly at almost 20% since 1996. Increased test anxiety at a much earlier age cries for the need for stress management earlier than ever. The half-century old "test anxiety, poor test performance downward spiral" effect is presented, along with the Test-Anxiety-Scale for Children (TASC). We explored why males may well need school stress management more than females to keep schools safe. Since school can be a successful and satisfying 12-year career, some tips on how to "make it so" are provided. The Goldilocks principle of providing "just the right amount of stress for school success" is presented.

We discussed the risks and results of misdiagnosing anxiety disorders as ADHD. The reasons why school stress management are so important for children are presented in the incidence and impact of school stress. The role of stress in childhood obesity is also discussed. The five benefits of managing school stress are addressed with several tips on helping to curb school stress through the W.A.L.K.E.R. program (Walking, Attitude, Laughter, Keeping up and Expressing stress, Rewarding) which can be used at home or school.

The President of Columbia University's top-rated Teachers College presents lessons to be learned (and taught) from the 9/11 terrorists' WTC bombings. Written only a week after the suicidal bombings, this "letter" provides lessons to be taught in our nation's schools to reduce the chances of further senseless violence.

The best of biofeedback devices (the computer program called *Freeze-Framer*™) is briefly reviewed for use as a classroom teaching tool for stress management. This stress-management unit could be incorporated into various curricular areas such as P.E., health, biology, psychology, or test-taking skills. Contact <www.freezeframer.com> for more information.

As stated before, the best way to handle stress is to treat the root-cause. When polled, most children cite tests as one of their top stressors. Therefore the next chapter deals with tips on how to do well on tests.

FOR FURTHER READING

ADHD Report (2000). ADHD and post traumatic stress disorder. Barkley, R. (1998). *Attention-deficit hyperactivity disorder, a handbook for diagnosis and treatment.* New York: Guildford.

"Biofeedback stress monitor." This easy-to-use device allows you to listen to your physical stress converting your stress to sound. $13.99. Locally available. Radio Shack, Fort Worth, TX 76102.

"Biodots." (100 for $10.00) adhesive, heat-sensitive 1/4-inch dot converts your stress. A teacher lesson guide included in price. Phone 1-800-272-2340.

Blank, A.S. (1994). Clinical detection, diagnosis and differential diagnosis of post-traumatic stress disorder. *Psychiatric Clinics of North America,* 17, 315-38.

Freeze-Framer™ emotional management enhancer. (2001). Boulder Creek, CA: HeartMath LLC & the Institute of HeartMath. Heartmath, Phone 1-800-372-3100 or email: <info@heartmath.com>, <www.freezeframer.com>.

Institute of HearthMath, PO Box 1463, Boulder Creek, CA 95006, Phone (831) 338-8500, Fax (831) 338-9861, or <http://heartmath.org>.

Levine, A. (2001, Tuesday, September 18). The lesson to be learned. *Alumni Letter,* <GothamGazzette.com>.

Mandler, G., & Sarason, S. (1952). A study of anxiety and learning. *Journal of Abnormal and Social Psychology,* 47, pp. 166-173.

Nunn, R.O., & Gallaher, J. (2001). *Inspiring tranquility: stress management and learning styles in the inclusive classroom.* Washington DC: NEA Professional Library. <www.nea.org/books>. Phone 1-800-229-4200 (120 pages, $10.95 NEA members).

Zaslow, J. (2002, March). When little kids take big tests. *Time* (New York: NY) 159, 10, p. 71.

17

SCORING BEST ON ALL LIFE'S TESTS

BY USING YOUR "WHOLE BRAIN"

If stress is sand in the machinery of thought then relaxation is the oil.

Advice from the world's-highest IQ holder: repetition and relaxation (R & R)

Scoring best on tests — from one who has scored best on tests: In line with Dr. Richerson's tip to repeat what has to be learned, (see side story), Marilyn vos Savant, who possesses the highest-recorded IQ, echoes this advice, that repetition is the best way to learn. Repetition even helps improve understanding, just like seeing a movie more than once, helps us pick up more details and remember what happened better.

Relax: Test anxiety impairs test performance

Ms. Savant points to test anxiety as the culprit in why many don't do well on tests. Ms. Savant, who is on the advisory board of the National Association for Gifted Children, on February 18, 2001 answered this question: "Do you think that being good at testing (the kind needed to suc-

---

Bob was amazed as he casually looked at the books the thirty-three-year-old neurosurgeon had in his study. These foot-thick books had titles such as Gray's Brain Anatomy. Bob could hardly lift the books much less understand their contents. When Dr. Richerson came in from his yard to visit with Bob in his study, Bob asked, "How on earth did you ever learn all this material?" Keith smiled and shook his head, saying, "Repetition. I just kept going over the material, over and over again, until I had it. That is the key to my success." Dr. Richerson was right, of course, having passed his "Boards" and every requalifying test since. But it took him years to memorize all this material.

As a neurosurgeon intern, he did not even have a car until he was 32 years-old, devoting all his life to memorizing and practicing his craft. After his first year of practice as a brain surgeon, however, he made one-million dollars, and his income has climbed ever since. The lesson to be learned — Repetition is the way to master material.

---

ceed in school) is an inborn talent?" Ms. Savant, who truly does best on tests, responded: "Assuming you mean tests of learning, I don't believe such a talent as 'being good at taking tests' exists. However, plenty of people receive inappropriately low scores (that is, they have the knowledge but don't show it) on tests because they're 'bad at testing.' The most common reason is anxiety, which often impairs intellectual functioning."

Memory problems? Tips on having a razor sharp memory

Memory problems? Stress may be short-circuiting your short-term memory. Do you forget an important name or phone number at the worst times (when you are under pressure to remember, during tests, during important meetings)? It could be as simple as being distracted by something else, so you don't remember where you put your keys, because you had your mind on something else. Under stress, our attention will be drawn away from what's important to what seems important at the time. It's impossible to remember what you don't pay attention to.

Again, if you can't remember information long enough to maintain a conversation or write it down, chances are you are stressed out! Your short-term memory is designed to help you remember up to seven bits of information (as long as a telephone number without the area code) and to keep up a conversation with someone. Have you ever been so overwhelmed with information that you came into a room and you could not remember what you came there for? Unfortunately, one of the most important intellectual functions to short circuit under stress is short-term memory. If you can't remember something for even a few seconds, how are you going to retrieve it later? Not to worry, once you've learned to relax that information may come to you. And there are strategies to help "cement in" those short-term memories into long-term, almost unforgettable, memories. These strategies will be presented later in this chapter.

Go in for your 50,000-mile brain check-up. Having senior moments

According to Dr. Gayatri-Devi, a specialist in memory, the hormones estrogen and testosterone play a very significant role in memory or loss of it. The hippocampus, the "memory" center of the brain, is greatly affected by decreases in these hormones (estrogen in menopausal women, testosterone decrease in men as they age). Successful hormone-replacement therapy, with memory skill training, has successfully helped people sharpen their memories. Contact your local family practitioner: At a university hospital memory clinic you can even ask for an MMSE, a ten-minute test. Many people become depressed or even fearful when their memory starts going. So see your doctor, chances are it is not Alzheimer's disease. Before we forget, let us look at some tips on how to have a razor sharp memory.

EIGHT GENERAL TIPS FOR HAVING A RAZOR SHARP MEMORY (Left brain)

A normal memory problem is when you can't remember where you put your car. A serious memory problem is when you can't recall how to drive home. In either case, you should go see your doctor. (See Chapter 22 for the only herbal remedy that is clinically-proven to improve memory.)

Simple memory boosters include:

1. "The palest ink is better than the best memory," so put it in writing.

Write notes to yourself. If you have to, use hyper notes (those small, yellow sticky notes that allow you to cover an entire desk top or refrigerator with reminders). Leave messages to yourself on your answering machine. Like location, location, location, remember, "repetition, repetition, repetition."

2. Play with your brain, that is, keep your brain in tune by playing games.

3. Bridge the gap.

(One of the brightest people this author knows plays bridge expertly and technically qualifies for AARP membership.) *Games* magazine is great, which emphasizes word play. Maybe the *New York Times* crossword puzzle is not your style, but any crossword puzzle will do. You can even get crossword puzzles that deal with a hobby interest of yours. Even playing checkers exercises your brain better than playing your TV remote.

4. Remember the old saying, "A place (and time) for everything and everything in its place."

It may be boring, but learn to routinely put your keys (wallet, etc.) in one place. That will be one less thing you have to remember. It takes about three weeks to a month for your brain to reroute to a new routine. So remind and reward yourself for the first month in retraining your brain.

5. Tell jokes (to tested audiences, like your best friends).

This requires timing and remembering the punch line. If you can't remember punch lines, write them down.

6. Communicate.

If you are not computer phobic, join a chat room (There are even chat rooms devoted exclusively to standard poodle lovers). Get on the Internet, or if nothing else, write a letter to your friends, using snail mail.

7. Take up a course that has nothing to do with what you have to do, but something you want to do (painting, coin collecting).

You probably don't need the extra credit but it will give you something to look forward to. Even your classmates can keep you young.

8. Exercise by taking a brisk thirty-minute walk, three times weekly. (Always get your doctor's permission first.)

Mental decline over age is blamed to a degree on decreased circulation to key parts of the brain. Exercise supplies these deprived key areas with freshly oxygenated blood (Duke University study, 2001).

Without the ability to remember, most other test-taking skills will not help much. Having covered memory basics, let us turn to testing realities for tens of millions of our children.

The "front-page" news item read, "Pretest jitters will try to be soothed by schools"

The article continued: At 7:30 A.M. on Thursday, students will enter the classroom as usual. At about 8:00 A.M., the test booklets will be taken from the locked, secure room down the hall to this unusually quiet classroom. The 10- to 11-year-old students will then begin the nearly two-hour-long test. These test results will help decide whether these children will pass the fifth grade. The teacher of this class, interviewed by the newspaper stated, "I'll be a nervous wreck. I'll be eating antiacids like candy." Fortunately this teacher instituted pregame practice sessions with volunteers drilling students with flashcards "prepping" them for EOG (End of Grade) testing.

For many, test is a four-letter word. The threat of a test may well be like our fear of getting pulled over for going 70 in a 50 mph zone. Tests can lead to stress or success. The choice is yours.

Tests are not life or death. There is "life after tests." Because of a terrorist anthrax scare of November 2001, a very large batch of college aptitude tests never arrived in New York for scoring. According to a November 18, 2001, news report, the considerably large group of just-taken aptitude tests probably got lost in "a post office in Jersey due to anthrax quarantine of mail." The highly-reputable company giving the test indicated that all these thousands of students would have to retake this college admission test; one of the most important tests universities review as part of their admissions packages. Many students studied for months and spent hundreds of dollars preparing for this test – just to have to do it all over again. So getting stressed out over a particular test is not only unwise and unpleasant, but may be just a waste of time, because things can happen to even the best of test companies. Save some energy for your "life after tests" with your family and friends.

This chapter looks at the why's and how-to's of test-taking, which involves left brain (head) and right brain (heart) skills. A concise test-prep checklist is provided at the end of the chapter (section 8) for those interested in "just the facts."

Other important points we will look at include:

- Why take tests? It's the law. Landmark legislation was passed by the U.S. Senate, June 2001, mandating annual reading and math tests.

- Why do well on tests? Test-taking skill mastery can make a test-score gain of 15% on standardized tests (from high average to gifted performance), or at least one whole grade.
- Why reduce test anxiety? It is even "front-page" news; it causes student boycotts, sabotage and reduces parent panic.
- The $64,000 question: Why should my child take recommended test-prep courses?
- Just spell SAT — $AT. Colleges will pay to have high SAT scorers attend because it improves the colleges' ranking.
- 27 tips: Thirteen tips on how to become "fact-smart," and possibly scoring "gifted" (p. 206), eight tips on "test-smartness," six activities to become stress-intelligent.
- Gifted performances: Earning top scores is no accident — a lesson from gifted test-takers (95% +).
- A concise test-prep checklist (p. 215).

---

1. Why take tests? It's the law.

On June 14, 2001, in an effort to improve public schools nationally, President George W. Bush pressed for and was successful in passing a legislative bill requiring all third through eighth grade students to take reading and math tests. Poor-performing schools would get additional aid, but if enough progress was not shown after two years, low-income students could transfer to another school if they so wished. After three years of poor performance at a school, these same low-performing students could use federal funds for transportation or actual tutoring.

---

2. Why do well on tests?

Tests are here to stay

One-hundred-million standardized tests are administered for elementary and middle school children yearly, according to Dr. Peter Cookson, Director of the Center for Educational Outreach and Innovation. Doing well on tests is an area of increasing concern both for students and educators. Since tests (which are better than guessing what a person might know) are obviously here to stay, we might as well learn how to master them. Other important reasons to do well on tests follow.

Enjoying a successful 12-year career

Tests are "success benchmarks" during everyone's 12-year academic career. Used correctly, tests actually serve as "success stepping-stones" rather than as stumbling blocks. Enjoying "test success" both satisfies basic self-concept/ achievement needs and motivates a student to strive for personal excellence.

Triumphing over fear of failure

Fear of academic failure was the leading "most difficult problem" American teenagers faced, according to a 1994 Gallup Poll. Equipping students with proven "test-taking tools" results in real success experiences to triumph over imaginary fears. The confidence built from doing well on tests can then be carried into life's arena with its many other challenges.

"Proving your knowledge" is power to succeed

The ladder of success is built with small but measurable steps. A famous scientist once said nothing is really that hard, there are just a lot of little parts. Tests can help measure readiness for the next step toward goals. Also, knowing someone has "proven her knowledge" through testing raises the level of trust in her. The days of self-proclaimed experts are gone. Who would trust a "self-proclaimed" surgeon?

---

3. Why reduce test anxiety? It is even "front-page" news; it causes student boycotts, sabotage, and parent panic.

Test Stress triggers boycott threat

As Delia was driving into school the morning before the big three-day-block of End of Grade (EOG) testing, to her amazement the radio blared, "Parents threaten to boycott EOG testing." Delia, in disbelief, was hoping it was not her school where the boycott was threatened. Never in the 110 year history of this school district had the elementary and middle school parents even talked about any kind of boycott, much less refused to let their children take a battery of tests. However, the stakes of these tests were higher than ever to the fifth graders. The results of these tests were used to help decide whether they passed their grade level and whether they had to go to summer school. The EOG results for each school were made a matter of public record by the local newspaper, which further increased the pressure on school personnel and students. To add to the stress, test scores determined school evaluations and even teacher salary bonuses.

Delia had conducted all the legitimate test-taking preparations, had held a booster session for her classroom, and had told them that the test would be the reward for their hard work. However, she was working against the tide of panic about these tests in the community. As a teacher she had taken and mastered numerous tests to be credentialed, and she knew many of her students would be successful. But in 2002, testing pressure started earlier and the consequences were greater. Delia had heard from counselors that children were becoming test anxious three weeks before the actual event. The counselors had told the children that you "can't be scared and smart" at the same time. Last year several students were even physically sick on test day, but still insisted on taking the tests.

Delia knew that the test pressure cooker of the classroom was merely a laboratory for what her students would be facing in the work world. Getting a grip on performance anxiety now would prepare them for success later in their jobs. Proving competency through performance was just a reality of the 21st century world-community. Fortune 500 corporations had begun applying a policy of automatically firing the bottom ten percent of performers in the company. Even though she knew that these children had to be "toughened up," it still broke Delia's heart to see tears well-up in the eyes of her favorite, but perfectionistic, student. Delia's job was to create a great sense of desire in the students to do well, rather than to fear failure. She did her best to instill feelings of hope rather than despair.

Student sabotage

On the day of testing, two students, standing outside the classroom where End-of-Grade testing was to take place shortly, were planning to "do everything they could to put irregularities on the End of Grade tests they were just about to take." Test anxiety had made them desperate to the point that rather than trying to do their best, they would engage in the self-defeating activity of losing by default. They would go through the motions of taking the test, and that was it. Again, they were reacting to the testing situation with despair rather than hope. Studies show that when people don't feel they have a chance to succeed, they sabotage their own efforts.

Parents catch test-anxiety panic; they give children offers they can't refuse and wait outside the classroom during testing

Delia was performing her "car-rider student pickup" duty at the school entrance when she couldn't believe her ears. The well-meaning parent shouted kindly to her daughter as she dropped her off at school on test day, "Remember, dear, if you pass both these tests I will give you $100.00." To a fourth grader, $100.00 might as well have been a million. The child's face grimaced in determination as she entered the testing room. Delia had recommended as a reward for "trying hard" a trip to a popular hamburger place, *which had as its motto, "Over twelve-billion hamburgers sold, feeding the entire world twice." This "well-meaning" parent didn't realize that the child would now expect ever-increasing rewards, since the "bar" had been set so high. The child will probably expect a car if she does well on the SAT in high school. Fortunately the child did well, and would have done just as well with going to "McBurgers" as a reward.*

Delia was in the classroom on Thursday, the last day of EOG testing. A large sign on her classroom door prominently displayed, read, "Testing, Please do not disturb." Delia heard a knock at the door as she was collecting the completed EOG test materials. As she opened the door, she saw the flushed face of one of her student's parents. Forcing a smile on his face he asked desperately, "Did he pass?" Delia assured the "test-anxious" parent that Richard had done his best. She assured him that as soon as she received the results she would share them with Dad, when she shared them with the other children's parents. The father pleaded, "Isn't there any way you can estimate how Richard did?" Trying to calm this very conscientious parent, Delia said, "Richard worked hard, so he will do well! "But how did you get to my room without getting a visitor pass at the front desk?" He said, "I told them at the office I wanted to see how Richard did, and I just took off toward your room. Sorry, but I have been so worried about my son's test results I didn't sleep a wink." This was a first for Delia, having a parent expecting test results immediately on conclusion of the day's testing. This was a panicked parent. And his child was only nine-years-old.

A 100-point SAT score increase: the bottom line for reducing test anxiety

According to a Columbia University study conducted by Dr. C. H. Faigel, a 100-point gain in taking the SAT (Scholastic Achievement Test) was realized by students whose test anxiety level was clinically reduced. Numerous other studies demonstrate score gains as test anxiety is reduced. As stated above, Ms. Savant lists anxiety as the leading cause of doing poorly on tests even when you have the knowledge.

As mentioned in the previous chapter, a great resource for keeping a calm and cool classroom climate is *Inspiring Tranquility: Stress Management and Learning Styles in the Inclusive Classroom,* by Rebecca Nunn and Janet Gallaher. The National Education Association, (NEA), the major clearinghouse for educational materials, endorses this book which can be ordered at <www.nea.org/books> or 1-800-229-4200.

4. The $64,000 question: Why should my child take recommended test-prep course?

The answer to this question is simple: The students winning the $64,000 scholarships take test-prep courses. Even if your child is very "fact-smart," if he is not "test-smart" and "stress-smart," he is at a disadvantage. So get professional help to even the playing field. No competent coach would ignore loosening, strengthening and stretching exercises before the "big game." It is important to stretch (but not snap) a student's skill areas weeks before a test.

Kaplan, the company famous for preparing children for the SAT, is now looking at North Carolina's fourth and fifth graders, who could possibly be held back a grade if they score too low on the state's End of Grade tests. In North Carolina, EOG tests are partially used for entrance into gifted programs and grade promotion. Like an experienced athlete going out for the "varsity," our intellectual athletes need warming and stretching mentally to give their best on tests. Gifted programs are designed to stretch and strengthen a child's success and satisfaction in school, which prepares him or her for formal testing.

Kaplan, in cooperation with Simon and Schuster, has just published a 52-page *Parent's Guide to N.C. Tests: 4th and 5th Grades.* This guide provides test-taking tips designed for End-of-Grade exams for fourth and fifth grades. This guidebook is being prepared for other states — Texas, Florida and New York. One of the guidebook's tips is to start reading children's magazines with your child. The guide suggests that students guess on questions they're unsure of.

Another route to consider is one-on-one attention from private tutors available at businesses like Sylvan Learning Centers. As of 2001, Kaplan's North Carolina guide offers only test-taking tips; it doesn't provide sample tests on which students can practice at the elementary grades. However, as of February 2002, Kaplan provides actual practice tests for the GRE, LSAT, MCAT and GMAT at various locations. You may call 1-800-KAPTEST or go to the website, <www.kaptest.com/testdrive>. Most importantly, Kaplan, within a week of the practice tests, provides each student with a profile of his or her strengths and weaknesses to help them prepare for the actual tests.

Officials at *Princeton Review,* by contrast, will create End-of-Grade practice tests for 3rd through 8th grade, using the same language the North Carolina tests use. The *Princeton Review* materials precisely focus on those skills covered on the test, according to Stephen Kutno, vice-president of educational policy. The website is <Princetonhomeroom.com>. Your state department of public instruction provides a list of the skills and goals for which the exams test.

An excellent resource for parents is the 13-page booklet, *Studying for and*

Taking Tests, available from The Parent Institute, P.O. Box 7474, Fairfax Station, VA 22039-7474 (phone 1-800-756-5525). This booklet provides clear, practical tips on the why's and how-to's of doing well on tests for children. It talks about how to get rid of test stress, how to make memorizing easier, and how to study smart, not just hard. It gives pointers on what a child should do when they get to the actual test. Their website is <http://www.parent-institute.com>. A minimum order is for 25 at only 99 cents each, so it would be worthwhile for a PTA or test-prep group to order a quantity.

A 100-point SAT gain realized from SAT prep course

Matt Oeschli of Greensboro, North Carolina, is a national consultant who offers proven SAT preparation. In his book, *Mind Power for Students* by St. Martin's Paperbacks, he provides methods that can raise SAT scores by 100 points. The Matt Oeschli Institute can be contacted at (336) 273-6582.

An excellent online resource for specific SAT preparation is located at the website <www.collegeboard.com>. Once at this home page, click on The College Board — 100 years of connecting students. Then click on Prepare for SAT. Free preparation materials are provided in terms of an online SAT sampler, a diagnostic Mini-SAT and SAT preview software. Specific packets are provided to help you prepare in your area(s) of weakness on the SAT for a nominal fee ($10/packet at this writing).

Go to the source: The SAT writers

An associate director of public affairs for the College Board (which directs the SAT) said familiarization with the SAT is critical. She also said that there are two main phases in readying for the SAT, long term and short term. Under long-term SAT preparation, she indicated it is important to build one's vocabulary, read widely, take as many college preparation courses (including math) as possible. The student should find what the colleges are looking for in terms of admission.

The short-term preparation, which could start as early as three months before the actual SAT, should include familiarization with the SAT by studying such books as "Ten Real SATs." This 2000 edition book includes a CD-ROM. See "For Further Reading" at the end of this chapter for ordering information. Short-term preparation is not a substitute for long-term preparation. The key to doing well on the SAT, from those who bring you the SAT, is familiarization with the tests through long-term studying over years and short-term advanced practice.

---

5. Just spell SAT – $AT. Colleges will pay to have high SAT scorers attend because it improves the colleges' ranking.

The Princeton Review provides a detailed listing of the average SAT scores for the country's best universities. Your child may want to do well on the SAT for bragging rights, but it does not hurt to spell SAT as $AT, after they have received their SAT scores. Your child may win thousands of dollars in scholarships by doing well because high SAT students improve a university's standing. Don't tell your child ahead of time about the $AT angle; it may create additional, unneeded pressure, which will actually decrease your child's score.

Aim high

In February of 2002, nationally only 587 students received a perfect 1600 on their SAT's. The average SAT score for Harvard is 1495 and MIT is 1454. An SAT Score of 1394 (693 verbal/710 math) may win a scholarship to Columbia University, the most expensive university in the nation, at $29,057 per year just for tuition, ("College Rankings by Annual Tuition," *Providence Journal Research*, 2000). Columbia has been ranked the number one university in the country at least twice in the last decade ("America's Best Graduate Schools — Exclusive Rankings," *U.S. News & World Report,* March 18, 1996).

What is a parent to do? Relax!

Sixteen-year-old Andrew Shoffner obtained a perfect SAT score of 1600. He is also an avid musician. He said he takes classes that interest him and he is not particularly competitive academically. He joked about his perfect SAT performance by saying, "I must have had a good day." Ms. Ann Barr, a leading authority on gifted education, suggests pursuing the possibility of taking some early college courses while the young man still is attending high school.

---

6. How to do your best on tests: 27 tips.

Why does gold medallist test performance take triathlon training?

Gold medallist test performance (or a gifted performance) demands triathlon-like training. Imagine if you will, that an athlete competes for the gold in a triathlon, consisting of swimming, tennis and soccer. Being naive, he says to himself, I am strong in soccer, but really need to work on my tennis game. Swimming, so what! I was part of the tennis and swim club as a child, so I know swimming that mile will just come back to me even though it's been a decade. Unsurprisingly, on the last leg of the triathlon competition, his overall score sank faster than he did, in the final, and most important leg of the triathlon, swimming. No matter how smart you might be, gifted performance on tests requires a triathlon of training for three types of smartness.

You must be "fact-smart," "test-smart" and "stress-smart." In fact, if you are really "test-smart" and "stress-smart," you can do well on tests you know nothing about. Don't try this at home, or do only under professional supervision, for fun. Details on triathlon training for testing follow.

Peak test performance requires today's students to be "smart" in three ways. "Fact-smartness" is mastering what you need to know, which is a left brain skill. "Test-smartness" is knowing how to use facts on tests. "Test-smartness" involves both left brain and right brain thinking skills. "Stress-smartness" is learning how to think calmly under test pressures, which calls into play the right brain's emotional/positive visualization skills.

Twenty-first century testing also measures the child's "whole-brain thinking" skills. "Whole-brain thinking" goes beyond traditional left brain (verbal, factual, logical) thinking, tapping also into the right brain (creative problem-solving abilities, visual, emotional) thinking. To train their whole brains, we look at left brain skills ("fact-smartness" — which in school receives the most emphasis), combined left/right brain skills ("test-smartness" plus creatively solving abstract questions to provide the correct answers), and right brain skills ("stress-smartness" — keeping your whole brain working smoothly by relaxing.)

THIRTEEN TIPS FOR HELPING STUDENTS AND ADULTS TO BECOME "FACT-SMART"

(Mastering what needs to be known, a left brain skill.)

1. Get the "big picture." Encourage students to read summaries, questions, headings and look at any graphs, drawings or pictures before reading the assignment. Have students call the "Homework Hotline" from home.

2. "Seeing is believing" for most students. "Teach smart" by using graphic organizers such as Venn diagrams, flowcharts and mapping. Since elementary grade children are mostly visual learners, the best way to get the "visual basics" of any subject is to go the library and ask where the elementary grade section is. Then, look for the topic you want. If they don't have it in the elementary grade section, go to the secondary grade section and ask for the "visually-illustrated version" on the topic. The following table provides a mini-lesson plan on whole-brain teaching, entitled, "The Anti-Boredom 'Whole-Brain' Balanced Approach to Curriculum."

ANTI-BOREDOM "WHOLE-BRAIN" BALANCED APPROACH TO CURRICULUM 2003

© Dr. Ron Rubenzer, Thinking Dynamics (1-336-282-4539)

Content	left brain	Integrated	right brain
Arithmetic	Calculation drills.	Graph presentation of calculation results (pie graphs with different colors).*	Determine number of different shapes that can be made from limited number of cubes. Relax **
Science	Prepare experimental report write-ups.	Develop hunches--hypotheses. Generate methods of investigating hunches. Conduct actual experiment. (Relax students!)*	Build a model demonstrating procedures and dramatize results of experiment (science fair). Relax.
Language Arts	Write topical paper.	Conduct "newspaper interview" with tape recorder and write human interest story with accompanying photographs.	Communicate pictorial messages in secret code relating important event(s). Relax.
Social Studies	Produce term paper on social structure of society X.	Create a weekly diary relating humorous, trying experiences living in the society. (Relax students!)	Develop artifacts of the society 50 years in the future. Relax.

Originally from CEC best-seller, *Educating the Other Half Implications of Left-right brain Research.* Winter 1983, Vol. 15, No. 2. 44 pages Stock 264. The Council for Exceptional Children Sales, 1920 Association Dr., Reston, Va. 22091-1539, $4.00. *Call BrainLink at 1-800-969-4996 for math, science, language arts units. **See HeartMath Products for Best of Relaxation Techniques and Materials.

3. *Make meaningful memories by connecting to students' current interests (e.g., teach how percentages work for predicting rain/snow days).* Let them know why they are learning something. (Learning to take tests will help them pass their driver's license test.)

4. *Teach memory mechanics.* The basic rule is repetition, repetition. Teach students that understanding a fact is not the same as mastering a fact. (e.g., one can understand how to shoot baskets without being able to do it). If you want to remember someone's name, repeat it to yourself several times and then write it down.

5. *Play tricks on your mind with games.* Make liberal use of word games, crossword puzzles. If you have the time, take courses having nothing to do with your main course work or job.

6. *Require students to develop their own flashcards and stack the deck with only the memorized facts.* Have them submit flashcards as an assignment immediately before the test.

7. *Encourage note-taking while students are reading or listening, especially if the test requires written responses.* Teach them "The palest ink is better than the best memory." Use "post-its." Develop as many helpful routines as possible, and even leave yourself notes or voice-mail. Regarding routines, always put your car keys in the same place.

8. *Divide and conquer information overload by encouraging students to study several short sessions over several days/weeks rather than cramming the night before.* Suggest a study calendar and weekly "progress check points" for students. Provide positive feedback on study progress.

9. *If appropriate, provide a test-specific diagnostic survey to pinpoint strengths and weaknesses.* This will help the student spend the most time on the weakest areas while building on strengths.

10. *As a reward, have students play "not-so-trivial pursuit" by making up their own questions about material and quizzing a rival team.*

11. *Celebrate "sticking to their test-prep schedule" by giving periodic rewards matched to the size of the efforts.*

12. *Make these tips part of each student's study habits by introducing them at the beginning of the year/course.*

13. *Scoring gifted — "varsity" tryouts for scholars.*

Just like their athletically-gifted peers (otherwise known as the "varsity") are afforded all types of special classes, equipment, privileges, trips, awards and fellowships, the intellectually gifted can earn prizes by proving intellectual "varsity" level skills. But the gifted athlete was not just born that way. It took him or her thousands of hours devoted to develop the exact skills to be selected as the best. Likewise, there is no magic to being selected for the intellectual "varsity," if a child is so inclined. Sometimes, if a child shows a strong interest in reading or using words at a preschool level, he or she may have specialized talents. Your encouragement and providing opportunities may just be her ticket into joining the "varsity" for scholars (And isn't that what school is also about?). Be careful however not to "burnout" your child with too much stimulation. An excellent book warning of the dangers of lopsided development is entitled, *Beneath the Wheel,* by Sidhartha. Only if your child hungers to climb the "intellectual mountain, just because it's there", should they be provided more work.

According to a major research study, strong verbal reasoning is the most important skill area for gifted students as measured by individual intelligence tests according to Kaufman (1990). Karnes and Brown also found that according to a study of 946 gifted students, the vocabulary area was the highest area of performance on an IQ test. Interestingly, these gifted students were weakest in a handwriting-symbol memorization related test (coding subtest). The message is if you want your child to show "what he/she knows," play word games (scrabble, etc.) just as you would play basketball in the backyard with a child showing great athletic promise. Parents of a gifted child are blessed with the burden of feeding a hungry mind. Some useful vocabulary builders would be: *Study Skills: Strategies and Practice* (Curriculum Associates), *The Dictionary Skill Box* (Troll), *Intermediate Dictionary* (Houghton Mifflin), and *Using Dictionary Skill*s (Instructional Fair). You may say, it's only words, but our constitution and laws, are "only words." The Library of Congress is only words. See your educational psychologist or counselor for sources of ideas and materials to build and stretch your child's mental muscle. See *WISC-Compilation,* by Whitworth, under "For Further Reading" for professional-use materials.

EIGHT TIPS ON IMPROVING "TEST-SMARTNESS"

Facts are necessary but not enough for top performance. Approved practice on such tests as the SAT can improve performance by 500 points. This 500-point improvement was realized by a young man who took the SAT over nine times since the age of twelve, finally achieving a nearly perfect SAT score of 1530.

Developing "test-specific" skills improves test performance by drawing attention to small but important details. Multiple–choice tests all vary greatly on how learned facts and skills are to be used. If you are unsure about the design of tests to be given this year, see your test coordinator. Some general guidelines are:

1. Answer the question. Answer the core question, without being tripped up by "word traps" (irrelevant details) or generalizations (always, never, everywhere).

2. *Teach students to "pace not race" through test items.* Encourage students to answer those questions they feel they know, marking those difficult questions to return to later.

3. *Emphasize that multiple-choice tests are not multiple-guess tests.* Teach students to choose, not to guess on multiple choices. This requires mastering problem-solving skills. When offered multiple choices, anticipate the most correct answer before reading available choices. Then look for the best answer among those provided. If all the choices appear to be correct, select the most correct answer by eliminating wrong answers. Develop reasons why the other answers are wrong. Again, students should mark and return to these most difficult questions after answering the more obvious questions. Teachers might effectively demonstrate or model this technique using examples.

An excellent resource is the book dedicated to all aspects of test-taking entitled, *Teaching Test Taking Skills: Helping Students Show What They Know,* by Scruggs and Mastropieri.

4. *Be clerically correct.* Develop the habit of having students build in enough time to check for wrong answers simply due to marking the wrong answers or misreading the questions the first time through.

5. *Provide "test rehearsals" if appropriate.* All great performances start with rehearsal. Practice any and only those approved practice tests weeks before the actual test takes place. See your test coordinator for approved pre-test activities. As stated above Kaplan, Inc. now provides actual practice test sessions for the GRE and LSAT.

6. *Study groups.* There is some evidence that hard-working study groups actually work in helping high school students improve test scores. At the high-school level, conscientious study-group students will study harder to contribute to the group, and will be exposed to more questioning than they might have thought of on their own. Advanced Placement students have found study groups to be most helpful. Be sure, however, to avoid having students develop "test-banks" by not allowing previous examinees to provide questions they had memorized from actual exams.

7. *Money back guarantee that test scores will improve.*

Frank E. Ferguson, president of Curriculum Associates, assures that test scores will improve using the well-researched materials offered by Curriculum Associates®.

The Curriculum Associates Company® offers materials developed by teachers for teachers in the Test Ready series. Curriculum Associates offers diagnostic tests, to highlight strengths and weaknesses to help each child prepare for upcoming tests. This excellent test-prep series covers grades K-12, in critical subjects such as Reading, Vocabulary, Mathematics (including take-home tests)

Spanish, Algebra, Science and Social Studies. It is claimed that test scores can significantly improve with only fourteen days preparation. Testimonials from top administrative personnel and classroom teachers revealed up to seventeen-percentile point gains on EOG testing using these materials. This before/after percentile score increase is in range of what top researchers predict. Call 1-800-225-0248 or order online at <www.curriculumassociates.com>.

Only a few days are needed between your ordering the materials and your receipt of materials. Also, upon request, an entire series of research and testimonials are provided supporting the test-score gains predicted by Curriculum Associates. Teacher preparation materials and actual student workbooks are, of course, provided. Finally, the use of these materials by Curriculum Associates is endorsed by school systems.

A resource, specifically designed to meet North Carolina's testing needs, is *Preparing for the North Carolina Competency Test in Reading,* by Stephen Feinstein and Rubi Borgia Pinger. These materials, published by Amsco School Publications, Inc. (1999), provide an actual sample state-competency test. Amsco School Publications, Inc. can be located at 315 Hudson Street, NY, NY 10013. Contact Amsco to find out if competency-testing guides are provided for your state.

8. Get high school students used to taking tests on computers because computers will be testing them.

Bob had studied for months for his nine-hour licensure exam to practice financial management. Being old-fashioned, he expected to have a paper/pencil exam. To his surprise, he was in the first wave of examinees to take the completely computer administered — timed and scored tests. The proctor cooly sat him in front of the testing PC after Bob had given his testing entrance pass to the person outside the door. The only directions the human proctor gave were: This exam is broken up into 250 questions for the morning session and 350 questions after your lunch break. If you should need a break while the testing program is running, raise your hand and the proctor will stop your computer program and will start-up your computer program when you return. There is an automatic countdown clock in the lower right-hand corner of your monitor.

Any questions? The room was quiet except for the synchronized beeping of each computer's start-up programs being initiated. Bob swallowed hard. He knew the material but this computer administration was a wrinkle in his plan. He thought to himself, welcome to testing in the 21st century. No wonder our high school students have to pass computer literacy courses to graduate.

SIX TIPS TO BUILDING "STRESS-SMARTNESS"

(An emotional, right brain skill)

Relaxation is oil in the machinery of thought

Just like your car engine, your brain will soon "freeze-up" or "burnout" without the oil of relaxation. Strong emotions affect clear thinking. Calm, clear thinking is the key to "best test performance." Over a half-century of test-anxiety research reveals that excessive stress impairs test performance. Relaxation is a "must" for test-score improvement according to a test-preparation corporation that guarantees results (up to seventeen-percentile point increase). This is the difference between high average performance and gifted performance.

Herbert Benson, M.D., Harvard researcher who coined the term, "relaxation response," states that students inducing the "relaxation response" immediately before exams do better. He also found that professionals who relax immediately before brainstorming generate more solutions to problems than those who do not relax. As said before, scared students can't be smart students.

Preparation for the "big day"

Also, allow children to wear their favorite school outfit to the test. Have them eat fruit right before the test (Sugar is food for thought). Have them drink a bit of water to speed up the breakdown of the fruit to fructose, which is food for thought. Honey is an excellent source of fructose. Have your child eat toast with honey before they leave for the test site. Caffeine is at best a double-edged sword. Only if you are already a "caffeinist" (Caffeine is the most popular drug in the U.S.) will caffeine help your mental performance. While it can sharpen your thinking (no more than two cups of coffee), you pay for it with caffeine jitters. If you don't use caffeine, don't start. Avoid having children drink sugary drinks or eat candy bars right before testing because of the unsteady flow of sugar provided by these foods.

The following suggestions may be useful to reduce excessive stress:

WEEKS BEFORE THE TEST

1. *Conduct a "reality checklist" of what the student can expect in the testing situation.* This will reduce stressful "surprise or shock reactions." (Always follow pre-test restrictions on what can be shared with students prior to testing.)

2. *Prior to the testing situation, provide a "relaxed exposure" to these "test reality conditions" as much as possible.* That is, see your test coordinator on legitimate practice materials, and have students relax just before and during the "test warm-up" sessions.

3. *Accentuate the positive: Expect your best but respect the test.* Think of the test as a reward to show off your hard work and knowledge. It is important for the student to have a positive attitude but this attitude must be combined with positive action, (i.e., thorough study beforehand).

4. *Positive peer pressure: Use the power of peer pressure to develop a "pre-game" winning spirit toward an upcoming test.* Students could create posters on the rewards for doing well on tests. Have students bring in appropriate cartoons about test-taking.

5. *Good modeling by all adults: Students will catch adults' anxiety about tests and this "secondary stress" can hamper their peak performance.* Even the tone of voice used in reading pre-test and test instructions will raise or lower test anxiety. Modeling "grace under pressure" in front of students will show it is possible to stay calm and succeed under stressful conditions.

6. *Relaxation training: See your mental-health professional on relaxation-training tips or methods to identify children at risk for excessive test anxiety.* It typically takes several weeks to learn how to relax under testing conditions.

The best way to learn relaxation is through biofeedback. Biofeedback works like training wheels to help you keep your balance when you are first starting. Biofeedback gives you live, scientific feedback on whether you are "centered" in terms of relaxation. HeartMath, in Boulder Creek, California, provides the best personnel, training and tools to teach and learn biofeedback. Other forms of relaxation training, such as progressive relaxation, breathing relaxation, autogenic training, systematic desensitization, visualization and other techniques are available from appropriately trained mental-health personnel. It usually takes several weeks for your muscle memory to learn to relax, so if a test is given in October, start teaching relaxation in September. Think of relaxation training as learning an athletic skill. Just because you understand the concept doesn't mean you have mastered the skill.

---

7. Gifted performances: earning top scores is no accident — a lesson from gifted test-takers.

The top 95% scorers on the SAT work on staff to coach student on test-taking

The *Princeton Review* indicated that the average SAT I score gain was 140 points compared to prior best SAT score or prior PSAT/SAT. It is guaranteed in writing that the student will gain at least 110 points from his previous SAT score or the first diagnostic test if the student has not yet taken the SAT test. The *Princeton Review* offers *Inside the SAT,* which has won awards as a CD Rom program that is also interactive. It is highly recommended that any parent who wants his or her child to do best on tests contact the Princeton Review Program at <www.PrincetonReview.com>, <chaphill@review.com> or 1-800-2Review/ (919) 967-7209, America Online: Keyword "Princeton." Testimonials by students having taken the course revealed score gains of 190 to 300 points.

All Princeton Review teachers have scored at the 95th% or above on the SAT.

The classes are small to provide for more individualized attention. Even the conservative *Wall Street Journal* considers the *Princeton Review* most effective in any ETS exam. Students who were able to win entrance into Ivy League schools through their SAT scores are quoted.

The *Princeton Review* offers free SAT and College Admission Seminars at such top-tier universities as Duke, Wake Forest, and Chapel Hill. One Princeton Review office is located at 1525 East Franklin Street, Chapel Hill, NC 27514. Call 1-888-755-PREP for other national locations. The *Princeton Review* has a fifteen-year track record of improving SAT scores on the average of 140 points. As stated previously, this test-prep service even lists the average entrance SAT scores for three-hundred of the nation's top schools.*

*The *Princeton Review*, February-October, 2001, pp. 1-15.

For information on specific details on any standardized test, log on to <http://www.unl.edu/buros/>. This will link you to the best "test" review resource: Buros Institute's *Fourteenth Mental Measurement Yearbook* (MMY) published in 2001. They have been reviewing tests for over 60 years.

A brief note about stress and gifted performances

By most authorities, gifted performance is at the top 2 in 100. Children with IQ's of 130 or above could have stress-related social-emotional problems because they usually don't have a classmate to talk to or play with. Occasionally, have these like-minds interact, through clubs, playing with older children (if the younger children are accepted), etc. It is also extremely important to enroll gifted children in courses on common sense so they know how to relate to the rest of the 98 out of one-hundred people. It is even more important for brighter children to be blended with "birds of a feather" occasionally. Try to imagine having friends if your IQ is 145 (one out of a thousand), IQ of 152 or 2.3 out of 10,000, or an IQ of 167 (3 in 1,000,000). If your IQ is 190, you will have to search the world for the 5 other people you can relate to (IQ of 190 is 1 in 1,000,000,000). [A.J. Tannenbaum, 1983].

Stress tests: Relax to "show what you know." (By 15% better!)

For the well prepared and motivated, relaxation will help "show what you know" better on tests. Think of a teeter-totter relationship between stress and tests. As stress goes down, test performance goes up. William James, the father of American psychology in his 1899, Harvard lecture-series on teaching said, "The teacher who succeeds in getting herself loved by pupils will obtain results which one of a more forbidding temperament finds impossible to secure," (p. 45). To put modern numbers on this educational principle, Scruggs & Mastropieri of Purdue University in 1992, concluded that a fifteen-percentile point test-score increase, or a whole letter-grade improvement, results from learning test-taking skills for students. This 15% point advantage can make the difference between a "gifted performance" or an above average performance.

---

8. Pre-test checklist.

GENERAL TIPS FOR HELPING STUDENTS TO BECOME "FACT-SMART"

- Make these tips part of each student's study habits by introducing them at the beginning.
- Get the "big picture" (Overview first, read end of chapter questions first).
- "Seeing is believing" for most students. "Teach smart" (visually). See "Anti-Boredom 'Whole-Brain' Balanced Approach to Curriculum, (p. 207).
- Make meaningful memories.
- Teach memory mechanics. Repeat info at least seven times.
- Students develop flashcards. Submit flashcards as an assignment immediately before the test.
- Encourage note-taking while students are reading or listening.
- Divide and conquer information using more frequent, shorter, study periods spread over time.
- If appropriate, provide a test-specific diagnostic survey.
- As a reward, have students play "not-so-trivial pursuit" by making up their own questions about material.
- Celebrate "sticking to their test-prep schedule."

TIPS FOR IMPROVING "TEST-SMARTNESS"

- Answer the questions (Multiple-choice tests are not multiple-guess tests, but use creative problem solving if needed).
- Be clerically correct.
- Provide practice sessions (with time limits) if appropriate.

BUILDING "STRESS-SMARTNESS"

Weeks before the test:

- Conduct a "reality checklist" of what the student can expect to avoid shock on test day.
- Prior to the testing situation, provide a "relaxed exposure" to these "test reality conditions."

- Positive attitude: Expect the best but respect the test. The test is the reward to prove your knowledge. "Inch by inch anything's a cinch." "Yard by yard, life is hard."
- Use positive peer pressure: Bring in cartoons about testing stress — I took an IQ test and the results were negative.*
- Good modeling by all adults.
- Relaxation training (See your mental-health professional. Clear this with administration first).
- Food for thought — natural sugars. Honey on toast will give your brain a natural boost. Any sweet fruit (peaches, oranges, melons) followed by a glass of water will provide your brain with a natural power boost.
- Caffeine is at best a double-edged sword. Only if you are already a "caffeinist" (caffeine is the most popular drug in the U.S.), will caffeine help your mental performance. While it can sharpen your thinking (no more than two cups of coffee), you pay for it with caffeine jitters. If you don't use caffeine, don't start.

*Used by permission, as seen in Interfax Daily, March 2, 2001, Vol. WZ1V795.
Call (336) 397-0000 for a Free-Daily humor fax.

SUMMARY

One-hundred-million tests are administered each year at the elementary and middle school levels. This figure does not even include high school, much less higher education. Tests are here to stay, so we have to learn to tackle them and use them as stepping-stones rather than stumbling blocks. Yale research reveals that children are smarter today (higher IQ's), but not wiser. They are more likely to "burnout" because they are forced to learn more-faster-earlier compared to any other generation. Two stories reveal the secret to doing best on tests, repetition. Test-taking tips are provided from Marilyn vos Savant, who has the highest IQ on record. Using an R & R approach (repetition and relaxation) is what Savant recommends.

Direct resources for EOG preparation and the best SAT preparation are provided. Tips from the SAT test-makers are provided. Several reasons for mastering test-taking skills are discussed plus practical tips on what to do to become "fact-smart," "test-smart" and stress-intelligent in the 21st century. Proven "foods for thought" (honey, fruits followed by drinking water) are provided, plus the "good news — bad news" about caffeine on performance. Scoring gifted is discussed for those having a potentially gifted child, trying to make the intellectual "varsity" (i.e., advanced learner or gifted program). The stress from isolation of gifted performers is addressed. Children with an IQ of 130 are two out of a hundred, or one in every three regular classrooms. It's almost as if gifted children speak a language of their own, which seems foreign to others, and are subject to rejection and ridicule.

These tips take advantage of using the child's whole brain, not just the left brain emphasis of facts only. Perhaps equipping students with the right tools will enable them to enjoy their twelve-year careers. Specific references for parents are also provided to help them help their children. A national expert on gifted education, Ann Barr, provides advice on what to do when high school students get that perfect score of 1600 on their SAT. The potential use of study groups for mature high school students is explored. The wave of computers testing us is also discussed. A point-by-point checklist is provided to help organize test-taking skills in all three areas: "fact-smartness," "test-smartness" and "stress-smartness." The combined strength of all three types of smartness spells success.

FOR FURTHER READING

America's best graduate schools - exclusive rankings. (1996, March 18). *U.S. News & World Report.* (Columbia ranked No. 1).

Benson, Herbert, M.D., Harvard researcher who coined the term "Relaxation Response."

Buchanan, Bruce, (2002, February 5). The perfect performance. Greensboro, NC. *News and Record.* B1. Perfect SAT score.

College rankings by annual tuition, (2000). *Providence Journal Research.* Columbia University, Highest tuition.

Columbia University (2000, Summer). *TC Today,* p. 20.

Flynn, J.R. (1987). Massive IQ gains in 14 nations. *Psychological Bulletin.* 101, 171-191.

Kaplan, S., et. al. *Parent's Guide to NC tests: 4th and 5th grades.* This guide provides test-taking tips designed for End-of-Grade exams for fourth and fifth grades.

Matthews, J. (2001, May). Sharing knowledge: study groups may boost performance. *Washington Post* as cited in Greensboro, NC. *News & Record.* p. 1, Section D, p. D3.

National Association for Gifted Children. February 18, 2001.

Neisser, U., (Ed). (1998). *The Rising Curve.* Washington DC: American Psychological Association.

The Princeton Review Program at <www.PrincetonReview.com>, <chaphill@review.com> or 1-800-2Review/, Phone (919) 967-7209, America Online: Keyword "Princeton."

A Princeton Review office is located at 1525 East Franklin Street, Chapel Hill, NC, 27514. Phone 1-888-755-PREP for other locations.

The Princeton Review, (2001, February-October). pp. 1-15.

SAT preparation is located at the Web site <www.collegeboard.com>. Once at this home page click on The College Board - 100 years of connecting students.

Scruggs, T.E., & Mastropieri, M. (1992). *Teaching test taking skills: helping students show what they know.* Cambridge, MA: Brookline Books. Order at (617) 868-0360 or 1-800-666-2665 or <Amazon.com>.

Sternberg, R. (2000, Fall). Wisdom as a Form of Giftedness. *Gifted Child Quarterly,* 44. (4), pp. 252-260.

Studying for and Taking Tests available from The Parent Institute, P.O. Box 7474, Fairfax Station, VA 22039-7474. Phone 1-800-756-5525.

Tannenbaum, A.J. (1983). *Gifted children: psychological and educational perspectives.* New York: Macmillan. p. 69.

Ten Real SATs. (College Boards, NYC) 2000. Includes CD and actual questions from the SAT test designers (The College Board). For further information call (212) 713-8175.

Whitworth, J.R., & Sutton, D.L., (1993). *WISC-III Compilation.* Novato, California: Academic Therapy Publications.

For the Reader's Convenience

STRESS/TEST-PERFORMANCE HISTORICAL BIBLIOGRAPHY DATING BACK TO 1899 WITH WILLIAM JAMES (FATHER OF AMERICAN PSYCHOLOGY)

Anastasi, A. (1971). *Psychological testing.* New York: Macmillan.

Anthony, E.J. (1970). Two contrasting types of adolescent depression and their treatment. *Journal of the American Psychological Association,* 18, pp. 841-859.

Bovilsky, D. (1982). Up against the ivy wall. *Independent School,* 41(3), pp. 51-55.

Brotman, P. (1980). *EMG instructional manual.* New York: Biofeedback Instrument Co.

Brown, B. (1977). *Stress and the art of biofeedback.* New York: Harper and Row.

Budzynski, T., & Stoyva, J. (1972). Biofeedback techniques in behavior therapy. In D. Shapira (Ed.) *Biofeedback and self-control.* Chicago: Aldine Press.

Cacioppo, J.T., & Petty, R.F. (1981). Electromyograms as measures of extent and affectivity of information processing. *American Psychologist,* 36(5), pp. 441-445.

Campbell, D.T., & Stanley, J.C. (1963). *Experimental and quasi-experimental designs for research.* Chicago: Rand McNally College.

Carlson, J. (1983). Levels of cognitive functioning as related to anxiety. *Journal of Experimental Education,* 37(4), pp. 17-20.

Carter, J. (1983). Better writing reaps rewards. *National/State Leadership Training Institute on the Gifted and Talented Bulletin,* 10(3), p. 3.

Carter, J., & Russell, H. (1980). Biofeedback and academic attainment of LD children. *Academic Therapy,* 15(4), pp. 483-486.

Chaffee, E.E., & Lytle, I.M. (1980). *Basic physiology and anatomy.* Philadelphia: J.B. Lippincott.

Chaney, D.S., & Andreasen, L. (1972). Relaxation and neuromuscular tension control and changes in mental performance under induced tension. *Perceptual and Motor Skills,* 34, pp. 677-678.

Cohen, J. (1977). *Statistical power analysis for the behavior sciences,* (Rev. Ed), Chapter 7. New York: Academic Press.

Cohen, J., & Cohen, P. (1975). *Applied multiple regression/correlation analysis for the behavioral sciences.* Hillsdale, New Jersey: Lawrence Erlbaum Associates.

Counts, D.; Hollandsworth, J.; & Alcorn, J. (1978). Use of electromyographic biofeedback and cue-controlled relaxation in the treatment of test anxiety. *Journal of Consulting Clinical Psychology,* 46(5), pp. 990-996.

Danskin, D.G., & Lowenstein, T.J. (1977). *Biofeedback application in Counseling and education.* New York: Biomonitoring Applications, Inc., Tape T114.

Davis, R.C. (1957). Response patterns. *Transactions of the New York Academy of Sciences,* 19, pp. 731-739.

Davitz, J.R., & Davitz, L.L. (1977). *Evaluating research proposals in the behavioral sciences.* New York: Teachers College Press.

Deffenbacher, J.L., Mathis, H., & Michaels, A.C. (1979). Two self-control procedures in the reduction of targeted and nontargeted anxieties. *Journal of Counseling Psychology,* 26(2), pp. 120-127.

Dentler, R.A., & Mackler, B. (1964). Originality: Some social and personal determinants. *Behavioral Sciences,* 9, pp. 1-7.

Deslisle, J. (1982, September/October). Striking out: Suicide and the gifted adolescent. *G/C/T,* pp. 16-19.

Dreger, R.M. (1978). The state-trait anxiety inventory. In O. K. (Ed.), *The eighth mental measurements yearbook,* Vol. 1. Highland Park, New Jersey: Gryphon Press.

Elkind, D. (1981). *The hurried child: Growing up too fast too soon.* Reading, Mass.: Addison-Wesley.

Endler, N.S. (1978). The state-trait anxiety inventory for children. In O. K. Buros (Ed.), *The eighth mental measures yearbook,* Vol. 1. Highland Park, New Jersey: Gryphon Press.

Feldhusen, J.F.; Denny, T.; & Condon, C. (1965). Anxiety, divergent thinking and achievement. *Journal of Educational Psychology,* 56, pp. 40-45.

Feldhusen, J.F., & Klausmeier, H.J. (1962). Anxiety, intelligence and achievement of low, average, and high intelligence. *Child Development,* 23, pp. 403-410.

Ferner, K., & Heck, S. (1983). Causes and cures of damaging stress. *Gifted Children Newsletter,* 4(7), pp. 3-4.

Frey, H. (1980, May). Improving the performance of poor readers through autogenic relaxation training. *The Reading Teacher,* pp. 928-932.

Gallagher, J.J. (1975). *Teaching the gifted child.* Boston: Allyn and Bacon.

Getzels, J.W., & Jackson, R.W. (1962). *Creativity and intelligence: Explorations with gifted students.* New York: Wiley.

Gowan, J.C. (1964). *The education and guidance of the ablest.* Springfield, IL: Charles C. Thomas.

Grollman, E.A. (1971). *Suicide.* Boston: Bacon Press.

Guilford, J.P. (1967). *The nature of human intelligence.* New York: McGraw-Hill.

Guilford, J.P., & Fruchter, B. (1973). *Fundamental statistics in psychology and education.* New York: McGraw-Hill.

Hadley, D.J. (1965). Experimental relationships between creativity and anxiety. *Dissertation Abstracts International,* 26, p. 2586.

Halitsky, S. (1976). *Cognitive style variables as related to compensated and uncompensated dyslexia in emotionally disturbed adolescents.* Unpublished doctoral dissertation, Teachers College, Columbia University.

Hayes, D.G., & Levitt, M. (1982, September/October). Stress: An inventory for parents. *G/T/C,* pp. 8-12.

Hinsie, L.E., & Campbell, R.J. (1960). *Psychiatric dictionary.* New York: Oxford University Press.

Hudesman, J., & Wiesner, E. (1979). Desensitization of test-anxious urban community college students and resulting changes in grade point average. *Community/Junior College Research Quarterly,* 3(3), pp. 259-264.

Hughes, H.; Jackson, K.; DuBois, K.E.; & Erwin, R. (1979). Treatment of handwriting problems utilizing EMG biofeedback training. *Perceptual and Motor Skills,* 48(2), pp. 603-606.

Jacobson, E. (1938). *Progressive relaxation.* Chicago: University of Chicago Press.

Jacobson, E. (1973). *Teaching and learning new methods for old arts.* Chicago: National Foundation for progressive Relaxation.

James, William. (Copyright, 1899). *Talks To Teachers on Psychology: and To Students on Some of Life's Ideals.* Published 1915, New York, Henry Holt and Company.

Kelly, E.L. (1959). The IPAT anxiety scale. In O. K. Buros (Ed.), *The fifth mental measurements yearbook.* High Park, New Jersey: Gryphon Press.

Keys, N., & Whiteside, G.H. (1930). The relation of nervous-emotional stability to educational achievement. *Journal of Educational Psychology,* 21, pp. 429-441.

Kinsman, R.A.; O'Banion, K.; Robinson, S.; & Staudenmayer, H. (1975). Continuous biofeedback and discrete postrial verbal feedback in frontalis muscle relaxation training. *Psychophysiology,* 12, pp. 30-35.

Kirk, R.E. (1968). *Experimental design: Procedures for the behavioral sciences.* Belmont, CA: Brooks/Cole Publishing Co., Inc.

Kisker, G.W. (1964). *The disorganized personality.* New York: McGraw-Hill.

Lanyon, R.E. (1978). The IPAT anxiety scale questionnaire. In O. K. Buros (Ed.), *The eighth mental measurements yearbook,* Vol. 1. Highland Park, New Jersey: Gryphon Press.

LaVallee, Y.J.; Lamontagne, Y.; Pinard, G.; Annable, L.; & Tetreault, L. (1977). Effects on EMG feedback, diazepam, and their combination on chronic anxiety. *Journal of Psychosomatic Research,* 21, pp. 65-71.

Malmo, R. (1966). Studies of anxiety. In C. D. Spielberger (Ed.), *Anxiety and behavior.* New York: Academic Press.

Mancini, P. (1977, November 14). School for whiz kids. *New York,* p. 76.

Mandler, G., & Sarason, S. (1952). A study of anxiety and learning. *Journal of Abnormal and Social Psychology,* 47, pp. 166-173.

Marland, S.P. (1971). *Education of the gifted and talented,* (2 Vols.). Washington, DC: U.S. Government Printing Office.

Matthews, D.B. (1981, November 18-20). *Biofeedback: Its uses in education.* Denver: Ninth Annual Association for Individually Guided Education Conference. (ERIC Document Reproduction Service, No. ED 217 338).

McReynolds, P. (1978). The IPAT anxiety questionnaire. In O. K. Buros (Ed.), *The eighth mental measures yearbook,* Vol. 1. Highland Park, New Jersey: Gryphon Press.

Meeker, M.N. (1969). *The structure of intellect: Its interpretation and uses.* Columbus, Ohio: Charles E. Merrill.

Meeker, M.N. (1980, May). Personal communication.

Meeker, M.N. (1982). *The structure of intellect (SOI) screening form for the gifted.* El Segundo, CA.

Nunberg, H. (1955). *Principles of psychoanalysis.* New York: International Universities Press.

Omizo, M.M., & Michael, W.B. (1982). Biofeedback-induced relaxation training and impulsivity, attention to task, and ocus of control among hyperactive boys. *Journal of Learning Disabilities,* 15(7), pp. 414-416.

Patten, M.D. (1983). Relationships between self-esteem, anxiety, and achievement in young learning disabled students. *Journal of Learning Disabilities,* 28, pp. 43-45.

Raskin, M.; Johnson, G.; & Rondestvedt, J. W. (1973). Chronic anxiety treated by feedback-induced muscle relaxation. *Archives of General Psychiatry,* 28, pp. 263-267.

Reinking, R.H., & Kohl, M.L. (1975). Effects of various forms of relaxation training on physiological and self-report measures of relaxation. *Journal of Consulting and Clinical Psychology,* 43(5), pp. 595-600.

Richardson, E.R.; Beall, S.; & Jessup, G.T. (1983, January/February). The efficacy of a three week stress management unit for high school students. *Health Education,* pp. 12-15.

Ringlaben, R.P. (1981, October). *Relaxation exercises for exceptional children.* Paper presented at the meeting of the Idaho State Council for Exceptional Children. Boise, Idaho.

Roeper, A. (1982). How gifted children cope with their emotions. *Roeper Review,* 5, pp. 21-24.

Rothman, H.S. (1979). Electromyographic biofeedback relaxation training versus progressive muscle relaxation training in the treatment of test anxiety. (Doctoral dissertation, Washington State University). *Dissertation Abstracts International,* 40.

Rotter, J.B. (1966). Generalized expectancies for internal versus external control of reinforcement. *Psychological Monographs,* 801, Whole No. 609).

Sabourin, M., & Riouz, S. (1979). Effects of active and passive EMG biofeedback training on performance of motor and cognitive tasks. *Perceptual and Motor Skills,* 49, pp. 831-835.

Sarason, I. (1956). Effect of anxiety, motivational instructions, and failure on serial learning. *Journal of Experimental Psychology,* 51(4), pp. 253-260.

Sarason, S.B.; Davidson, K.S.; Lighthall, F.F.; & Waite, R.R. (1958). Classroom observations of high and low anxious children. *Child Development,* 29, pp. 287-295.

Sararon, S.; Hill, K.; & Zimbardo, J. (1964). A longitudinal study of the relation of test anxiety to performance on intelligence and achievement tests. *Monographs of the Society for Research in Child Development,* 29 (7, Whole No. 98).

Sassenrath, J.M. (1958). Anxiety, aptitude and achievement. *Psychology in the Schools,* 56(6), pp. 472-477.

Schuchman, M.C. (1977). A comparison of three techniques for reducing scholastic aptitude test anxiety. *Dissertation Abstracts International,* 38(4-1), p. 2010.

Schultz, J., & Luthe, W. (1959). *Autogenic training: A psychophysiological approach to psychotherapy.* New York: Grune & Stratton.

Sheldon, C. (1969). The effects of positive and negative reinforcement and test anxiety on the reading performance of male elementary school children. *Genetic Psychology Monographs,* 80 (1), pp. 29-50.

Sieber, J.E. (1969). A paradigm for experiment modification of the effects of test anxiety on cognitive processes. *American Educational Research Journal,* 6(1), pp. 46-61.

Smith, R.C. (1974). Response bias in the state-trait anxiety inventory detecting the exaggeration of stress. *Journal of Psychology,* 86(2), pp. 241-246.

Spielberger, C.D.; Gorsuch, R.L.; & Lushene, R. (1970). *State-trait anxiety inventory (STAI).* Palo Alto, CA: Consulting Psychologists Press.

Standish, R.R., & Champion, R.A. (1960). Task difficulty and drive in verbal learning. *Journal of Experimental Psychology,* 59, pp. 561-565.

Stanford-Binet Intelligence Scale. (1960). New York: Houghton Mifflin.

Straughan, J.H., & Dufort, W.H. (1969). Task difficulty, relaxation, and axiety level during verbal learning and recall. *Journal of Abnormal Psychology,* 74(5), pp. 621-624.

Tannenbaum, A.J. (1983). *Gifted Children: Psychological and educational perspectives.* New York: Macmillan.

Thought Technology, Ltd. (1980). 2193 Clifton Avenue, Montreal, Canada H4A2N5.

Tobias, S. (1980). *Overcoming math anxiety.* New York: Houghton Mifflin.

Townsend, R.E.; House, J.F.; & Addario, D. (1975). A comparison of biofeedback-mediated relaxation and group therapy in the treatment of chronic anxiety. *American Journal of Psychiatry,* 132(6), pp. 598-601.

Treffinger, D.; Pyryt, M.; Hawk, M.; & Houseman, E. (1979). Education of the gifted and talented: Implications for school psychology. *School Psychology,* 30, pp. 191-231.

Tuckman, B.W. (1972). *Conducting educational research.* New York: Harcourt Brace Jovanovich.

Tuttle, K.C. (1977). EMG biofeedback training: Its impact on test anxiety and locus of control. (Doctoral dissertation, University of Michigan). *Dissertation Abstracts International* (University Microfilms, No. 78-4918).

Wechsler, D. (1955). *Wechsler adult intelligence scale* (WAIS). New York: Psychological Corporation.

Wechsler, D. (1975). *Wechsler intelligence scale for children* (WISC-R). New York: Psychological Corporation.

White, K. (1968). Anxiety, introversion-extroversion and divergent thinking ability. *Journal of Creative Behavior,* 2, pp. 119-127.

Whitmore, J.R. (1980). *Giftedness, conflict and underachievement.* Boston: Allyn and Bacon.

Wolfe, R.M. (1979). *Evaluation in education: Foundations of competency assessment and program review.* New York: Praeger.

Wolpe, J., & Lazarus, A.A. (1966). *Behavior therapy techniques.* New York: Pergamen Press.

Yadusky-Holahan, M., & Holahan, W. (1983). The effect of academic stress upon the anxiety and depression levels of gifted high school students. *Gifted Child Quarterly,* 27(1), pp. 42-46.

Yates, A.J. (1980). *Biofeedback and the modification of behavior.* New York: Plenum Press.

18

Relaxation: The Fourth "R" for Educators

How to Improve Your Satisfaction and Success in School

Without teachers I would not, could not, have become an astronaut. How else do you think I got here?

- Captain Sonny Carter, astronaut addressing the North Carolina Association for Gifted and Talented Conference. Wilmington, NC, March 21, 1987

What lurks in the "Dark of the Desk?" — One teacher's story

Delia came home that night from school, looking ashen and a bit shaken. She usually came home with a smile on her face, having enjoyed doing what she loves best — teaching sixth grade. Bob asked, "Did you have a bad day, dear?" She replies, "You could say that! You know how I hate snakes. Well, to start the school day, Donna, that sweet but talkative girl, suddenly started screaming at the top of her lungs. I thought to myself, this must be bad. I hadn't told you, but our class pet, Oscar, is a 6-foot boa constrictor on loan from the Natural Science Museum. As always, first thing, I glanced at Oscar's cage, and noticed no movement. I assumed Oscar was sleeping in the warm sun under the shavings in his aquarium. Actually he had slipped out of the makeshift glass aquarium through the hole in the top of the netting that night. Unknown to all, he was blissfully sleeping curled up in an empty desk all morning long."

"Donna had dropped a pencil behind her desk and was quietly retrieving it, when she came eye-to-eye with Oscar, the boa constrictor, compactly curled up in the storage compartment of the desk behind her. His forked tongue flickered out of curiosity at Donna. After Donna's blood-curdling scream, I knew in a flash it might be Oscar after glancing over again at his empty cage. Donna was pointing at Oscar with her hand over her mouth, her dark brown eyes as large as saucers. I immediately came over to Donna and hugged her shaking body, and we both looked at Oscar. He had only half opened his eyes, being rudely awakened from his siesta. All students were glued on Donna, and since she started laughing, so did all the other students."

"To make matters more interesting, the classroom PA system in the corner clicked on saying, 'Delia is everything OK in there? This is Ms. Inquisitive. I heard this shout come from your classroom next door, followed

by laughter.'" Delia continued with her story to Bob and said, "I then got to the PA and said, 'Ms. Inquisitive, could you please send down Mr. Ajax, our custodian? Thank you for your concern, Ms. Inquisitive. Everything is OK.' Within fifteen minutes Oscar was back in his cage, and the excitement must have worked up his appetite, because the boys in the classroom gleefully said, 'Good, it's time to feed Oscar. He's looking for his breakfast.' Well, you know Oscar's feeding ritual, kind of like one of Speilberg's dinosaur-feeding episodes. Things finally settled down after we fed Oscar. Needless to say, Bob, we are taking Oscar back to the Natural Science Museum tonight if you don't mind. Since I am already in my robe and you still have your work clothes on, be a dear and take Oscar back to the Natural Science Museum before 6 P.M. They are expecting him. Oh, on top of everything else, we have our practice writing exam tomorrow. Too bad they have to stick to writing prompts, they'd have a great Oscar the snake-tale to write about."

Although Delia's school day was higher on the stress barometer than usual, teaching today is more stressful than ever. On a February 7, 2001 *ABC Nightly News Special,* teaching was put in the same stress category as being a policeman. The need for teacher stress management is greater than ever.

Stress is blamed for a 30% new teacher dropout rate. The rate is much higher in poorer urban areas. According to the May, 2001 issue of the NEA newsletter, one out of three new teachers quits within their first five years. A leading reason cited was the stress of the job. This author knows of no teacher preparation courses that deal with the "heart" aspect of teaching. Losing one out of three professionals within a five-year-period strongly supports the need for teaching teachers to manage their own stress. Losing so many teachers breaks up continuity for their students and certainly does not make teaching a very attractive career goal for the young and energetic.

Every school day across America, 52-million children are greeted by about 3-million teachers. Many teachers and pupils pass through metal detectors to get to their rooms. Most are under intense test-score improvement pressure. Job-stress topped the list of teacher-stressors in an international study conducted by this author. School can be stressful, but it doesn't have to be.

Stress is not only contagious, but it flows downhill, from adults to children. Teachers are climate-controllers. For their own sakes, and for the benefit of the children, they need to preach and practice what they know about stress and its role in disrupting learning and relationships.

Currently there are 3,071,000 public- and private-school teachers. As stress builds throughout the school year, so does the volume of these teachers' voices. The noble profession of teaching is becoming less attractive to young people because of the high degree of stress from behavioral problems and ever-escalating accountability from test results. In praise of teachers, an astronaut once said, "How do you think I got to be an astronaut? I got from there to here through dedicated and inspiring teachers."

It's hard to be dedicated, though, when you feel battle-fatigued at the end of each day.

An NEA publication reveals that teachers who are calm and relaxed are more effective in helping children with ADHD symptoms and learning differences. Relaxed teachers are more likely to use strategies with these children that are more effective, without burning themselves out by expecting the unexpected. Applying these stress-management tips will not only make you feel better, but you will also perform better. Many teachers are among the "working weary," becoming colorless achievers even though they try to be enthusiastic. In this chapter we will look at:

- The two faces of stress.
- Distress is sand in the machinery of thought.
- Stress makes you fat, say Harvard researchers.
- Test scores rise as performance anxiety falls.
- Crossing the won't/can't let go line.
- Stress-management tips: paying the PRRICE of peace (p. 233).
- "What to do tomorrow" – tips for the lounge and breaks.
- The future of computer-assisted relaxation is here with *Freeze-Framer*™.
- How to have less-stress tomorrow: a checklist.

STRESS BASICS

Stress is simply energy, so stress management is merely energy conservation. We need to spend our stress-energy on important events.

---

1. The two faces of stress:

Good stress (eustress) keeps us motivated toward goals and helps us concentrate. Stress helps get us out of bed in the morning. The excitement we feel when our favorite team is winning is eustress. Eustress actually keeps us mentally and physically healthy. Euphoria is a type of eustress.

Distress is negative stress. Distress is when we are forcing ourselves to go on. Fear, frustration, fatigue, and frenzy are the most common forms of negative stress. Unrelieved distress makes us sick. A recent study shows that people under excessive stress are twice as likely to get colds.

2. Distress is sand in the machinery of thought.

Anyone (including students) who was ever in the grip of test anxiety can attest to this fact. By contrast, reducing stress significantly improves performance on IQ, creativity, and achievement measures. Stress triggers the right brain at the wrong time. The right brain is good for "flight or fight," coming up with many creative and general ideas, whereas most tests want calculating, left brain, single correct answers. Our mental machinery runs roughly when you feel like running out of the testing room. Right brain emotions tend to be negative, when you need left brain optimism to do your best.

3. Stress makes you fat.

The *Harvard Health Letter* revealed that stress promotes obesity. Many people are stress-eaters. Eating is a convenient, fast and effective (but not healthy) way to reduce stress. What does getting fat from stress have to do with teaching? Not only is getting fat upsetting, but putting on as few as ten pounds can increase diabetes, hypertension and heart attack risk. The snack industry knows full well the power of stress-relief eating. Have you ever seen a teachers' lounge without a snack machine? In Denmark they even have beer-dispensing machines in the teachers' lounges, which would seem a highly counterproductive practice. So stress-eating indirectly leads to robbing our energy and health. You can't work well if you don't feel well.

4. Test scores rise as performance anxiety falls.

Tests can be a source of stinging stress or great satisfaction. Using both your "head" (facts) and "heart" (feelings) assures better test scores. Marilyn vos Savant, who possesses the highest-measured IQ on record, revealed that a little relaxation goes a long way in reducing performance anxiety to improve memory. Performance anxiety can block you from remembering the most basic information (even your own phone number) under stress. Columbia University research provides a solid, half-century bedrock of support for the fact that lowering performance anxiety improves test performance. So to reduce your "test-results anxiety," lower your students' performance anxiety in addition to focusing on standard test preparation.

When we desire to go to work, we are experiencing eustress. Dreading to go to work is distress. The view you choose is up to you.

When we refer to stress in this chapter, it will be distress. A stressor will refer to anything that causes you to feel frustrated, fearful, fatigued, or frenzied.

Stress is not a neutral force. Either you control it, or it will eventually control you. Xanax (a tranquilizer) is the fifth most-prescribed drug in the United States, powerfully showing that many people are wrestling with excess stress. Common headache remedies now include sleeping agents, because of increasing sleep disorders. One out of three people has trouble sleeping, mostly due to stress.

---

5. Crossing the won't/can't let go line.

If you won't let go of stress willingly, you may reach the point when you can't let go of stress. Stress has a grip on you when: you can't relax without "stress-relief-overindulgence"; you can't sleep; you get tension headaches, backaches, or dental problems because you can't relax your muscles; you can't enjoy life because you are caught up in hurry and worry. The good news is that your stress habit is reversible and all you need to do is cut back (not cut out) your stress. Within a few weeks you will be firmly in the driver's seat, controlling stress to make it work for you. Reversing the word stressed will give you a pleasant result (the word "desserts"), just as reversing your actual stress will improve the quality of your life and productivity.

---

6. Stress-management tips: paying the PRRICE of peace.

Try this simple **PRRICE** of peace stress-management program. (The **PRRICE** acronym stands for Prevent, Relax, Reduce, Ignore, Communicate and Escape.)

P-REVENT the causes of stress

Use the **SOS** approach: Simplify, Organize, Sensibly prioritize. You can simplify things by eliminating those things which are not important or central activities to your job or life. "Just say no" pleasantly to requests that are not really important. Organize what is important by developing systems through time-and clutter-management. Sensibly prioritize your life. Do you work to live or live to work? Keep things in perspective. Will this worry be important five years from now? If not, don't worry about it as much.

R-ELAX. Muscle relaxation

It is impossible to have relaxed muscles and feel tense at the same time. Learn progressive muscle relaxation. It may take two or three weeks to acquire the habit because muscle relaxation is a neuromuscular skill. Relaxing your neck, shoulder, jaw, and scalp muscles hourly will eliminate most stress headaches and nocturnal teeth grinding.

Simply wanting to relax is not enough, just like wanting to play a sport well without practice is not effective. Practice relaxing in calm situations. You wouldn't build a house in the middle of a storm, so don't wait until your stress storm starts to practice relaxation.

Sighing is nature's tranquilizer. If you can sigh, you can relax. Breathing is the only autonomic (and automatic) response you can control. A basic technique is to breathe in as deeply as you can through your nose while mentally saying, "In relaxation." Then breathe out slowly through your mouth mentally saying, "Out tension." Do this three or four times while letting your jaw, facial, and neck muscles relax. Doing this exercise whenever you find yourself sighing or before and after stressful events (presentations) will discharge stress build-up. This technique will become "second nature" after about three weeks of daily practice.

R-EDUCE the impact of remaining stressors

Lower your "stress reactivity" by exercising, getting enough rest, cutting back on caffeine (two or less cups of coffee) and taking breaks at work. Join a wellness program if available. Learn how to be assertive (not angry). Practice a systematic group management method, which includes rewards for good behavior. Often, the reward aspect of most discipline plans is dropped, rendering them as only punitive.

I-GNORE unimportant irritations

Who cares if someone has "blue hair" or still wears "bell-bottom jeans?" Don't let rude people get to you. Learn to use waiting time effectively rather than fuming.

C-OMMUNICATE, COPE, AND HOPE

Talk out your problems with trusted friends. Seek out solutions. If you're beginning to feel overwhelmed by stress (experiencing insomnia, excessive worry, headaches), see your doctor. After receiving your clean bill of health, you may want to consider counseling to help you cope. Try to keep a positive attitude. Reading or listening to motivational material will bolster your ability to cope and hope until you improve or change your situation.

A useful phrase to help you cope is: "Let it go" or "Go with the flow." That is, know what you can and cannot change. If there is something you cannot change, then let it go. If you can't let it go, (i.e., You have to stay in this situation), then go with the flow. Take each day by itself.

Keep your eyes on the prize!

If you have a difficult work situation, try to find meaning in your work. Ask yourself, why am I working? What are the rewards for working? Who am I helping? What am I learning? Is this just a stepping-stone to something better? Derive satisfaction from doing the best you can where you are. If you do the right thing long enough, you will be successful. Replace the phrase, " I have to" with "I want to." This increases your sense of control over events.

Have an attitude of gratitude toward your job situation. Talk to a friend who has been out of work six months to help you gain a more realistic attitude toward your job.

When dealing with criticism, consider the source. Is this person critical with everyone? Is there a kernel of truth to the criticism? What can you learn from this situation?

- Smile. The act of smiling will actually lift your mood.
- Have heroes and try to be around people you admire.

E-SCAPE

Take your breaks away from your desk. Enjoy "get-away" weekends. Planning for regular renewal is a hallmark of outstanding achievers. Physical energy is absolutely necessary to cope with stress.

If confronted with a very difficult situation, take a five-minute break every 50 minutes. At least take your lunch breaks.

---

7. "What to do tomorrow" tips.

LOUNGE TIPS

- Offer three choices of coffee: Leaded (full-caffeine), Unleaded (decaffeinated) and half & half blend (half-caffeine, half-decaf, for those trying to withdraw). Try green tea.
- Drink something warm. This relaxes your throat and hands. Have fruit/vegetable choices available instead of those traditional high-sugar snacks which can increase stress.
- Have a humor board with cartoons and jokes. Humor releases the stranglehold of stress.
- Have posters or books that encourage rather than discourage (e.g., The poster: "**Twelve Commandments** for People Who Work With People" by Ann White [1996]; The books: *Seeds of Greatness* by Denis Waitley, *Meet You at the Top* by Zig Ziglar).
- Put a TGIE poster up (Thank goodness I'm employed). The only thing more stressful than job-stress is JOBLESS STRESS.
- Provide pleasant music. Research reveals that the heart rate paces itself to the music we hear. Your favorite music directly stimulates a pleasure center in your brain according to the Proceedings of the National Academy of Sciences.

BREAK TIPS

- Take your breaks. Try to be around adults.
- Walk outside during lunch if at all possible. Sunlight has a "mood-elevating" effect. If you cannot walk outside, try to use the gym or any available large space.

- Avoid "pity parties." They often make you feel worse. Talk with people who are positive. Venting negative feelings without any eye toward improvement often strengthens feelings of frustration.

BUILD IN STRESS BUFFERS

- Cultivate strong work friendships.
- Have your "pleasure islands" at work. Take out a minute or two to look at or think about something pleasant.
- Have a fish tank in your classroom. Watching fish has a calming effect on most people. Posters of nature scenes soothe nerves also.

---

8. The future of computer-assisted relaxation (CARS) is here with *Freeze-Framer*™.

Combating CyberStress (computer phobia) or fighting fire with fire

Every other adult has little liking or even dislike for computers, which we have coined as CyberStress. CyberStress affects about one out of every two adults. The incidence of CyberStress increases among women and older individuals. CyberStress is least likely to occur for young males. A form of CyberStress depression has been discovered in individuals whose entire waking hours are spent on the computer. Since many professional licensing/certification exams are now being given by computers, it would behoove professionals to overcome their computer phobia. Fighting fire with fire, a good way to overcome computer phobia or CyberStress, is to use the computer-assisted relaxation system (CARS).

The future of stress management is here in the form of Computherapy. We will address, in general, how to use computers to cure (not create) stress through the computer-assisted relaxation system (CARS).

The computer-assisted relaxation system (CARS) is an easy-to-use, entertaining, and highly-effective stress-management system designed for teachers and students. CARS uses a computer-biofeedback program. The user simply sits in front of a computer with his/her hand on a device that feeds stress level information directly into the computer. The computer displays this "live" biofeedback information on the screen, enabling the user to actually "see" his/her fluctuating stress level. (Numbers are also provided for the more research-oriented.) This computer biofeedback is very effective in helping teachers relax (within a few minutes) after training. It is also helpful in teaching students to overcome test anxiety, anger or impulse-control problems. Reducing students' stress-related overactivity will lower the teacher's stress level.

Freeze-Framer™ and CARS

On February 7, 2001, the *ABC Nightly News* aired a feature viewed by 22 million on the latest in biofeedback technology called *Freeze-Framer™*. This prime time event showed a child smiling, saying that after he used the *Freeze-Framer™* device, the bad feelings he had before went away. The teacher using the *Freeze-Framer™* computer-assisted relaxation program for her class was smiling at the calming effect the program had in reducing problem behaviors so she could actually teach.

CNN, in April 2001, highlighted the use of *Freeze-Framer™* from a student's point of view. One particular high school student said that *Freeze-Framer™* actually helped him concentrate during tests better.

Freeze-Framer™ is a simple-to-use, entertaining but highly-effective, computer-biofeedback program that is so field-tested it is even used by police departments to reduce the number one danger to policemen — stress. *Freeze-Framer™* teaches you how to get better control of your heart rhythms to calm yourself.

Using the *Freeze-Framer™* device could be easily integrated into a health, wellness, PE, science, psychology or test-taking unit. It could also be used in a stress-control coaching setting for children plagued with performance-robbing test anxiety. It could also be used as a support tool for anger management training.

Many highly-stressed teachers use this *Freeze-Framer™* to calm down the chaos they experience daily.

For more information on *Freeze-Framer™*, call Heartmath, 1-800-372-3100 or email <info@heartmath.com>. This enjoyable, but highly accurate and effective biofeedback product makes relaxation training fun and fast in almost any setting, (business, school, stress-control coaching setting or home).

---

9. How to have less-stress, tomorrow: a checklist.

THE PRRICE APPROACH

- **P**-REVENT the causes of stress.
- **R**-ELAX your jaws, neck muscles, hands and breathing.
- **R**-EDUCE the impact of remaining stressors.
- **I**-GNORE unimportant irritations.
- **C**-OMMUNICATE, COPE, AND HOPE.
- **E**-SCAPE.

LOUNGE TIPS

- Offer decaf coffee. Try green tea.
- Drink something warm.
- Have a humor board with cartoons and jokes.
- Put a TGIE poster up (Thank goodness I'm employed).
- Provide pleasant music. It can directly stimulate the brain's pleasure center according to the 2001, study in the proceedings of the National Academy of Sciences.

BREAK TIPS

- Take your breaks. Be around pleasant adults.
- Walk outside during lunch if at all possible.
- Avoid "pity parties."

BUILD IN STRESS BUFFERS

- Cultivate strong work friendships.
- Have your "pleasure islands" at work.
- Have a fish tank in your classroom.
- Posters of nature scenes soothe nerves also.

SUMMARY

Teachers are the architects of the future. Through their calm example they provide today's students with the attitudes and skills to be the leaders of the 21st century. Teachers owe it to themselves and their students to take time to add Relaxation as the fourth "R" in this "turn-of-the-century curriculum." One-third of new teachers drop out within five years partly due to unexpected levels of stress encountered in the classroom.

Many use stress-eating to calm down. Harvard has cited stress as a major promoter of overweight. So excess stress not only makes you feel bad, it makes you think you look bad and contributes to life-threatening illnesses. Gaining as few as ten pounds increases your risk of hypertension, diabetes and heart attack. Have you ever seen a lounge without a snack machine?

We briefly look at how to combat computer phobia or CyberStress by "fighting fire with fire." In other words, the use of the computer-assisted relaxation system to calm computer phobia (affecting about 50% of the teaching population) is addressed. More specifically, *Freeze-Framer™*, a state of the art computer-assisted relaxation device, is presented, having already been proven effective for education on CNN to millions of viewers.

For the time-starved educator, a one-minute checklist is provided to help you have less-stress by tomorrow. We now turn our attention from helping at school to helping our mates at home, which is obviously the stress-intelligent thing to do. The benefits of reversing the word stressed to desserts was humorously pointed out, to encourage readers to take a lighter look at stress management. The next chapter will attempt to help us understand or at least accept and respect brain-based differences we will always encounter. You will be offered a brief "Brain Scan," which can also be given to your significant other. Strategies to help us see eye-to-eye will be provided, which should help keep peace on the home front.

FOR FURTHER READING

Freeze-Framer™ call Heartmath, 1-800-372-3100 or email: <info@heartmath.com>.

Jehlen, A. (2001). An open secret: why teachers leave the profession and what can make them stay." *NEA Today,* 19, 8, 8-9.

Zatorre, R., & Blood, A, (2001, September). Research proves that music soothes. *Proceedings of the National Academy of Science,* reported by Recer, Paul (2001, September 25) (Associated Press) Greensboro, NC. *News and Record,* p. A2.

19

THE "RULES"

MEN AND WOMEN AREN'T FROM DIFFERENT PLANETS, BUT FROM DIFFERENT HEMISPHERES (OF THE BRAIN)

The sole purpose of the body is to support the life of the brain.
- Thomas Edison

"At home it is better to be happy than right;
At work it is better to be right than happy."

Take the five-minute Brain Scan

Since about every other person you meet on earth will be of the opposite sex, it would be good to be aware of the real anatomical and functional gender differences in our brains. Each person's brain is as different as his or her individual facial features. "Can the brain understand itself?" is an age old question. In order not to create too much stress in "thinking about thinking," we will take a lighthearted look at some possible thinking-style differences. Since it is hard to get volunteers for an anatomical study of brain differences between males and females, a five-minute paper and pencil Brain Scan has been provided in this chapter. Take a Brain Scan yourself, then give it to your significant other. The gap between your thinking styles may be as wide as the Grand Canyon, which could be stressful when you're trying to see eye-to-eye.

Your thoughts imprint your brain

A major brain research discovery is that maintaining anxious/depressed thoughts for as little as two weeks depresses the production of our major natural antidepressant, serotonin. The use of antidepressant medication merely "jump starts" the brain's production of serotonin again. As stated earlier, always see your doctor first when experiencing unusual emotional discomfort. It could be another gland that's not working correctly (e.g., thyroid). A 2002, *Scientific American* special publication on how the mind makes the brain examines how your thoughts form your physical brain, and how your physical brain shapes your meta-physical (beyond the physical) mind.

Some research suggests that females use both right and left brain hemispheres when thinking because they allegedly have a thicker neural bridge (corpus collasum) between the left and right brain. They are more adept at talking to several people at once, and are more sensitive to subtle emotional cues. This supposed ability to switch between left and right brains may result in better intuitive thinking. It is believed that males are more single-minded, making it easier to make decisions (which may or may not be wrong, we just make them faster). Hormone differences, jokingly referred to by many women as "testosterone poisoning," may also affect the force with which we deal with things and ideas. It is also held that the brain doesn't totally integrate until about 40 years-old. Therefore, it may be that the other person can't see things your way, rather than refusing to see things your way.

The "so what" bottom line of all this brain/hormone research is that there may be unchangeable brain-based or gender-linked differences in how we view and interact with the world. Differences often create sparks and tension. Just knowing that the other person's view may actually be valid, even though it is not the way we look at things, may provide some understanding in becoming stress-intelligent. It should be noted that you can reroute your brain's physical operation in as little as two weeks by being negative and depressed.

The "Rules for the sexes." Thanks to Bill Flynn, prominent radio personality, hundreds of thousands of listeners know about the survival manual, *Rules for husbands.* Written by comedian Jim Dale, this manual takes some of the mystery out of trying to figure out what women want. Mr. Dale, also wrote a companion book, *Rules for wives.*

The related topics that may help you learn your brain-base of operation and how to cope with others' styles follow:

- Brain Scan (Five-minute).
- Change your mind to change your life.
- Male aggression-Female expression: Possibly different brain styles.
- Brain-based communication gaps. Won't versus can't remember.
- Seeing eye-to-eye: Making it work. A woman's work is never done.
- Correctivitis (over-correcting compulsion), or anything you can do, I can do better.
- Unplanned, unexpected but "on-target" gifts to show good intent, including in-home "room service," with a smile, and "I owe you a favor" coupons. Surprise her with a gift of manners.
- Rules for husbands and Rules for wives. The unwritten laws are now written.

BRAIN SCAN: A FIVE-MINUTE EXERCISE

I have half a mind to . . .
This is a no-brainer . . .
He is so scatter-brained . . .
If I only had a brain . . .

---

1. Brain Scan.

Some of the characteristics that correspond to left-right brain thinking styles are listed in the table below. Of course, we always use more than "half a brain" when thinking, just as we actually use more than one hand [even back muscles] when we pick up a soda to drink. For the overly left brained, a set of serious resources is provided in the text for follow-up.

How to do your own Brain Scan:

- Casually read each left brain/right brain style choice.
- Circle the one that seems more like you.
- It is all right to circle corresponding opposites if both describe you.
- Add the column totals (Write L= [for left brain column total]; R = [right brain]).
- The column (left or right) with more items circled suggests your tendency or thinking style (left or right brain).
- Have your partner (child, etc.) take the Brain Scan.
- See if you are on the same "brain wave" length. If you have all L's and your partner has all R's, this could create stress. Opposites may attract, but may also result in thinking the other person is only using half their mind.
- Learn to compromise and use both your brains.

---

2. Change your mind to change your life.

"At home it is better to be happy than right;
At work it is better to be right than happy."

The only adult's mind you can really change is your own. If you are constantly in a state of agitation because everyone else seems scatterbrained, you might consider consciously trying to change your mind. Using the Brain Scan below, you may wish to take a couple of the items that you feel you can't give up (which you are "urgently addicted" to) and try to change them.

An excellent way to start to change your mind is to read pages 58 to 65 in

Chapter 3, "Getting Back to the Moment," of the excellent book, *Living at the Speed of Life.* Solid reasons and methods are provided to help you shift your thinking into a more balanced, productive, satisfying and sociable gear.

Two different worlds; like light oil and water. Brain styles separate eventually

Brain styles differ. In real life, brain style differences can cause real problems.

A person who plays house, will never understand a person who plays at writing.

Opposite brain styles are like trying to mix lightweight oil and water. No matter how you stir them up, they always separate.

If you are really interested in an educational analysis of four basic thinking styles, please see the book and materials in the 4Mat series. (Just ask your local media specialist).

Also see the 2000 edition of an *Annotated Bibliography: Brain Research* by Marny Sorgen. It is an excellent review of over forty books and articles on the brain.

BRAIN SCAN© (Circle characteristics more like you)

LEFT BRAIN	**RIGHT BRAIN**
Early bird	Night owl
Analytical (breaks things down)	Analogical (makes connections)
Prefer clarity	Prefer vagueness
Prefer correct answer	Seek alternative responses
Doer	Dreamer
Exactness and precision desired	Tend to exaggerate
Structured, forced	Unstructured, free
Intellectual	Artistic
Test ideas	Make ideas
Serious	Jokester
Logical	Intuitive
Motivated by external rewards	Motivated by satisfaction
Focused, narrow	Nebulous, diffuse
Makes Order out of Chaos	Makes Chaos out of Order
Opinionated	Open-minded
Planned	Directionless
Ask factual questions (what, when, who, etc.)	Ask speculative questions (what if, why not)
Rule maker	Rule breaker/bender
Interested in science fact	Interested in science fiction

By the clock (Lunch is always at noon)	Timeless (Lunch is "whenever" you are hungry)
Uptight	Uninhibited
Verbal	Visual
Task oriented	Idea oriented
Enjoy complicated	Keep it simple
Astronomy buff	Astrology fan
Loathes surprises	Loves surprises
Total your left brain column descriptors __________L's	Total your right brain column descriptors__________R's

---

3. Male aggression — Female expression: possibly different brain styles.

Seeing eye-to-eye is difficult

There is some research that suggests that the male brain is more designed for aggression. The female brain may be better designed for expression. One brain style wants to aggressively get to the bottom line, the other wants to talk in a free-flowing stream of words. For example, Delia presents a problem. Bob poses a solution. Delia actually only wants to express her frustration, not necessarily solve the problem. Bob aggressively tries to get to the "heart of the matter" by taking care of business and solving the problem. To Delia, expressing herself about the problem is part of the solution and not just describing the facts of the matter.

Here's another example of the different styles

Bob, aggressively driving as if he were in the Indy 500, refused to "express" his need for directions by stopping at the local 7-11 store to ask for directions. His patient wife in the passenger's seat voiced her concern over his obviously (to her) heading in the wrong direction at a breakneck pace. Bob's male brain, in the flight mode, felt that if he went faster maybe he would get to the next correct exit more quickly. As time, and fifty more miles of wandering proved, he found that if he had overcome his aggression tendency and had humbly tried to shift into the expression mode to ask directions, he would have been better off. The happy ending to this story is that neither one pushed the other from the flight mode into the fight mode of the stress response.

An excellent guide to helping us navigate through the opposite sex's thinking style is a book by Dr. Deborah Tannen, a communications expert. Her book, *You*

Just Don't Understand (Ballentine Books, 1990), will not only smooth the way across the gender gap, but also helps in bridging the age gap between parents and their children.

The summer trip through "mental pause"

Have you heard the one about going through "mental pause?" When the teacher asked students to volunteer who had traveled the farthest that summer, Suzy's hand right hand shot up. The blond haired, blue-eyed seven-year-old, Suzy, said excitedly, "I didn't go there myself but Granny went through 'mental pause' this summer, even though she didn't take me. I don't know where 'mental pause' is, but my grandfather just kept saying to my Granny this summer, I thought you already went through 'mental pause' by now." Suzy continued by asking innocently, "Ms. Didactic, where is 'mental pause?' I can't find it anyplace on my state map. Can you tell me what state it's in?" The teacher, biting the inside of her cheeks to keep from laughing out loud said, "Suzy, menopause is a state of mind."

4. Brain-based communication gaps. Won't versus can't remember.

"You never listen to me! It seems like you are only half-paying attention to whatever I say," said Delia, as Bob once again forgot half the items on the "mental" shopping list he had made. Delia continued saying, "Furthermore, you completely forgot about that dinner we set up with the Epicures."

It may be biological: brain-based communication gaps

Men may only be "half-listening" when women are trying to communicate. A November, 2000, brain study conducted at Indiana University School of Medicine by Dr. Joseph T. Lurito, shows that men may only be half-brained listeners. When listening to a story, men used only the left side of their brain, whereas women used the left side and the right side of the brain (associated with more abstract reasoning). There seems to be a biological brain-based difference between the sexes in information processing. Other related studies suggest that women are better at listening to two conversations at once, which may be overwhelming for men. In phone conversations, it would probably be annoying to most males if you try to talk to them while they're talking on the phone, since they devote one brain to one conversation at a time. Also, don't try to talk to a male while expecting him to navigate onto complex highway exits. He will have to make a choice of either listening to you and missing the exit, or getting the exit and giving the speaker surface attention (what, huh, oh yes). Since listening differences are probably hard-wired in the brain, don't get stressed out over communication glitches. It is not a matter that the opposite sex won't think like you do, it's that they can't think like you do.

To narrow the communication gap and reduce the stress between the sexes when communicating, simplify the amount and details of the message, and have the receiver rephrase the message to make sure it just didn't go in only one brain, and out the other.

Since the right side of the brain, which women also use to communicate, is more sensitive to the tone of voice, make sure your tone of voice matches the intent of your message. The right brain is also responsible for reading facial expressions, so once again, try to make your facial expression match your verbal expression. In other words, if you are communicating with someone who uses both sides of their brain, then you have to speak to both sides of the brain through words, tone and gesture.

---

5. Seeing eye-to-eye: making it work. A woman's work is never done

On the home front, remember
it is better to be happy than right.

Don't fight battles you won't win. It is not "stress-smart"

Seeing eye-to-eye may require holding back on what seems natural. Of course, until we know better, we think everyone thinks as we do. Nothing could be further from the truth. Trusting the value of the other person's thinking style and realizing that he or she did make it this far using that style, it may be necessary to show a little respect, back off and listen to the other person. This may reduce a lot of stress from unchangeable brain-based communication gaps.

A woman's work is never done. You better believe it

In some cultures there is the belief, "A woman's work is never done." This is the "mantra" that some grow up with. If you are going to help someone who has this belief, then understand that "your work will never be done." It's not a good or bad belief, it's just if you expect closure on helping out, you probably need help yourself (which this book aims to do). So get ready for "work without end," and get a grip.

---

6. Overly correctness (correctivitis) or anything you can do I can do better.

"And always is heard a discouraging word and the skies are cloudy all day."
(The theme song of victims of correctivitis, sung to "Home on the Range.")

Correctivitis is the obsession with being right, having the last word and dominating. This common malady is highly stressful to surrounding people. Every single time you try to make a point they always counterpoint, to the point that you don't even try to talk around them. Get the point? In our parents' day, there was a song, "Anything you can do I can do better," which is a good example of two people dueling it out through one-upmanship. People with correctivitis just have to be a little more "righteous." Those who need to be correct are left brained to a fault. Being a target of someone with correctivitis is like jarring over unnecessary speed bumps when you are trying to talk. People with correctivitis are always interrupting and correcting you, whether they know what they're talking about or not. They look for any loophole to unravel your thread of thought until you completely lose your train of thought. These are the people you hear say, "I don't need to read — just ask me." They are the first to say, "I don't need stress-control coaching, more education, etc." In the old days these people were the bossy "know-it-all's." Since we can practically access the Library of Congress with our computers, it is unlikely that anyone will "know-it-all" and get away with it. But that has never dawned on those afflicted with correctivitis.

If you feel you can't even open your mouth without being criticized, you should try the book, *I Only Say This Because I Love You,* by Deborah Tannen, who was mentioned previously as an expert in communication.

I was looking for "Mr. Right." Once we hooked up, he turned into "Mr. Always-Right"

Annoying "know-it-alls" somehow remember minute details of events that often didn't even happen, confident in their enlightened knowledge. If you try to talk with someone inflicted with correctivitis, they'll always punctuate what you say with "Yes, but did you know" or "No, it really wasn't that way or "That's not what I heard." They even say, "What she means to say is." These people don't waste time gathering facts. They are planning ahead as you speak, just waiting for you to inhale so they can talk again. As if we are completely lacking direction without their guidance, they fill our day with often pointless and endless lists of tasks. On top of everything else, these people are often loud and annoying. If you ask how these people are, they'll always answer with an IT (It's too . . .) It's too hot, cold, slow, expensive here, etc. You usually don't want to take these people out to dinner (service is too slow), a movie (it's too cold in here), or on a picnic (it's too sunny out here).

Sometimes, people with chronic correctivitis are well-meaning, hoping to save you from yourself by protecting you with valuable (and endless) lessons from their lives. However, they may "cry wolf" so much that when they do hit the nail on the head with an important suggestion or warning, no one listens to them. Sometimes, however, people with correctivitis are the human relations equivalent of "fingernails being scratched across a chalkboard." They never feel good and are always negative. You say, "It's going to be a great day," They'll say, "What makes you think that? You obviously have not heard about the latest _______." You will never please these people. So often, people start avoiding the "overly correct." It is draining being around these "emotional vampires" who suck all the joy out of your life because you know what's coming next, some criticism or unpleasantness.

A cure for correctivitis: Try the NAG approach. "No action gear"

You don't want to reward "know-it-all" behavior or efforts to control your very life by people who (think they) know what's best for you. The best way to curb, but not cure, correctivitis is to take the "No action gear" approach (NAG for short) and wait a while before you comply with their endless requests or before you respond to questions they, of course, already know the answer to. This is a good time to try the "In one ear out the other" technique if you can. Smile if you can manage it. Do take notes if it's appropriate to review later. Even better, have them write down their suggestions.

Her bumper sticker read: "My wish is your command"

Correctivitis has probably dissolved more relationships than anything else. Overreacting to correctivitis has probably strained many work relations. If you are pointing a finger at a person who has correctivitis, remember that your other fingers on your accusing hand are pointing back at you.

An excellent book for those afflicted with correctivitis is *Living at the Speed of Life*, by Richard Carlson, author of the best-selling series, *Don't Sweat the Small Stuff.* In *Living at the Speed of Life,* he and his co-author, Joseph Bailey, talk about shifting from the analytical (critical) thinking mode to the free-flowing processing mode to actually reduce your stress and get along better. This book would make a great anonymous contribution to your work library.

Try tolerance for a change. When you are tempted to correct someone's life (overeating, overindulgence, sloppiness, poor grammar, senseless chatter, driving, the list could go on forever), say this to yourself:

> My love for them is not affected by their self-abuse.
> - *William Joyce, 2001.*

If you are courageous enough to look at yourself under the "Miss Martha S. Manners" microscope, just change this saying to:

> My love for myself is not affected by my self-abuse.

After forgiving yourself, concentrate on improving that behavior (e.g., being overly critical, overspending, looking for faults, not listening).

7. **Unplanned, but "on target" gifts. "Room service," and "I owe you a favor" coupons.**

"On target" gifts

Folks who use their right brains actually like pleasant surprises more than a left brained person would ever imagine. Right brainers love surprises; left brainers loathe surprises (even good ones). It never dawns on a Mr. Datum type "left brainer" that a person who has access to both sides of thinking (left and right brain) may really enjoy a surprise. Providing unplanned gifts will actually force the overly left brained person to pay attention to his or her significant other. The flip side of the coin is if you forget to give a gift to this person when they expect it (e.g., birthday) this person will be very upset. It's a great idea to have a "gift/card drawer for any occasion," which you can use to pull gifts and cards from if you should ever accidentally forget that special occasion. If this idea has never occurred to you, you are probably a strong left brainer, which is good for running the world's military campaigns but not your family.

"Room service" — at home, with a smile

Provide your partner with "room service" for a predetermined time. This includes the amenities you'd find at a nice hotel (breakfast in bed, massages, baths, getting the newspaper, slippers, good movies, flowers, pleasing conversation). People consider these amenities so important they are willing to pay a lot for them. Hotels have spent millions on research about what makes people happy. Take advantage of the research they have already done for you.

"I owe you a favor" coupons

For the person who has everything, you could give her a " I owe you a favor" coupon. A "favor coupon" is a coupon that can be redeemed any time, anywhere, for you to do her a favor (without whining or questioning).

Surprise her with a gift of manners

Missed Manners: If someone chronically forgets to say please, please yourself.

Forgetting he was no longer in the military, the drill sergeant barked to his young bride, "Get that document out of the trash bin. I don't care if you were president of your grammar school class." In anger she fired back, saying, "Honey, didn't you forget to say something?" He growled back, "Get that document out of the trash bin. NOW." The verbally-bruised bride then rephrased his command, and with a tear in her voice mumbled to herself, "Please, get that document out of the trash bin." She then said, "Honey, remember, please is not a four-letter word!!" Muttering to himself, the ex-drill sergeant actually started counting out the letters to the word "please," and after five minutes of strainful calculation, and double checking his work, he said to himself, "Golly, she's right. Please is not a four-letter word."

---

8. Rules for men, and Rules for women — "Rules for the sexes."

The unwritten laws are now written. Top radio personality, Mr. Bill Flynn, brought these survival manuals to light for hundreds of thousands of listeners on December 5, 2001, in the North Carolina area. This author had to pull his car over (safely) to the side of the road to fully enjoy Mr. Flynn's revelations from the books, *Rules for husbands,* and *Rules for wives.* These companion books, written by comedian Jim Dale, are the true relationship-survival manuals, which should be part of every pre-nuptial, pre-house sharing agreement. The abbreviated list below paraphrases Mr. Bill Flynn's "read" on Mr. Dale's books.

Rules for Men:

- Apologize — even though you don't know what you've done wrong.
- Don't count her shoes. Pointy toes, square toes, round toes, no toes. It will never make sense to you.
- Don't burp and then laugh about it. Only men and their sons think that burping is funny.
- Don't make fun of Oprah.

Rules for Women:

- No trick, "Am I fat?" questions.
- Beer is to men what flowers are to women.

Thank you, Mr. Bill Flynn. Sometimes it takes more than a lifetime of trial and error, especially for men, to learn these tried and true rules for pleasing the opposite sex. And men, if you think you know the rules, think again. Even Einstein did not know the "Rules for the sexes" as testified to by his far less than ideal marriage.

When a hormone avalanche thunders your way, don't argue, but run for your life.

Ignorance of the law does not excuse you from following the law. There is no excuse now. Of course this is all "tongue-in-cheek" to relieve stress.

SUMMARY:

A lighthearted look at the possible brain-based differences between thinking styles is provided in this chapter. You are given the opportunity to take a five-minute Brain Scan. Also give the Brain Scan to a "significant other" with whom getting along is important. Hormone-based differences in how we deal with life (through aggression or expression) are briefly discussed. Correctivitis, a "tongue-in-cheek" look at the highly stress-producing practice of constantly being corrected, is briefly discussed, with the suggestion of using the "No action gear" approach (NAG) to reduce the recipient's stress level and give some kind of control. Seven tips to bridge the gap between hard-core left brainers and hard-core right brainers are suggested. Six important Rules for husbands, wives and partners are listed and are considered survival tips for reducing relationship stress and "uncivil" wars.

The next chapter deals with How the Best Handle Stress. This left brained, research-based author asked a co-researcher a question, which she quickly answered, using her right brain intuitive powers. Her answer was right-on, which gave this author renewed respect for her brain-based thinking style. This question, "How do astronauts deal with stress?," leads into our next chapter. This question is very important with the recent 2002 discovery of life-supporting ice on Mars. Astronauts will be compelled to go there just "because it's there."

FOR FURTHER READING

Andrews, S.B., & Dale, J. (2001). *Rules for wives.* Kansas City, MO: Andrews McMeel Pub.

Dale, J., & Small, E. (2001). *Rules for husbands.* Kansas City, MO: Andrews McMeel Pub.

Lurito, J. (2001). Men may only be half-brained listeners. Indiana University School of Medicine.

Rubenzer, R. (1985). Which thinking style do you have? Left meets right in whole brain thinking. *Gifted Children Monthly.* 6, 7, 1-3.

Rubenzer, R. (1982). *Educating the other half: implications of left/right brain research.* Reston, VA: ERIC Clearinghouse on Handicapped and Gifted Children, Council for Exceptional Children.

Rubenzer, R. (1978). Bridge the gap between "unfeeling knowledge" (primarily left-hemisphere development) and "mindless arousal" (primarily right-hemisphere development only) in Tannenbaum, A.J., (1983). *Gifted children: psychological and educational perspectives.* New York: Macmillan Publishing Co., p. 122.

Tannen, D. (2001). *I only say this because I love you.* New York: Random House.

20

How The Best Handle Stress:

Lessons from the Top

How do astronauts handle stress? They rise above it
- Donna O'Dell Rubenzer

After several unsuccessful attempts by her research-based husband to contact NASA in answer to the question, "How do astronauts handle stress?", his wife quipped, "They rise above it." No truer words could be spoken. By relaxing and letting the right side of her brain work at the right time, she hit the nail on the head.

How do astronauts handle stress — NASA style?

To answer this question, we will look at the cures, causes and costs of stress in astronauts. We earthbound citizens can learn valuable lessons from humanity's pioneers of outer space. Since the dramatic discovery of life-supporting ice on Mars (March, 2002), there will definitely be future flights to search for life on our nearest neighboring planet. Practical spin-off from this research may be that we can learn how not "to go into orbit" by keeping our calm. Space travel has no place for the stress prone or stress overreactors. Lessons on how these "best handle stress" follow:

CURES

Most of these five tips are not "out of this world."

- Take the day off. Astronauts in space "took the day off."
- Get a hobby.
- Provide your own quiet space you can escape to.
- Personalize your own space (pictures of loved ones and favorite books).
- Watch the company you keep. Surround yourself with winners.
- Calm leadership can be learned, so the government bet!

Three-million-dollar stress cure

The National Space Biomedical Research Institute, with NASA's support, plans to spend about three-million-dollars to look into the psychology and behavior of isolated groups. This study will be done to develop objective ways to recognize failing performance.

CAUSES

The 1998 Mir Space Station stressors were:

- Autocratic Russian leadership,
- Egos of the American astronauts.

Other astronauts' sources of stress:

- weightlessness,
- lack of privacy,
- work,
- cabin fever, and
- the fear of not returning from a mission (which lowers immune system).

Interpersonal conflict tops the list of problems reported in the diaries of personnel at remote posts on earth to study effects of isolation in potential space disasters.

COSTS OF STRESS TO THE SPACE MISSION

- Performance problems,
- Contagion of diseases leading to sick astronauts in space.

CURES, CAUSES AND COSTS OF SPACE-STRESS FOLLOW: A DISCUSSION OF CURES FOR STRESS USED BY THE ASTRONAUTS OR PLANNED BY NASA

1. Take the day off. Stressed-out astronauts took a day off from work (in rebellion against mission control) to relieve job-stress in space. This happened on the U.S. space station, Skylab, during the third and final crew rotation, which began in November, 1973.

2. Get a hobby. Astronaut Andy Thomas, brought along pencils and paper, making sketching his new hobby for his five-month stay on MIR with two cosmonauts. "It's a psychological escape when you can't get away physically," he explained. Astronaut Thomas is leading the development of a new NASA training program, making astronauts sensitive to the psychological challenges they will face in space.

3. Provide your own quiet space you can escape to. When completed, the space station will have individual collapsible cubbies that are soundproof.

4. Personalize your own space (pictures of loved ones and favorite books).

NASA's working with architects who are helping engineers design individual crew quarters for the International Space Station. Astronauts will be able to personalize their quarters with photographs held in place by Velcro and books held in place with bungee cords and straps.

5. Watch the company you keep. Surround yourself with a team of winners. Most NASA experts agree that above all, crew selection is key to mission success. Looking at a person's track record in her ability to get along may provide hints to her ability to endure difficult times.

6. Since calm more effective leadership can be learned, the government bet on it with millions of your dollars.

Calm leaders are more effective. A calm, effective leadership style can be learned. The government bet on this fact with millions of your taxpayer dollars funding the N/SLP or National/State Leadership Project. The 1980's National/State Leadership Project head, Professor emeritus A.J. Tannenbaum of Columbia University, described that program as follows:

". . . Columbia University was provided with [federal] support to coordinate efforts by seven universities in recruiting and training graduate students to become seminal figures in the field. It was seen as a long-range investment in the careers of men and women who had shown promise for making significant contributions" (p. 37).

Did the investment pay off or what ever happened to the "most likely to succeed nationally" class of 1984? Who knows? This class however, was taught two important things: 1) Effective leaders show grace under pressure, and 2) One has to produce knowledge rather than just consume knowledge. It is probably about ten times more stressful to write than read, to create than criticize. It was drilled into these people that the sting of short-term self-imposed success stress is worth long-term success. Their motto was "unwarranted optimism."

Interestingly, once in this national leadership program, there were no tests. With emphasis on production of knowledge, these leadership students were graded on how many publications they had during their course work. Rather than just take tests, they had to produce something useful to others which was much more stressful than taking a paper and pencil test. That was the true test of their competency.

The cost for being highly productive is a shorter life. Even race horses die earlier than other horses. So get a grip on your "success stress," and pull in the reins if you are galloping out of control.

It is now time to see what "these people with promise for making significant contributions," have actually done. Unfortunately "educated fools" abound in our society. They hide behind many degrees and bore people with their senseless and useless chatter. These people create more stress than they relieve.

CAUSES

After five months of living in a Winnebago-sized capsule circling the earth, with at least two other cosmonauts, the 1998, Mir space station stressors were:

Autocratic Russian leadership. Our astronauts visiting MIR had great difficulty coping with "bossiness." In fact, that was their main complaint, in addition to the stress caused by language and cultural differences between the Americans and Russians.

Egos of the American Astronauts. The Russians complained of the Americans' "big gun" cowboy attitudes.

Only the first source of stress is unique to astronauts:

1. weightlessness,
2. lack of privacy,
3. work,
4. cabin fever, and
5. the fear of not returning from a mission (which lowers immune system).

Sources of stress are also associated with long periods of isolation in related NASA studies. In preparation for the upcoming eight-month (one way!) Mars flight, prospective astronauts are isolated for months in a frozen tundra-like area with no contact from the outside. On the upcoming round-trip Mars mission, astronauts could be cooped up in space for two and a half years.

With the March 2, 2002 breakthrough discovery of life-supporting ice on Mars, it is inevitable that there will be an expedition to Mars. Science fiction is being replaced by science fact. Instead of a gold rush, the 21st century will be heralded by a martian ice rush. Who ever gets there first can stake their claim.

Interpersonal conflict tops the list of problems reported in the diaries of personnel at remote posts on earth to study the effects of isolation in space. Things that might seem trivial at home, (e.g., feelings of exclusion from a clique or even the irritation of hearing a mate's jokes over and over) can blister in tight quarters. During a Mars flight, a dysfunctional crew could spell disaster.

COSTS

A stressed-out crew could result in performance and illness problems. The results of unmanaged space-stress are:

1. Performance problems due to lack of team work.
2. A sick crew due to stress-suppressed immune systems.

Now to get our feet planted firmly on the ground, we will look at world-class leaders and their tips on how to win success in spite of stress.

HOW THE BEST HANDLE STRESS ON PLANET EARTH

Tips from the top: using stress for success.

You can learn how to have success without distress.

Life in the fast lane may be the only way to stay ahead. Deadlines, lack of time, competition, difficult people, and criticism are roadblocks that are common to everyone. While these may be obstacles for some, the "best" actually use these stressors as stepping-stones rather than stumbling blocks to get where they want. What separates the whiners from the winners? Each of the following fourteen "top guns" has developed individual coping techniques to thrive on stress, rather than just survive .

Those best at handling stress included: an Emmy award-winning writer, a top Nielson-rated TV personality with an earned doctorate, an Olympic pretrial competitor, a world leader in stress management, a former Ranger, now English professor, a *Sports Illustrated* photographer, a federal judge, a top radio personality, the Executive Director of the North Carolina Writers' Network, a Yale educational consultant/retired interim superintendent of a 62,000 student school system, and a private-school teacher from Australia. One of their personal formulas, listed below, could just work for you. Their winning tips are summarized below and detailed later in the "rest" of their stories.

- Enjoy all aspects of your life.
- "Stress management is thought management."
- It is the strength and focus of the mind that allows one to overcome fear, pain and doubt. Do something physical, tedious and repetitive.
- Meditate, exercise, enjoy and achieve.
- Have fun in all you do, and leave a legacy.
- Forget yourself by serving others.
- Keeping calm to help others under adversity.
- Using a proven technique.
- "Get physical" and focus on family.
- Making the right decision.
- Tips from our Australian neighbors: Meditate, exercise and dine.
- "Creating what makes one happy."
- Providing the most good for the "cause."
- Walking, massages and movies.

The "rest" of their stories

It may be of interest to match the above stress-management techniques with the names and jobs of those who were deemed to be best at handling stress. Their most interesting stories of success over stress follow.

---

1. Enjoy all aspects of your life.

"I don't practice any specific stress-reduction technique. I find that good social support from friends and family, and enjoying and being able to derive pride of accomplishment from what I do are powerful stress busters. I derive a lot of fun from my work, which I consider to be more like play . . ., I also have fun playing golf.

I can't wait to get up in the morning, including weekends and holidays, to continue with any one of a number of exciting projects and assignments at work. I believe much of the satisfaction derives from the fascinating people I meet, and the opportunity to keep learning."

- *Dr. Paul J. Rosch, M.D., President of the American Institute of Stress in Yonkers, New York and Clinical Professor of Medicine and Psychiatry at New York Medical College. He is also an author and frequent contributor to publications such as* Reader's Digest, *which is read by more than twenty-two-million people.*

---

2. "Stress management is thought management."

"Stress management is thought management. . .. Control is ultimately the answer to stress; the more control you have over your life the less stress you should experience. Regardless of whom we work for we should all consider ourselves "self-employed" and act and manage our lives accordingly. . .. Move away from the stressful orbit. So you need multiple strategies."

- *Winner of the 2000-2001 Toastmaster International Award for Leadership and Communication and top Nielson-rated local TV News anchor, Dr. Lee Kinard, developed the nation's most successful, longest-lasting local TV show in the nation. For forty years he has hosted the early dawn, "**Good Morning Show**." Remarkably, he has carved time out of his busy schedule to earn a doctorate and write a book entitled,* Good Morning, *that details the development of this top-rated TV show.*

---

3. It is the strength and focus of the mind that allows one to overcome fear, pain and doubt. The best technique I now employ is to do something physical, tedious and repetitive.

Former Ranger (the Army's elite special forces) during Vietnam, currently Professor of English, Dr. Jeffrey Parker (A&T University - University of North Carolina) talks of his stress during Vietnam when he was a Ranger: "I learned that the biggest thing I had to overcome was the stress of dealing with situations that were unpredictable, could drastically change in an instant, and could cause the death of team members and myself. . .. This is the purest form of stress I have ever experienced."

---

4. Meditate, exercise, enjoy and achieve.

"I have learned . . . through [daily] meditation how to better manage all the things one must manage day in and day out." This multiple Emmy-winning writer also jogs daily. For fun he reads, goes to the movies, and visits with friends as much as possible. His major job satisfaction is "the completion of a well-written scene or script."

- Two-time Emmy award-winner, Rex Best, writes weekly TV scripts for a top-rated show. The Nielson ratings are used to assess his performance. This former teacher is under great pressure to coordinate the TV scripts with other writers under tight deadlines.

---

5. Have fun in all you do, and leave a legacy.

". . . I make it my job to find fun in whatever I do. Clearly there are some limitations. Funerals, visiting the IRS, excessive dental work would all be beyond stress relief. But playfulness within the daily routines of life can be a life saver. Be on guard not to become too professional. Outright silliness can be very healthy and helpful to the bottom line.

Jobs allow the opportunity to positively touch the lives of co-workers, customers and others. To leave a human being progressed by an encounter with your company is the best of personal satisfaction."

- This is the stress-management advice of Bill Flynn, host of a long-running and highly-successful daily morning radio show on WMAG, High Point, North Carolina. Bill also writes a weekly newspaper column and recently wrote a book.

---

6. Forget yourself by serving others.

"I forget myself by serving others. I like to read and play with my three-year-old. My major job satisfaction is service to others. Provide service to others without concern for outcome and your stress will evaporate."

- Dr. Sanford Danziger, M.D., and Director of TRP: Training for the Totally Responsible Person as a way of eliminating "victim mentality" in the workplace. Danziger is recipient of the highest award for training, innovation and creativity from the American Society for Training and Development. Co-author of the successful book, Better than Money Can Buy, *Danziger practices in Winston-Salem, North Carolina.*

7. Keeping calm to help others under adversity.

"I keep myself calm in order to control any adversity. I read and watch soccer on TV. My job satisfaction is helping members of the San Marino community in New York. (San Marino, Italy, holds the world record for countries with the highest life expectancy for men [77.2] and women [85.3].)"

- This is the stress-management advice of Jose Riba, K.M., Honorary Consulate General of the Republic of San Marino, Italy, assigned to New York.

8. Using a proven technique.

"I use *Freeze-Framer*™, a five-step, scientifically proven, one-minute technique to clear thinking and calm down. I play, hike in nature, dance, 'explore the heart' daily. My major job satisfactions are finding new ways to share Heartmath relaxation techniques with people, seeing their lives improve, seeing my staff's lives improve and having fun staff meetings."

- Thus advises Dr. Deborah Rozman, Executive Vice-President, Heartmath, Boulder Creek, California. Heartmath programs focus on business-stress training to improve productivity, and have been featured on national TV programs and presented at the 1997 International Congress on Stress, Montreux, Switzerland.

9. "Get physical" and focus on family.

"I manage stress with physical exercise three or four times per week for forty-five minutes. I also spend time with family. What I look forward to at work is satisfactory completion of projects such as negotiation of a new contract or meeting a deadline."

- So says Roy Bixby, M.B.A., Human Resources manager, R. J. Reynolds Corporation, Milwaukee, Wisconsin.

10. Making the right decision.

"My major job satisfaction is simply getting the right decision made (as often as possible) and doing so expeditiously," advises Judge Charles Biscoe, Administrative law judge, Southeast Region, Greensboro, North Carolina.

11. Tips from our Australian neighbors: Meditate, exercise and dine.

This Olympic pretrial gymnast states, "To manage stress, I practice yoga once per week, use meditation daily, and exercise three to four times per week. For fun, I have dinner with friends once a week."

- This advice is from the dynamic Rowena J. Robinson, B. Sc.Ed. PDHPE,

Dip. HM, Olympic pretri a competitor, Health and Fitness Consultant, Monte Sant'Angelo Mercy College (private school). North Sydney, Australia.

---

12. "Creating what makes one happy."

"For stress management I use music and dance. I read inspirational quotes daily and I exercise or do yard work three times a week. My major source of job satisfaction is creating a photograph that makes me happy," says Tim O'Dell, sports photographer for the world's leading sports magazine, *Sports Illustrated.* Mr. O'Dell has successfully broken into a highly-competitive field where only the best thrive. Albuquerque, New Mexico.

---

13. Providing the most good for the "cause."

"For stress management, in addition to other exercise, I walk three times per week. On Saturdays, I unwind by cooking and baking and listening to the Metropolitan Opera on the radio. My major source of job satisfaction is advising writers on their work and the completion of a newsletter for the North Carolina Writers' Network [NCWN] six times yearly. I also enjoy helping to organize two state conferences for NCWN," says Dr. Linda Hobson, professional writer and Executive Director of the North Carolina Writers' Network. She is the author of two scholarly books.

---

14. Walking, massages, and movies.

Yale consultant, and retired interim superintendent of a large (62,000 students, 5,000 employees) school system, Dr. Lillie M. Jones recalls that after more than thirty years of service as a teacher, she was promoted "from within" to the "top" in a North Carolina school system, which is a distinct honor. She was a very highly-regarded, unusually effective top-level administrator, who led her staff and students through positive leadership and no-fault administration.

STUDY SUMMARY AT A GLANCE

Outstanding achievers:

- Accentuate the positive.
- Take pride in accomplishing goals on the way to excellence (e.g., continual self-improvement).
- Possess a strong "service to others" orientation without undue concern over immediate rewards.
- Reduce one's "fun-deficit" by enjoying all aspects of life (e.g., music, dining, family, work).

- Exercise.
- Practice a proven relaxation technique.
- Calm, effective leadership can be learned.

Are you one of the "best" at handling stress? Grade yourself on this Leadership Report Card.

REPORT CARD
YOUR LEADERSHIP REPORT CARD © 2003
"A GREAT REPORT CARD IS YOUR SUPPORT TO OTHERS"

Eleventh Commandment (Not intended to be part of the Heavenly Top Ten Commandments.)

Know thyself & don't judge lest you be judged.

What does Your Leadership Report Card look like? Please spare five minutes to find out your LQ (Leadership Quotient) and Grade by taking the following Leadership Survey. Get your reality checked by having one other person rate you.

Your Name: ____________________________

Date: ________________________________

Rater: Yourself: ______________________(Use Code name)

"Reality Checker": ___________________(Use Code name)

Code Name should be used to protect the innocent from revenge.

Please make another copy of the rating sheet and a blank report card. Give blank rating sheet and this blank LEADERSHIP REPORT CARD© to your peer "reality checker" before you rate yourself. Both of you rate you. Compare notes afterwards with your "reality checker" maybe in a public place, if you often "fly off the handle."

HOW YOUR LEADERSHIP GRADING CURVE IS DETERMINED

LQ = 100 (Grade A) Best in class
LQ = 90 (Grade B) Most preferred co-worker, [MPC]
LQ = 80 (Grade C) The bland leading the bland
LQ = 70 (Grade D) The weakest link in the chain of command
LQ = 60 (Grade F) Least preferred co-worker, [LPC]
LQ = 50 (Grade F-) Anti-Leader

Best in Class is used for developing the required grading curve (A through F). The ceiling (highest point) is determined by comparing yourself to real leaders. For example just find out who was employee of the year. This person is the most preferred co-worker [MPC] in your field. For example: At Columbia University the Best in Class is Dr. Henry Kissinger, Nobel Peace Prize winner. On the low downside of the leadership curve is the least preferred co-worker or the weakest link in the chain of command. The bottom of the leadership "totem pole" is occupied by the anti-leader (one who actually repels people).

HOW YOUR LEADERSHIP QUOTIENT (LQ) IS DETERMINED

Simply take the number of positive leadership traits you think you have from the Power of Positive Leadership trait list found in Chapter one. Divide by 10 (e.g., 10/10 =1.0) Then multiply by 100 (1.0 x 100 = LQ of 100). Since the LQ is marked on a curve be sure not to over-rate yourself. An LQ (Leadership Quotient) of 100 (perfect) would go to Dr. Henry Kissinger, Harvard and Columbia Professor and Nobel Peace Prize winner. Just for fun, have someone else rate you and give you a report card grade of your leadership skills. Compare your "realty-checker's" report card to your own grade.

Having a "reality checker" rate a person is an excellent exercise for those "who are legends in their own minds." It may be a refreshing "wake-up call" so they don't drift into become anti-leaders without even knowing it. (Go to page 14, check off these traits you have under the ten traits to "Inspire Leadership.")

Number and Percent of Good Leadership qualities out of ten (p. 14):
10/100%
Grade: A
LQ =100
Descriptor: Most preferred co-worker (MPC). People seek leader out.
Example: Dr. Kissinger, Columbia and Harvard University Leadership Lecturer. Believes, "Don't judge lest you be judged."
Power Base: Faith.
Result: Nobel Prize 1973
Remedy: None needed. Natural born leader.

Number and Percent of Good Leadership qualities out of ten:
9/90%
Grade: B
LQ = 90
Descriptor: Most preferred co-worker (MPC).
Example: Solid, "inspired" leader.
Power Base: Faith and trust. Hope not despair.
Result: Employees stay because they feel hope rather than despair.
Remedy: None needed.

Number and Percent of Good Leadership qualities out of ten (p. 14):
8/80%
Grade: C
LQ = 80
Descriptor: Adequate, follow the leader.
Example: The bland leading the bland: Colorless achiever.
Power Base: By the book.
Results: Employees tolerate because of necessary evil (leader evaluates and/or signs pay checks, etc.).
Remedy: Leadership training courses.

Number and Percent of Good Leadership qualities out of ten (p. 14):
7/70%
Grade: D
LQ = 70
Descriptor: Ranting and raving.
Example: Barney Fife, (Fictional, bony-fingered character with squeaky voice, always ranting and raving; irritates like "fingernails on a chalkboard." Screeches out: "Let me tell you how it's done." Nitpicker, control freak); loud and annoying mannerisms, ruled by "administrivia."
Power Base: Despair rather than hope. Distrust rather than trust. "Watch your back."
Results: Employees endure, stay only out of dire financial necessity. Excessive but real sick-of-work days. Workers four times more likely to suffer colds/flu. Slower recovery time from surgery. (Harvard Medical School, 2002)
Remedies: Leader to take "Dale Carnegie" course on winning friends, influencing people. Speak in lower, slower manner. To lower irritating

voice, enjoy warm, decaffeinated drinks. See doctor about possible anxiety disorder treatment.

Number and Percent of Good Leadership qualities out of ten (p. 14): **6/60%**
Grade: F
LQ = 60
Descriptor: Least preferred co-worker (LPC).
Example of Peter's Principle: Promoted to level of incompetence. Toxic because makes others sick.
Example: CHICKEN LITTLE: Constantly is saying, "Sky is falling. Keep your head down so it won't get cut off."
Power Base: Fear — distrust. Wants to be the "fly in the ointment."
Results: Employees pity. Abnormally high turnover; Leader is least preferred co-worker (LPC).
Remedies: Go back to school; Join ASTD or Toastmasters to learn how to talk so people listen.

Number and Percent of Good Leadership qualities out of ten (p. 14): **5/50% or less.**
Grade: F-
LQ = 50
Descriptor: Anti-Leader, Little Hitler (Term used by Dr. Jay Carter, 1989*), (Bottom one percent).
Example: Captain Blah. Begins yearly kick-off speech with: "Let the suffering begin," "It's my way or the highway." Practices twisted belief that it is: Kind to be cruel. Lower than least preferred co-worker.
Power Base: Ruthless control and criticism. Despair rather than hope.
Results: Employees jump ship as soon as possible; loathe rather than love their jobs.
Remedy = Intensive Care from Center for Creative Leadership.

---

*Sadly, one to twenty percent of people are nasty according to Counseling psychologist, Dr. Jay Carter. His 1989 book, *Nasty People,* is a must read if you are going to work with nasty people and remain calm.

The best leadership measure

The Campbell Leadership Index™ (CLI®), is the best way to see if a leader measures up to this ruler of true leadership. The CLI® consists of 100-single phrase descriptors, and is probably the most valid, reliable and most researched instrument available. For more information on the CLI® contact the Center for Creative Leadership, Greensboro, North Carolina, with other training facilities in San Diego, Colorado Springs and Europe. For program information, call (336) 545-2810. CCL's head office is located at 1 Leadership Pl. Greensboro, NC 27410. Visit their website at <http://www.ccl.org/search>.

SUMMARY

This chapter looks at how "out-of-this-world" leaders handle stress by answering the question: How do astronauts handle stress? To answer this question, we looked at the cures, causes and costs of stress in astronauts as reported by NASA. Their stress cures included: Take the day off; get a hobby; provide your own quiet space; personalize your own space and surround yourself with winners. Causes of space-stress were: autocratic leadership and egos. Calm leadership is more effective leadership. This chapter looks briefly at a million-dollar leadership project designed to educate leaders to produce knowledge rather than merely consume knowledge. The stress level between consuming knowledge and producing knowledge is probably about tenfold, which is common sense. It is much more stressful to write than read, to create than criticize. These "supposed leaders" in this 1970's leadership project were taught to endure self-inflicted short-term "success-stress" to get long-term success to improve their field. The phenomenon of undisciplined intelligence, resulting in the abundance of educated fools was presented. Educated fools are extremely stressful to be around.

Interpersonal conflict tops the list of problems reported in the diaries of personnel at remote posts on earth to study possible effects of isolation in space. The major cost of space-stress is "mission failure" because of sickness being spread among the astronauts from their stress-suppressed immune systems.

To keep our feet firmly planted on the ground, we then looked at "world-class leaders."

To get at the real winners, an original, international study was conducted to learn personal stress-management tips from world-class-achievers that you could apply. Emphasizing pride and enjoyment in their work appears to be a characteristic of leaders in their field more than any other characteristic. In general, it appears that exercise, using a relaxation technique, and having more fun in life are powerful stress busters used by "the best to handle stress." A quick LEADERSHIP REPORT CARD© is provided to help rate one's leadership skills. Like the real business world, the grading system is marked on a curve. The Campbell Leadership Index™ (CLI®) is presented which is probably the best instrument to see if a leader measures up to this "ruler" of true leadership. This "ruler" for comparison is one-hundred items long and is the best measure of its kind.

In the next chapter we will look at how to deal with stress when it gets under our skin. People are less happy and more stressed than they were thirty years ago, especially after the 9/11/01 terrorists' bombings. More people are angrier than ever. The next chapter deals with the consequences of taking stress personally, such as anger, worry, headaches and insomnia.

The level of lethality of anger is illustrated by the fact that Anger spells Danger, without the D. Insomnia is on the rise. The good news is that the cures for these modern maladies are within our reach.

FOR FURTHER READING

Danziger, S. (2001). *Better than money can buy.* Winston-Salem, North Carolina. Director of TRP: Training for the Totally Responsible Person.

Kinard, Lee, Ed.D. Lee Kinard on May 5 received the 2000-2001 Toastmasters Communication and Leadership Award as voted by the 2,200 members as one of the most outstanding leaders in the world. *People and Places: College Section* (Greensboro, NC. *News and Record,* May 20, 2001, p. 4).

McFarling, U.L. (2002, March 2). Spacecraft detects ice on Mars. *Los Angeles Times.* (Greensboro, NC. *News and Record*, p. A-9).

Satish, M. (1999, Nov.). A sick crew can't work well in space. *Odyssey.* 8, 8, p. 2.

Simpson, S. (2000). Staying sane in space. *Scientific American.* 282, 3, 61.

21

When You Take Stress Personally:

Conquering Anger, Worry, Headaches and Sleepworking (Insomnia)

"Genius is eternal patience." - *Michelangelo*

WHY CONTROL YOUR ANGER?

Anger is the worst stress-reflex because it is doubly destructive. Your anger destroys your health and your relationships. Getting angry is like a scorpion stinging itself. It will kill you. Anger hangovers are a bad way to start your day. An anger hangover is simply waking up mad from the fight you had the previous night.

"I will not let any man diminish my soul by making me hate him."
- George Washington

Dr. Redford Williams, M.D., Director of the Behavioral Medicine Research Center at Duke University, is the author of the book, *Lifeskills* (Times Books, 2000). He states that people today appear angrier than ever. Anger, whether inner- or outer-directed, can kill you. According to the *Journal of the American Medical Association,* men with higher-hostility levels were 2½ times more likely to have evidence of developing heart disease. Postmenopausal women who were angry also had increased heart disease symptoms. Men are more prone to react to anxiety with anger and hostility because a surge of testosterone is added to the stress hormone cocktail (adrenaline and cortisol). As mentioned previously, cortisol causes cardiac racing, getting your heart ready for "flight or fight."

Dr. Williams listed job-stress, being socially isolated, and depression as key factors linked to anger and heart disease. A double "whammy" would be a man who is hostile under great job-stress where he has little control and high demands.

Too much technology, too little time, fuel the rage of anger

C. Leslie Charles, in her book, *"Why is Everyone So Cranky?",* emphasizes that much of today's unhappiness comes from the collision of too much technology with too little time.

Four topics that relate to understanding anger will be discussed in this chapter. These are:

- Anger is Danger without the D.
- Trading clubs for pencils: Why Anger spells Danger.
- Holes in the block of wood.
- What we say or do in the heat of anger may endanger careers/relationships.

To cool down anger from becoming a raging emotional firestorm, we will look at six major techniques to manage anger:

- Move out to a different city. Go to your room for quiet time.
- Gaining self-control: What the American Psychological Association says.
- Getting along with others.
- Fighting fair.
- Writing "things you hate" mail, then destroying it, undelivered.
- Be a good sport: Follow your dream team.

Long-distance dating: A story about going overboard

"How well can you date my daughter from a hospital bed, you degenerate low-life?" shouted the red-faced middle-aged man as he shook his fist. Shocked, the young man carefully let his girlfriend off the back end of the motorcycle. He backed down the driveway and gave Mr. Stroke a single digit sign-language goodbye. "How could you, Daddy?," asked the sobbing sixteen-year-old girl. That was just the beginning of the wedge that Mr. Stroke drove between himself and his daughter, a bright, very attractive and caring young girl. Eventually Mr. Stroke blew a gasket, when he heard that after moving to Texas, she had starting dating "some cowboy" who rode horses and branded cattle. Before he blew his top, his anger had developed a "hate triangle." His wife hated him, his daughter hated him and any suitor of his daughter learned to hate him. By the way, the biker became a U.S. Senator and now makes $180,000,000 per year with his Internet highway connections called "free ride" (using a motorcycle logo).

---

1. Anger is Danger without the D.

To put anger in perspective, remember that the word danger is made up mostly of anger. Lethal levels of anger, carried by one of out five people, cause heart and blood pressure problems.

Anger: adding gasoline to the fire

Becoming angry is like throwing gasoline onto a smoldering fire, triggering a dangerous explosion. We may already be smoldering from built-up resentment, and the smallest event can fuel the firestorm. When mad, we often add our own fuel to the fire by bringing up the past.

---

2. Trading clubs for pencils: Why Anger spells Danger.

Fighting when angry worked successfully until we traded ancient clubs for pencils. The motto, "Speak softly but carry a big stick," shows our obvious comfort with clubbing our threats. Generally, today's stressors demand cool, precise responses such as thinking quickly, or using a computer. Yet once frustrated we angrily clench our teeth and fists, just as our ancestors did getting ready to use their handy club.

---

3. Holes in the block of wood.

It has been said that in anger we "nail" our victims with sharp words like driving nails into a block of wood. When the heat of our anger subsides, we pull out the nails, but the holes in the wood remain. The permanent holes in our relationship are often not worth the satisfaction we derived when we attacked our victim. This wisdom was shared by Al Pecor, a philosopher and mentor.

---

4. What we say or do in the heat of anger may endanger careers and relationships, so we repress our anger.

Pent-up anger can kill you. So wrestling to control your anger deserves your attention. Road rage, workplace violence and school violence are all examples of unmanaged anger.

George Washington was credited with saying, "I will not let any man diminish my soul by making me hate him." By allowing someone to make you angry, you give someone control of you. Cut the strings of other people's controlling you like a puppet. It will be difficult because the bonds of habit are very strong. But character is nothing more than lifelong habits and with practice you can prevent anger from robbing you of control of situations.

MANAGING ANGER

---

1. Move out to a different city. Go to your room, for quiet time.

There is a strong link between hostility and death rates. Cities reporting the lowest levels of hostility enjoyed much lower mortality rates than high-hostility cities. Honolulu, having the lowest self-reported hostility level, also had the lowest death rate. Mainland cities reporting low hostility rates included Seattle, Minneapolis, Denver, and Des Moines. Merely living in high-hostility environments increases your chances of shortening your life.

Go to your room for quiet time

When you get heated up, just go to an agreed upon "quiet room." It doesn't matter who's wrong or right. Have an agreement that this room or floor is like Switzerland, a neutral corner, where you won't be hounded. About 20 minutes should be enough time to cool down. A "tongue-in-cheek" research project would be to see if two story homeowners have a better rate of staying with their living partners, compared to those in cramped quarters. Even astronauts don't get along perfectly well with their fellow space travelers when in cramped quarters. Their biggest complaint was personality clashes. You'd think they'd be more fearful of the mission.

---

2. Gaining self-control: what the American Psychological Association says.

The American Psychological Association suggests that you calm down by deep breathing and creating pleasant images; change your thinking when mad (attitude); plan problem solving without self-blame; communicate better, apply humor; improve your surroundings and schedule your time better. A free brochure on controlling anger is available from the APA.

---

3. Getting along with others:

We need to learn to make decisions when we get mad. We need to ask ourselves whether this irritation is worth our attention. Is our anger justified or not? If our anger is not justified, we should try to talk ourselves out of anger. If self-talk does not work, use meditation or some type of distraction. If we are justified in getting angry, we need to think of a sensible response, and deliver our message calmly and respectfully.

---

4. Fighting fair:

Dr. Paul Coleman offers the following tips:

Do not use name-calling, do not try to psychoanalyze the other person, and do not fight the last thing at night or right after getting home from work. He also suggests that both parties sit down to keep cool. Young males are at risk for learning anger, therefore anger management should be taught early. There is a good game called "Keep Your Cool." Learning to prevent or control anger impulses is what separates us from the animals. Learning to make the right choices under stress can be started even at the preschool level. Simply count to ten before you respond.

---

5. Writing "things you hate" mail, then always destroying it, undelivered.

If your anger has gotten the better of you, you may have to lance it "like a boil." Express your "anger glands" through writing, listing what really makes you angry about a specific thing. Then destroy the angry letter, without sharing it with anyone. Seek help from a mental-health professional if your anger keeps coming back or is so intense you have irrational intents about someone. Crimes of passion are still crimes.

---

6. Be a good sport: Follow your dream team.

Sporting events let us be aggressive in a socially approved way. This indirect expression of aggression, by watching sports, is so highly valued that many professional athletes make more than the President.

WHY GET ABOVE AND OVER YOUR WORRIES? ADVICE FROM EINSTEIN

We cannot solve problems at the same level they were created.
- Albert Einstein

To solve problems we must get above the worries that we attach to problems. Learning to relax will help us see that many of our worries are unfounded, never come true or are exaggerations.

So that you worry less about worrying, let's dissect this almost universal stress trait by addressing the following issues.

- Worry and GAD (general anxiety disorder).
- Benefits of managing your worries.

Cutting your worries in half

Among the tips that we will look at to help you deal with worry, the following "baker's dozen" below are most helpful.

- Blocking your worry-urge can actually improve your physical health and emotional well-being.
- Remember: Your attitude is your stress-control gate.
- Don't bleed until you are cut. Worrying is 97% wasted mental effort.
- Throw your worries away. Actually, "Fire your worries."
- Dissect your real problems into solvable steps.

- Weave your own "psychological safety net."
- Use humor to whittle down your worry to size.
- Avoid "pity parties."
- Get or give help.
- Don't just worry — work (hard and smart).
- Engage yourself in physical activity.
- Learn to focus on today.
- Reward yourself for "stopping" your worry habit.

Before we begin to look at how to slow down your worrying (which is almost universal in all people), let's have a word about something to worry about – if it is unchecked.

---

1. Worrying and generalized anxiety disorder (GAD).

Unchecked, a worry habit can solidify into a generalized anxiety disorder requiring professional treatment, often using medication and talk therapy.

According to the *Diagnostic and Statistical Manual IV* (DSM-IV), excessive anxiety and worry happening the majority of days for at least six months about various activities or events, signals a possible generalized anxiety disorder. The worry is far out of proportion to the chance of the event occurring, or to the actual effect of the event that is feared. The person's worries keep him or her from concentrating and the person has problems stopping worrying.

Adults with a generalized anxiety disorder worry often about typical life activities like their jobs, money, health of family members, and safety of their children. They even worry greatly about minor things such as being late for appointments, chores around the house, or routine car repairs.

Don't worry about worrying. Consult a doctor if the above description sounds like you or a loved one. **"Don't borrow sorrow."**

---

2. Benefits of reducing your worrying.

Worrying and stress are inseparably woven together. Worrying causes physical stress, and physical stress (e.g., drinking too much caffeine, alcohol, fatigue) can cause us to worry. By breaking the worry-stress cycle, physically dangerous aspects of stress can be reduced. Many people worry themselves sick. Worrying actually short circuits your brain's smooth operation, impairing productive problem solving. Tension from worrying raises blood pressure. Recently, stress has been shown to actually kill brain cells in the hippocampus, the memory center of your brain. Extreme worry retards learning and will bring about that which you are fearing the most, failure.

CUTTING YOUR WORRIES IN HALF

---

1. Blocking your worry-urge.

This can actually improve your physical health and emotional well-being. Realistic trust in what is trustworthy is the best antidote to fretting and worrying about things that will never happen. Trusting in your ability to deal with problems will improve your chances of solving the problem!

---

2. Remember: Your attitude is your stress-control gate.

Your attitude is your first line of defense against worry. Always "crying wolf" mentally will leave you battle-fatigued at the end of the day. Practice positive mental toughness. That is, believe things will turn out for the best even if you do not feel that way. Picture yourself succeeding in the difficult situation.

If you feel anxious, you are much more likely to worry. Scientific studies prove that people who are made to feel stress (through stress-inducing chemicals) find reasons to justify their nervousness. In other words, they worry because they feel tense. Exercise replaces stress hormones with endorphins (a natural tranquilizer). Reduce or avoid these "stress amplifiers": caffeine, nicotine, excess sugar, and withdrawal from excess alcohol. Tense muscles produce stress chemicals, therefore, learn to relax your muscles, particularly your jaw, neck, and shoulder muscles. Get enough rest. Anxiety is caused by alcohol withdrawal and caffeine withdrawal.

---

3. Don't bleed until you are cut. 97% of worry is wasted.

According to Reverend Fred Warnecke, in a sermon on reducing worry, we should not anticipate the unpleasant before it happens. Worrying is 97% wasted mental effort. Worrying is mostly negative advanced rehearsal about events that never happen. To prove this fact, get out a calendar. Write down all the major things you are worried about for the next two weeks. Put the calendar away. After two weeks have passed, check what your "worry prediction hit-rate" was. For example, if you predicted ten agonizing events would happen over the next two weeks, and only one event was truly agonizing, your "worry hit-rate" would only be 10%. The three percent hit-rate is generally the rule. We waste about 97% of our mental resources worrying about things that never happen, or were not as bad as we feared.

---

4. Throw away your worries. "Fire your worries."

Write down your irrational worries on a sheet of paper. Throw the piece of paper away. Better yet, "Fire your worries." Dispose of them safely in a campfire. If you are worried about "Firing your worries," then simply dampen the area around your fire source first, then light the fire. Use common sense precautions. If you think you have so many worries you'd set off a nearby smoke detector, it may be time to get professional help.

---

5. Dissect your real problems into solvable steps.

The first step might be talking with someone who is knowledgeable and sympathetic about your problem.

Know the difference between worrying and planning. Worrying is blowing the problem out of proportion, and feeling overwhelmed or trapped. Tell yourself, "Plan it, don't panic."

Face your fears with faith. A deep positive faith in something or someone beyond yourself will conquer your fears. Remember the saying, "Fear knocked at the door. Faith answered. When the door opened, nothing was there." Even our federal currency system is based on faith, "In God We Trust." After the September 11, 2001 suicidal plane bombings, return-to-church attendance was the highest it has been for decades. Replace your "false sense of insecurity" with calm confidence based on the fact that with proper preparation you will succeed. Review your relevant past successes.

---

6. Weave your own "psychological safety net."

Be realistic about the worst thing that can happen if Murphy's Law kicks in. Study the situation, talk to others. There may be unexpected solutions or escapes.

Now list the positive things that you would still have left even if the worst happens: your life, your health, loved ones, your friends, pets, the club/organization, your "psychological safety net." Everyone has a "psychological safety net," but most people forget it is there until after they've been saved by it. If you remember it is there before you start across the tight wire, you will worry less.

---

7. Use humor to whittle down your worry to size.

Your sense of humor is your sense of balance. There is even a website called <pinkslip.com> to help those afflicted with job loss to see the funny side.

---

8. Avoid "pity parties."

Stress, worry and fear are contagious. If you hang around "Chicken Littles" (the sky is falling), you will undoubtedly become more worried. Follow the lead of calm, organized people who are sympathetic to your cause.

9. Get or give help.

Ask for help from people you trust. Most people like helping others but they cannot "mind read." If you do not ask for help, do not be surprised if you never get it. Giving help to others will get your mind off your problems and get you committed to something beyond yourself.

Get things in perspective. If you are feeling sorry for yourself, visit a nursing home, go see an unemployment line, visit a cemetery. Downward comparison (comparing your situation to a dramatically more "down and out" situation that you or someone else overcame) can provide some relief to your worry.

Remember: Bad news has a bad effect on the worrisome. A popular motto for the media is: "If it bleeds, it leads." The most stressful situation is worrying about things you have no control over. People can become bad news-junkies. Winston Churchill said, "You are what you read." You can be totally informed by listening to a few-minutes "news capsules," or reading the "front-page" of the newspaper, or watching the nightly news once. You will have more energy to cope, console, and help with problems your friends or business experience if you choose your worries wisely. Corporately, your boss will usually keep you informed about realistic concerns.

Use your "right brain at the right time." Left/right brain research clearly shows that the left brain makes order out of chaos, while the right brain makes chaos out of order. Your right brain is responsible for negative emotions, while your left brain is responsible for positive emotions. When our energy is low we often "shift" to right brain thinking that is disorganized and negative. Reading/ listening to positive material will keep you in a left brain mode. Keeping your energy level up will also keep you in a positive left brain gear.

10. Don't just worry — work (hard and smart).

Equip yourself with the tools to deal with your circumstances effectively. Learn how to manage your money, time, clutter, and difficult people before they manage you. Master the science and art of problem solving. Learn the art of forgiving yourself and others for mistakes.

11. Engage yourself in physical activity.

Do something constructive, requiring concentration, to distract you from useless worrying. A detailed hobby, yard work or exercising while watching TV will get your mind off your problems.

12. Learn to focus on today.

Many worries come from mental "double vision." Looking back to the past, while previewing the future, blurs our vision of the "here and now." Time management experts assert that we should spend 90% of our time concentrating on the "here and now" and only 10% of our time planning the future.

Know that every day is new, with renewed energy. Proper sleep, nutrition and exercise will give you the energy to "bounce back" and handle your problems.

Focusing on the past is like driving while looking only in your rear view mirror. You'll crash eventually.

13. Reward yourself for "stopping" your worry habit.

Every time you start to worry, mentally picture a big red stop sign. Say silently to yourself, "Stop that," so no one else can hear you. If you say it too loudly you really will have something to worry about. Even more effective would be to find and cut out a miniature stop sign and place it where you can look at it every time you start worrying needlessly. Take pride in the fact that you can catch yourself worrying.

STRESS HEADACHES

Why prevent and relieve headaches

The headache is the most frequent single complaint of modern times. Most headaches are stress headaches. (Check with your doctor if you experience headaches often.) Headaches that occur at work make work even more stressful because you may anticipate getting a headache (which can actually trigger a headache). Headaches prevent you from concentrating well and can make the cause of your headaches (workload) even increase because of errors or sick-time due to headaches.

Possible causes of tension headaches

The exact cause of tension headaches is not clear, but the most likely culprits are: stress, muscle tension, restricted blood flow from sustained muscle tension, fatigue or too much or too little sleep. Other common causes of headaches include: holding a "frozen posture" for too long (e.g., looking at a computer screen too long), grinding one's teeth or even chewing gum too hard.

HOW TO PREVENT HEADACHES

- Regular exercise is the best way to prevent headaches.
- Practice muscle relaxation during your breaks.
- Take a warm bath or shower.

- Get a massage from a licensed professional.
- Smile more, frown less.
- Practice deep breathing.
- Reduce eyestrain.
- Maintain good posture.
- Eat properly.

To fill in the blanks on these tips listed above, read the following.

---

1. Regular exercise is the best way to prevent headaches.

The New England Center for Headaches explains how exercise prevents headaches. Exercise pumps blood through your body, delivering oxygen and eliminating waste more efficiently. Exercise brings about deep breathing, relieving strain on your neck and back muscles. Learning to stretch properly will reduce muscle tension.

---

2. Practice muscle relaxation during your breaks.

Stress accumulates in your jaw, facial, scalp, neck and shoulder muscles. Do "stress checks" in these areas periodically. You can "siphon off" painful muscle tension build-up so it never reaches the headache level.

---

3. Take a warm bath or shower.

A warm bath will relax your muscles. A bath that is too hot will actually tense you up.

---

4. Get a massage from a licensed professional.

---

5. Smile more, frown less.

The act of smiling and laughing will reduce your stress. Frowning tenses your forehead, leading to headaches.

---

6. Practice deep breathing.

Your brain requires one-fifth of your entire body's oxygen. Taking two or three slow deep breaths will relax you and improve your concentration.

7. Reduce eyestrain.

Hourly, focus your eyes at a far distant point. If you get eyestrain headaches, see your ophthalmologist or optometrist.

8. Maintain good posture.

Don't slouch when sitting. This puts strain on your spine muscles, which tightens your back muscles. Make certain your chair is adjusted to support your back, and your feet are flat on the floor. If you work on a computer or typewriter keyboard, adjust your chair height so your shoulders are not hunched or you have to reach down. If you stand at work, bend from side-to-side occasionally. Bend over forward, touching your knees. Every couple of hours, stretch, and if sitting, stand. If standing, sit.

9. Eat properly.

Some headaches come from hunger. Breakfast is your most important meal because you have not eaten since the night before. Also you need extra energy in the morning to give you the nutritional boost to energetically face the challenges of the new day. Eating a banana and having fruit juice along with some type of carbohydrate (e.g., cereal, bagel) with protein can get you off on the right foot. (There are cereals with no fat that contain protein.) Throughout the day, snack on bagels or dry cereal every few hours. Have a multiple-vegetable drink or orange juice in the late afternoon. You will feel and perform better with smaller, more frequent snacks rather than infrequent but large meals.

HOW TO DEAL WITH SLEEPWORKING (INSOMNIA)

Sleep disorders are increasing as stress is increasing. But don't lose any sleep over that fact. If you try to practice stress management (including anger and worry management) you may improve your sleep. Always see your doctor if you are having significant problems sleeping.

What is sleepworking?

Sleepworking is sleeplessness due to dreaming/worrying about work problems. Your sleep is invaded by unwanted thoughts. You sleepwork trying to solve problems or complete work. The problem with sleepworking is that you are only using half-a-mind. Your right brain, which functions at about a five-year-old level mentally and emotionally, dominates at night just as the stars come out at night when the sun goes down.

Useful and effortless tips to help you get to sleep are:

- Don't drink coffee or caffeinated drinks after lunch.
- Exercise no later than two hours before you go to bed.
- Shift into a relaxed gear about an hour before you go to sleep.
- Don't watch exciting sports shows or adrenaline-surging movies right before bed.
- Keep your room cool (about 68 degrees) and dark.
- If you eat before bed, eat lightly (e.g., a small bowl of cereal).
- Read something light and inspirational right before you go to sleep. Reading to your child may also help you get to sleep. Pull out an oldie but goody, such as, *The Little Engine that Could.*
- Use "emotional pacifiers" that worked on you as a child. Like, "I think I can; Everything is going to be OK; I have high hopes; Somewhere over the rainbow; When you wish upon a star; Time heals all wounds, Let go and let God; Love conquers all; Sticks and stones may break my bones but names will never hurt me; In one ear and out the other; Like water off a duck's back; Don't cry over spilled milk; Now I lay me down to sleep. . ., etc." It is amazing how these words of comfort said years ago by your loved ones can be revived to help you now. I would not recommend using your personal "emotional pacifiers" on other adults or saying them aloud.

If you don't have pleasant dreams try the following:

- Dismiss unpleasant dreams about work as just that, harmless, unformed thoughts. Bad dreams are to the brain, what Charlie-Horses (cramps) are to your muscles . . . , just a reaction to "overuse" or inadequate blood supply.
- Have pleasant dreams "at will."
- Go to sleep at the sound of the beach. More on becoming your own dreamweaver follows.

---

1. When sleepworking, dismiss unpleasant dreams about work as just that, harmless, unformed thoughts.

Try to remember you are only using half-a-mind. The right brain often apprehends (fears) while the left brain comprehends (understands and solves).

---

2. Have pleasant dreams, "at will."

You can actually direct your own dreams. If awakened at night, remember an enjoyable time or pleasant experience. Taking a few deep breaths may help you relax. Turn up the visual imagery of this pleasant dream experience. Make this experience as sensuous as possible, and add on pleasant features. It helps to review a pleasant experience before falling off to sleep, or you can watch a pleasant movie or read a pleasant book. You can make yourself the hero or heroine in your "dream replay."

3. Go to sleep at the sound of the beach.

Natural sounds are naturally relaxing. Hearing the soothing sounds of crashing waves with seagulls may lull you to sleep. Many radio-alarm clocks now feature nature sounds that turn off automatically after a preset time. Perhaps listening to chirping crickets, a running brook or other sounds will soothe you to sleep.

Bob, with dark circles under his eyes and looking like he hadn't slept in days, confided in his friend during his break at work. Bob said, "Like Hal, the uncooperative computer in the movie, 2001, the computer side of my brain refused to shut down, forcing me to be working on work even though I was trying to sleep. My mind kept going over the problem like a broken record, refusing to let me sleep. I was sleepworking instead of sleepwalking."

Irritable bowel syndrome; the bottom line of stress symptoms

Marcus Aurelius, the famous Roman philosopher and warrior king, said most people are mean out of ignorance. He started his very important book, *Meditations,* by saying, "Thanks" to everyone who helped him get control over his temper (p. 9, 1991, translation). His A-number one message to any reader down through the centuries was that before you can do anything useful, get a grip on your temper, first. He provided this advice as a guide to what he considered an "uncertain world," about 2,000 years ago.

Being irritable is ignorant and abnormal. To put it in 21st century terms, being irritable is as abnormal as the medical disease, irritable bowel syndrome (IBS). IBS is often just a physical manifestation of mental irritability. You can substitute many words in the IBS syndrome; for example IBS could be used (jokingly) to stand for irritable boy syndrome. Variations on the B in IBS bring up many interesting combinations (e.g., irritable braggart syndrome, irritable bore syndrome, irritable bigmouth syndrome). How many substitutions for the B in IBS can you come up with? Remember it's just for fun.

You may even know an adult who could be the "poster-child" for IBS (irritable blank syndrome), but be certain you are not the "poster-child" for IBS. You can avoid being the office IBS "poster-child" by complaining less than the next person. Suffering from medically diagnosed IBS is no joke unless you enjoy having diarrhea, abdominal pain and bloating. (Always see your doctor first). A leading cause of physical IBS is psychological stress; a leading cure for IBS is relaxing after eating according to the layman's *Medical Advisor* (1996). Harvard's Herbert Benson, M.D., who coined the "relaxation response," supports this advice (pp. 498-499).

SUMMARY

Anger, worry, headaches and sleeplessness can dominate and ruin our lives when we start to take stress personally. These symptoms are warning lights on our dashboard, warning us to slow down, take it easy, become stress-intelligent.

The why's and how-to's of dealing with these increasing modern maladies are provided in this chapter. The main idea is to ease back and try to relax. Basically, use the principle: "When upset-reset," discussed earlier in the book.

You can gain quick results within a short period of time, just by recognizing you are suffering from anger hangovers, which in turn can cause headaches and sleeplessness. Worry is the mother lode of stress. If you can work with worry, you will be able to rise above your problems, as Einstein suggested. Thirteen tips to deal with worry are provided in this chapter, including the use of tried but true "emotional pacifiers," which are heart-warming words your loved ones used to soothe you as a child. Using just a few of these stress-intelligent tips will help you prevent stress from getting under your skin (internalizing stress, like jumping on a hand grenade to "save" others). IBS or irritable bowel syndrome is when stress affects your physical bottom line. How not to become an IBS "poster-child" is presented.

The final chapter leads into the kind of "final chapter" we all hope to experience. This "final chapter" is about aging gracefully. The rewards and stresses of aging are discussed. We should face aging with "an attitude of gratitude," considering the cold facts our cave-dwelling ancestors lived to be about 18 years-old on average and that in 1900 the average life span, without today's medical advances, was 47. Infant mortality was 50%. If you are nearing or beyond 47, be grateful that you are on extended warranty! If you are 23 or older, be thankful you are not middle-aged (by 1900 standards).

FOR FURTHER READING

Coleman, P.W. (1989). *The forgiving marriage, resolving anger and resentment and rediscovering each other.* Chicago: Contemporary Books.

Craig, B., & Brandreth, G.D. (1981). *Amazing facts about the body.* Garden City, New York: Doubleday.

Keep Your Cool. Marco Products, Inc. 1443 Old York Road, Warminster, PA. 18974. Phone 1-800-448-2197.

Long, G. (1991). *Meditations - translated by George Long - Marcus Aurelius; Great Books in Philosophy.* (Buffalo, New York: Prometheus Books).

Piper, W. (1930). *The little engine that could.* New York: Platt & Munk Publishers.

Williams, R. (2000). *Lifeskills.* New York: Times Books.

22

The Young and the Rest of US

The Little Engine that Could - Adjust

You will never ever be younger than you are today - Enjoy this day.

Just the facts: Face aging with "an attitude of gratitude," considering that our cave-dwelling ancestors lived to be about 18 years-old on average, and that in 1900 the average life span, without today's medical advances, was 47. Infant mortality in 1900 was 50%. If you are nearing or beyond 47, be grateful that you are on extended warranty! If you are 23 or older, be thankful you are not middle-aged (by 1900 standards) or over-the-hill by cave-man standards.

In this chapter we will look at:

- The benefits of entering your golden years.
- Differing and common concerns for men and women:
  - Career focus,
  - Health issues,
  - Learning to live well with chronic illness.
- Being orphaned at 55, being widowed at 75. Dealing with loss.
- Tips on how to adjust to being among "The Rest of Us" (40 PLUS) including memory loss.

1. The benefits of entering your golden years.

To begin with, there are several advantages accompany aging. The elderly:

- Are less irritated by things,
- Become reflective,
- Grow wiser,
- Spend less time worrying and fighting,
- Improve mental performance especially in job-related and verbal skills,
- Report positive life satisfaction.

2. Differing concerns for men and women.

Career focus. Men in their fifties often reach their professional peak, with an eager eye toward retirement. Sadly, many in their fifties are put out to pasture, against their will. This is called "marginalizing." It means one is pushed so far to the edge of the margin at work, they quit. By contrast, women, after completing their child-raising work, often become interested in entering the work force or improving skills.

Health issues

Many women, as much as 50-85%, will experience mild menopausal symptoms. Many women actually become more energetic and assertive after menopause. The fear of sudden death from heart attacks surfaces for men in their fifties, as increasing numbers in their age ranks "fallout." Women are often concerned about being widowed.

It's a true gift to have time, money and health all at once.

Learning to live well with chronic illness

You can live a fulfilling life despite chronic illness by 1) joining a support group, 2) reinforcing your self-esteem, and 3) doing all you can to manage your condition. A very useful book on dealing with chronic illnesses is by Susan Milstrey Wells, *A Delicate Balance: Living Successfully with Chronic Illness,* (2000, Perseus Books.)

---

3. Being orphaned at 55, being widowed at 75. Dealing with loss.

Work with your local hospice, church, clinic, or call United Way to get help. Most funeral enterprises can connect you with ways to cope with loss. There is no reason to try to handle it on your own. It could shorten your life by years if you grieve beyond a certain point. Think of the loved ones you would leave behind by not taking care of yourself.

Remember that things may actually never get better, but with strength of will, you can become better. We can't control how things turn out, but we can control our thinking about how things turn out.

Dr. Victor Frankl writes about "tragic optimism" in the face of complete loss. A concentration camp survivor, he lost his father, mother, brother and wife to the concentration camps. This Vienna-trained medical doctor (neurology) with a Ph.D. in philosophy, forged his Logo-Therapy in the crucible of the Auschwitz and Dachau concentration camps.

If the book fits, read it. That is, Dr. Frankl's book offers hope to the hopeless. If there are still many rays of hope in your life, get strength from those factors. When hope seems lost, get professional help and read portions of Dr. Frankl's book. He proves over and over again that you can rise above your circumstances and you can change your attitude when you can't change your circumstances. Ask your mental-health professional to help you sift through the sometimes-complex lingo used in Dr. Frankl's book. The fact remains, if you need proof and the how to in getting through life's roughest spots, give this book a try. Again, if the book fits, read it. Survivors of the 2001 World Trade Center and Pentagon destruction may relate to Dr. Frankl's writing about hope and help during disaster.

Things may never be better in terms of permanent loss of loved ones, health or career. But you can become better, thus the saying, "Things aren't better but I am."

A very valuable resource for dealing with major life-altering health problems is *A Whole New Life — An Illness and a Healing* (Atheneum, New York, 1994), by Duke English professor, Dr. Reynolds Price. In this helpful autobiographical book, he provides a vivid account of his struggle with spinal column cancer that put him in a wheelchair. His insights would be most uplifting to those suffering from any catastrophic illness or accident.

Immediately relieving life's pain and suffering: advice from the Roman battlefield

Marcus Aurelius, one of the "good" Roman Emperors and one of the wisest men ever, said, "Pain is neither intolerable nor everlasting if you add nothing to it in imagination." He went on to say, "Neither the future nor the past pains you, but only the present . . . but this (pain in the present) is reduced to very little. Scold your mind if it is unable to hold out against even this." An excellent resource on how to keep chronic pain in its place is *Managing Pain Before It Manages You,* by Margaret Caudill, M.D., and Ph.D., Dartmouth Medical School. See "For Further Reading" for more information.

---

4. Tips on how to adjust to being among "The Rest of Us" (40 PLUS).

"The young and the rest of us" is a humorous phrase that reflects the age make-up of our modern society. This "young and the rest of us" slice of the pie is getting bigger. Seventy-six-million baby boomers have now joined the 40 to 50 year-old ranks. Early adulthood spans ages 20 to 40 years. In fact the entire baby boomer generation is rushing into the "rest of us" camp. Ten-thousand baby boomers a day are turning fifty and entering what has been called the "second adulthood." One of these baby boomers was already President, sending a clear message that the "young old" are becoming establishment. Even Bob Dylan, a legendary singer appealing to rebellious "youth," just turned 60 years-old on May 24, 2001. George Harrison, one of the "fab four" Beatles, died at age 58 on November 29, 2001, at a friend's house. He had battled cancer for three years.

Our society is aging, but gracefully. An individual's chances of living beyond 65 are four times greater than they were in 1900. Proper nutrition, exercise and medical attention are improving both the quantity and quality of our lives.

According to Dr. Ken Levinson, the mid-forties are visited by emotional turmoil. The struggle with shifting self-concept, career status, and body image is intensified during the mid-fifties. A 50th birthday party is typically unmatched in importance (and size) and confirms the arrival of middle age. The final symbol of middle age is undeniably sealed with grandparenthood.

Nine tips to deal with aging:

1. Using it or losing it — your memory.

As stated previously, mental abilities can actually increase as we age if we use our skills. Problems with memory and computation result more from lack of practice than change in our physical thinking equipment. Ninety-five percent of elderly DO NOT experience Alzheimer's disease. **"An idle mind is the devil's playground" (And that devil is Alzheimers).**

A recent article (June 2000) revealed that the best way to remember what you read or do is to concentrate on what you are doing or reading. Learning to concentrate on your breathing, discussed earlier, will improve your overall concentrating ability and therefore your memory. Also, repeating to yourself, silently, what you have just done (i.e., I turned off the stove, brought in the dog) will help you remember later that you did turn off the stove or brought in the dog.

Using it or losing it — Your memory. Go to Chapter 17, Scoring Best on All Life's Tests by Using Your "Whole Brain." A normal memory problem occurs when you can't remember where you put your keys. A serious memory problem happens when you can't recall what your keys are used for. In either case, you should go see your doctor.

Simple memory boosters include:

a. "The palest ink is better than the best memory," so put it in writing. Write notes to yourself. If you have to, use hyper notes (those small yellow notes that allow you to cover an entire desktop or refrigerator with reminders). Leave messages to yourself on your answering machine. Like location, location, location, remember, repetition, repetition, repetition.

b. Play with your brain, that is, keep your brain in tune by playing games.

Bridge the gap. One of the brightest people this author knows plays bridge youthfully and expertly, yet technically qualifies for AARP membership. *Games* magazine is great, which emphasizes word play. Maybe the *New York Times* crossword puzzle is not your style, but any crossword puzzle will do. You can even get crossword puzzles that deal with your hobby interest. Even playing checkers exercises your brain better than playing your TV remote.

c. Remember the old saying, "A place (and time) for everything and everything in its place." It may be boring, but learn to routinely put your keys (and wallet, etc.) in one place. That will be one less thing you have to remember.

d. Tell jokes to tested audiences, like your best friends. This requires timing and remembering the punch line. If you can't remember punch lines, write them down.

e. Communicate. If you are not computer phobic, join a chat room. There are even chat rooms devoted exclusively to standard poodle lovers. Get on the Internet, or write letters to your friends, using snail mail.

Take up a course that has nothing to do with what you have to do, but something you want to do (painting, coin collecting). You probably don't need the extra credit but it will give you something to look forward to. Even your classmates can keep you young.

Finally ask your doctor about ginkgo, the only clinically-proven herbal remedy that shows promise in truly improving memory. As with anything strong enough to alter your brain function, it has side effects. As of January 2003, it does not have FDA approval, but ginkgo is worth checking out in terms of what dosage (perhaps 120 mg or more daily) might be right for you and the warning signs of side effects to look for. Again, do not use this potential "memory enhancer" without the supervision of

Reality Check: It's not better, but I am.

As he sat in the doctor's office, Bob was still reeling from the traumatic and unexpected loss of both his parents within a year. Tears welled up in Bob's eyes as the team of doctors with clipboards entered the room. Adding insult to injury, he had to wear one of those gowns with the open backside and he could feel the air-conditioned air on his exposed backside. The diagnosis was grim, and basically the chief surgeon said to Bob and his wife that things are never going to get better. What Bob and his wife "heard at that moment" was that things are going to go from bad to worse with no hope for recovery.

Although not a terminal illness, adjusting to the self-administered medical procedure for life was highly distressing. The lead doctor calmly stated that this medical condition would require a "major lifestyle change." What an understatement.

Weeks after this medical bombshell someone asked Bob how he was doing. Struggling to practice what he preached in terms of being positive, he blurted out, "Things are not better, but I am getting better."

your doctor. It does have physical side effects for some people including bruising.

The best review of this and other remedies (e.g., St. John's wort) is available from "Herbal remedies…" Arch. Gen. 1998; 55: 1033-1044. (Website JAMA, *Journal of the American Medical Association*).

2. Use the real "fountain of youth" to add years to your life and life to your years.

Know that the true "fountain of youth" is sweat from exercise. Following an exercise prescription from your doctor will retard the aging process, make you feel better and improve your stress-coping abilities.

3. Make today count.

The "Make Today Count" national organization focuses on helping mature but troubled adults cope with aspects of aging. As the name of the organization states, enjoy each day you are given by maintaining an "attitude of gratitude."

4. Maintain a sense of humor to maintain your sense of balance.

Laughter is a potent medicine in counteracting stress buildup. In addition to its tranquilizing effect, laughter actually stimulates internal organs, making them work better. This finding is reported in Norman Cousins' 1989 book, *Head First - The Biology of Hope,* that explores the effects of positive attitude on aging and physical health.

5. Stay informed and in tune.

Become knowledgeable about the many advances being made in how to improve the quality of your life. Contact your local hospital for newsletters focused on health promotion for seniors. Consider membership in the American Association of Retired Persons (AARP).

6. Expand your friendship horizons.

The more friends you have the less likely you will experience anxiety and mood problems. Join a morning breakfast club. Become involved in a book club, or garden club if you are so inclined. Volunteer your services at a nursing home.

7. If alone, get a pet, even a wet pet (fish).

Investigate the chances of your dog's becoming a "therapy" dog at a nursing home. Many well-behaved dogs are welcomed. Being able to see and pet a dog can lift the spirits of many of these lonely people.

8. Remember, optimism is the breakfast of champions!

Force yourself to start your day off positively. Many positive thinkers read inspirational messages the first thing in the morning. Read the short poem, "Values," provided at the conclusion of this chapter, prior to the summary. It is short but powerful.

9. The Eden Alternative: Improving quality of life in elder-care.

A new philosophy and method of elder-care have been found to be effective in reducing illness and improving quality of life for those in nursing homes. The Eden Alternative offers unique environments for the elderly, including the presence of pets, lots of sunshine and plants and of course, children. It is the dawning of a new philosophy to help those at the sunset of their lives enjoy life more. To get more information on this rapidly growing approach, contact the Eden Alternative at (607) 674-5232, Fax: (607) 674-6723, Email: <info@edenalt.com> or their Website at <www.edenalternative.com>.

VALUES

The best day . . .
Today

The greatest comfort . . .
Work well done

The greatest handicap . . .
Fear

The easiest thing to do . . .
Finding fault

The greatest mistake . . .
Giving up

The worst bankruptcy . . .
Loss of enthusiasm

The best gift . . .
Forgiveness

(As provided by June Schutzberger, former "gifted" educator
[Author unknown].)

SUMMARY

Enjoy this day, for you'll never be younger than you are today. It was brought to light that our cave-dwelling ancestors lived to be about eighteen-years-old, on average, and that in 1900, the average life span, without today's medical advances, was 47. This "final chapter," looked at three major "aging" concerns for men and women. Six advantages of aging were identified. Nine tips on how to adjust to being among "The Rest of Us" (40 years plus) were provided including several ways to improve your memory. Also, the only clinically-proven "herbal ingredient" which shows promise to enhance memory is revealed. A new method of eldercare, called the Eden Alternative, is presented, which appears to have had success in improving the quality of life for the elderly in a more homelike environment. A final, comforting statement is provided to help us deal with "the end."

A Parable of Immortality

By Henry Van Dyke

I am standing upon the seashore, a ship at my side spreads her white sails in the morning breeze, and starts for the ocean blue.

She is an object of beauty and strength, and I stand and watch her until at length she hangs like a speck of white cloud just where the sea and sky come down to mingle with each other.

Then someone at my side says, "There, she's gone." Gone where? Gone from my sight — that is all.

She is just as large in mast and hull and spar as she was when she left my side, and just as able to bear her load of living freight to the place of her destination.

Her diminished size is in me, not in her, and just at the moment when someone at my side says, "There she's gone," there are other eyes watching her coming, and other voices ready to take up the glad shout, "There she comes."

That is dying.

FOR FURTHER READING

Caudill, M.A. (2001). *Managing pain before it manages you.* New York: Guilford Publications. <www.guilford.com> or Phone 1-800-365-7006.

Cousins, N. (1989). *Head first - the biology of hope.* New York: Dutton.

Eden Alternative at (607) 674-5232, Fax: (607) 674-6723, Internet – <info@edenalt.com> or their Website at <www.edenalternative.com>.

Levinson, K. (1978). *Seasons of a man's life.* New York: Knopf.

Price, R. (1994). *A whole new life - an illness and a healing.* New York: Atheneum.

Wells, S.M. (1998). *A delicate balance: living successfully with chronic illness.* New York: Insight Book.

Wong, H.C.; Smith, M.; & Boon, H.S. (1998, November). Herbal remedies in psychiatric practice. *Archives of General Psychiatry* 55. 11. pp. 1033-1044.

APPENDIX A

ONE-MINUTE ANTI-STRESS FACT SHEET ©

(Crib Sheets of the Complete Chapters)

Dr. Ronald L. Rubenzer, 2003

From: *How the Best Handle Stress*

This educational material is not intended in any way to be a substitute for professional treatment (psychological, counseling, medical) and should be used in addition to prescribed regimens. For classroom use: Enlarge the selected One-Minute Fact Sheet. Make transparency on topic. For counseling, give a copy of original sized Anti-Stress Skill-Builder Sheet for "homework."

Chapter One
Topic: WHY MANAGE STRESS?

The top reasons why it is important to be "stress-smart" are listed below

- The pursuit of happiness is your birthright. One out of three adults feel completely overwhelmed, according to a 2001 survey.
- Stress is fattening: and it's not just in your head. One in four adults is a victim of "stress-belly."
- The good don't die young. Optimists are healthier and outlive pessimists. Cortisol kills by stressing your heart.
- Life is at least 44% more stressful in the U.S. than 30 years ago, so you have to be thick-skinned yet tenderhearted. This was prior to the 9/11/01 suicidal bombings and anthrax anxiety. Depression has increased fivefold over ten years. "Weapons of mass destruction" was the phrase of 2002.
- Stress robs a dozen years off lifespan. Unwarranted feelings of stress are neurochemical lies.
- Making strong men faint: The "nocebo" effect has been proven hazardous to your health. (*Harvard Mental Health Newsletter* defined the "nocebo" effect as the expectation of negative health outcomes. Cortisol slows physical healing.)
- IOS, "Information overload stress," is a crime in New York ($100.00 fine for driving [right brain] and using a hand-held cellular phone [left brain] at the same time).
- P.S. Avoiding a nervous breakdown when your computer has one!
- Overcoming CSA, Computer-separation-anxiety, when 55-million obsolete computers are separated from their owners.
- Thirty seconds of insight into the 21st century "Rules for the sexes" saves thirty years of stressful living.

FOR THE CHILDREN

- Fifteen-percentile point test-score increase, or a whole letter-grade improvement results from learning test-taking skills for students. (Scruggs and Mastropieri, Purdue University, 1992). This can make the difference between your child's struggling through school or enjoying satisfaction and success (even scholarships). The U.S. Senate passed a bill on June 14, 2001, requiring **all** 3rd through 8th grade students to take math and reading tests.
- Stress stupefies through performance anxiety, according to the world's smartest person. Stress may be the leading contributor to impaired academic achievement (Eric Jensen, [1990], Association for Supervision and Curriculum Development).
- Thirty percent of 8,000 high school students report they are under great stress every day.
- Conquering your urgency addiction for Type A's, Type T's (thrill-seekers) and even some ADHD individuals.
- The shooter's stress syndrome: recognizing the warning signs in others who are about "ready to snap."
- The Character Education initiative depends on stress management.
- High-risk male stress syndrome: The triple threat to aggress under stress.
- Copy-cat suicidal/homicidal acts among youth is on the rise. Fifteen-year-old, ninth grader flies plane into building.

ONE-MINUTE ANTI-STRESS SKILL-BUILDERS ©

Dr. Ronald L. Rubenzer, 2003

From: *How the Best Handle Stress*

This educational material is not intended in any way to be a substitute for professional treatment (psychological, counseling, medical) and should be used in addition to prescribed regimens.

Chapter Two

Topic: ASSESS YOUR STRESS: Your Relaxation Quotient (RQ)

What is your RQ? Take the test

Your relax-a-bility quotient or RQ, is simply how well you can relax when it counts the most, under challenging circumstances. You will enjoy the personal, professional and health benefits of being able to relax by increasing your relax-a-bility. Below are the "dozen do's" of relax-a-bility. Take this brief quiz to determine your RQ. The more "yes'es" you have, the higher your RQ. The higher your RQ the longer and better you will probably live, if you also live a healthy lifestyle. (Always see your mental-health professionals for scientific assessment of emotional symptoms.)

YOU HAVE A HIGH RQ (Your RQ Quotient)

1. If you maintain a positive, can-do attitude, even on Mondays, and you usually do not complain much. [YES NO]
2. If you look forward to enjoying healthy pleasures daily. [YES NO]
3. If you generally feel in control of your life and trust that the future will turn out positively. [YES NO]
4. If you worry little, but work a lot, to patiently solve problems without feeling overwhelmed or impatient. [YES NO]
5. If you can relax enough under pressure to fully concentrate on what you are doing (phone calls, public speaking, taking tests, conflict, deadlines, and evaluations). [YES NO]
6. If you can accept, act and adjust appropriately to rudeness, mistakes, conflict, criticism and major changes. [YES NO]
7. If you know how and when to vent pent-up stress, resentment and anger (not ranting/raving at bad drivers, not unleashing fury at innocent loved ones, pets, etc.) [YES NO]
8. If you sleep with ease and generally feel energetic. [YES NO]
9. If you are generally headache/stomachache free. [YES NO]
10. If you can self-calm when faced with frustration, frenzy, or fear, using humor to keep your cool. [YES NO]
11. If you can fully live separate personal/professional lives, (not dragging shop talk home). [YES NO]
12. If you can "get-ready, get-set, and flow, powering-up your "second wind" to flexibly meet surprises and challenges. [YES NO]

ONE-MINUTE ANTI-STRESS FACT SHEET ©

Dr. Ronald L. Rubenzer, 2003

From: *How the Best Handle Stress*

This educational material is not intended in any way to be a substitute for professional treatment (psychological, counseling, medical) and should be used in addition to prescribed regimens.

Chapter Two
Topic: YOUR RELAXATION QUOTIENT (RQ)

She is wound up tighter than a cuckoo clock
And sadly
She goes off every fifteen minutes.

WHAT IS AN RQ (RELAX-A-BILITY QUOTIENT)?

Your RQ or relax-a-bility quotient is the portion of time you can relax under stressful situations. If you can calm yourself while waiting in endless lines you probably have a high RQ.

WHY IS YOUR RQ SO VITALLY IMPORTANT?

Benefits of a high RQ

Enjoy better relationships. High RQ improves your relationships because you are more likely to patiently listen to, accept and accurately act upon what an upset person is actually saying and feeling. High RQ people have more friends and get along better at work.

Become more promotable. Workers who are more relaxed and approachable are more desirable as leaders. Co-workers feel more comfortable communicating and cooperating with outwardly relaxed leaders.

Enjoy better health. Having a good RQ is so important that leading health insurance companies spend millions promoting stress management. And why? Because both you and the insurance companies win. Relaxing makes you healthier and the insurance companies wealthier. The insurance companies benefit from your making fewer unneeded visits to the doctor. (Stress symptoms can indicate the need for medical attention, so always see your doctor first for best treatment of anxiety).

Improved memory. Marilyn vos Savant, who possesses the world's highest-recorded IQ, states that performance anxiety occurs when you forget frequently used numbers (important dates, social security number, etc.) under pressure. She suggests relaxing to improve your memory.

Raising test scores by lowering test anxiety. The ability to wait (self-calming under stress) at four years of age was related to scoring 210 points higher on the SAT at high school compared to other high-schoolers who could not self-calm or wait at the age of four. Self-calming students were also more popular and well liked than impulsive students.

In a clinical study conducted at Columbia University, it was also discovered that students, scientifically taught to reduce their test anxiety, improved their performance on both IQ and creativity tests.

What is your RQ? *Take the test (See Skill-Builders, Chapter 2).*

ONE-MINUTE ANTI-STRESS SKILL-BUILDERS ©

Dr. Ronald L. Rubenzer, 2003

From: *How the Best Handle Stress*

This educational material is not intended in any way to be a substitute for professional treatment (psychological, counseling, medical) and should be used in addition to prescribed regimens.

Chapter Three
Topic: GAUGING YOUR STRESS. Are you speeding?

ISR (Inventory of Stress Responses, developed 1997, Switzerland, World Congress on Stress)

Simply answer YES if any part of each question applies to you. Total the number of YES answers, and place this score in the space provided. See the end of the inventory for the meaning of your YES score.

If you feel too pressed for time to take this survey, you REALLY need stress management!

1. Do you often feel angry, impatient or aggravated at yourself or others? EXAMPLES: You blame, complain, nag, boss, argue a lot or have anger hangovers (stay mad overnight, hold grudges). [YES] [NO]

2. Do you usually get very upset when you have to wait for things or people? EXAMPLES: You are impatient standing in line, waiting at stop signals. You often interrupt or finish people's sentences, complete their work or become quite upset when people are late. [YES] [NO]

3. Do you expect others or yourself to do everything perfectly? EXAMPLES: You get uptight when things don't go as planned or have a lot of regrets about bad mistakes (You should have done better; why didn't you?). You never seem to get things "clean enough," organized or planned enough. [YES] [NO]

4. Do you often feel "pushed around" by life, overwhelmed by all you have to do? EXAMPLES: I have to do everything, everyone else tells you what to do, or you never have enough time to catch up. [YES] [NO]

5. Do you like to do most things fast? EXAMPLES: You usually finish eating before everyone else. Like to drive fast, take shortcuts to get things done. You are usually early for things. [YES] [NO]

6. Do you often have sweaty palms, headaches/stomachaches, irregularity, heart palpitations, shortness of breath, vague pains or feel tired? EXAMPLE: You've had an exam revealing no medical reason for your complaints. [YES] [NO]

7. Do you worry a lot about things that often turn out okay? EXAMPLES: Most of your fears are exaggerated or never happen; You spend sleepless nights worrying. [YES] [NO]

8. Do you often make mistakes, forget or lose things because you're so busy? EXAMPLES: You're accident prone, clumsy, or feel your memory is not as good as it used to be. [YES] [NO]

9. Do you binge when under pressure? EXAMPLES: You overdo one or more of the following: eating, smoking, drinking, sleeping, watching TV, shopping, talking on the phone, gossiping. [YES] [NO]

10. Do you put off things or avoid certain situations? EXAMPLES: You're afraid you'll be embarrassed or you'll panic under pressure. You get very nervous over such things as math tests, being evaluated by your boss, working with computers, public speaking, crowds, high places, making phone calls. [YES] [NO]

11. Do you have nervous habits? EXAMPLES: You chew your nails, clear your throat, have tightly clenched fists, lock your legs and arms, run your hands through your hair, walk fast, gesture a lot when talking, sigh, frown, or clench your teeth. [YES] [NO]

12. Do you feel you are in a rut or are generally frustrated? EXAMPLES: You feel bored with the same old routine, experiencing little joy or excitement in life. [YES] [NO]

Total YES Score _____

Harvard Medical School. (January, 2003). Generalized anxiety disorder: Toxic worry. *Harvard Mental Health Letter*. Volume 19, Number 7. Author. <www.healthharvard.edu>.

ONE-MINUTE ANTI-STRESS FACT SHEET ©

Dr. Ronald L. Rubenzer, 2003

From: *How the Best Handle Stress*

This educational material is not intended in any way to be a substitute for professional treatment (psychological, counseling, medical) and should be used in addition to prescribed regimens.

Chapter Three
Topic: GAUGING YOUR STRESS. Are you speeding?

"Understanding lets me do by choice what others do out of fear."
- Aristotle

- What your ISR (Inventory of Stress Responses) YES score means. This was the survey on the previous page to look at symptoms only. It is not designed to be a clinical instrument. See your mental-health professional for clinical assessment using DSM-IV criteria or a validated, reliable scientific instrument. The higher your YES score, the more life's pressures are getting to you. The lower your YES score, the better you are at handling your stress. Stress management helps you lower your unpleasant stress reactions so you'll enjoy life more. Only Mother Teresa would probably have a score of zero "yes'es." The fictional, funny sheriff from Mayberry R.F.D., Barney Fife, would be a good example of someone with a YES score on the ISR of 12. The average score is about 9. As in golf, you should aim to have a lower score.
- Are you speeding? (Going ninety miles an hour in a 35 mph zone on mountain curves, [12 on the ISR]).
- Too much stress is like racing a car with no steering wheel, you will eventually careen out of control and crash into the wall.
- "Squeaky-wheel," "Old Faithful," "Mt. St. Helens," "Paddling Duck" — What's your stress-style? Which style is best?
- Sex and stress: Males tend to respond to anxiety with aggression, females with compassion.

ONE-MINUTE ANTI-STRESS FACT SHEET ©

Dr. Ronald L. Rubenzer, 2003

From: *How the Best Handle Stress*

This educational material is not intended in any way to be a substitute for professional treatment (psychological, counseling, medical) and should be used in addition to prescribed regimens.

Chapter Three
Topic: ADD, ADHD OR JUST ABB: Always bored/baffled

- Always see a qualified medical doctor or a clinical psychologist first if you suspect your child has ADD or ADHD. The best flag for ADD/ADHD is that the person always acts before he thinks, never follows instructions, interrupts, doesn't listen, takes on way too much and jumps from one task to the other, doing none of them very well, even if the activity is highly interesting. This is great if you work in a circus, and that's about all.
- ADD, ADHD are born, not made. ADHD/ADD adults are often merely labeled tireless, or actually called "Type T "(for thrill-seekers) for those who are pleasantly stimulated by a gush of incoming information. If there is not any trouble, they go look for it. Chances are many of the brave souls first coming to America had clinical levels of ADHD or ADD. However, untreated but diagnosed ADD/ADHD adults usually don't shine so brightly and without help, have difficult lives (far more likely to end up in institutions, be fined, fired, divorced, etc.). Many older but newly-diagnosed ADD folks are grateful to find out why life choices may be more difficult for them or why they own ten weed-wackers and are told they never listen.
- White flags on the fairway. True ADHD/ADD cases are clear. It's almost like a huge racing car with no steering wheel. Plenty of power, but they can't keep it on the road. To determine if the person won't vs. can't stay on the road, clinically eliminate the neurological reasons (which are brain based and hard-wired) before seeking non-medical treatment for ADD or ADHD. Brain-based hyperactivity, impulsivity or attentional problems require long-term medical and behavioral intervention, affecting only about six out of one-hundred people. (See the book, *Attention-deficit hyperactivity disorder, a handbook for diagnosis and treatment.* New York: Guildford, 1998, by Dr. Russell Barkley, a world leader in ADD/ADHD). Dr. Russell A. Barkley's monthly report: ADHD report (October, 2000) is a must read for concerned individuals.
- Again, only your medical doctors or (in North Carolina) your clinical psychologists are qualified to label and treat ADD, ADHD. If others tell you your child is ADD or ADHD, they are just guessing. The standard checklist for the school and the home is the "Conners' Checklist" available at most schools. Have an educational assessment to pinpoint the child's learning strengths/needs and interests. This educational assessment can be performed by a licensed or certified psychologist.

- "FIRE-READY-AIM" is the motto for those who can't vs. won't wait to take aim at what they want from life. They buy things they regret getting later. Whether the person can't vs. won't control his/her behavior, the sad results are about the same. In school it is the child who never checks his spelling in his assignment, or who answers the question even before it was completely given. On the road it's the guy who really steps on the gas pedal when the light clearly says slow down. These are your aggressive drivers. AAD/ADHD or ABB join motorcycle rallies and they simply act, then think. ADD/ADHD often act on impulse, often without remorse or regret. ABB (bored or baffled) knew that the graffiti they put up, or purse they snatched was wrong before they performed the act. The "multitasking" New Yorker will still get the same $100.00 fine for talking on his hand-held cellular phone while driving whether he is diagnosed as ADHD or not. The bottom line is the fire-ready-aim sequence must be turned around, whether it be through medical/behavior means (ADHD, ADD) or psychological/counseling needs. The world will be a better place with the person who is clearly in the driver's seat.
- ABB or Dysactivity, which is a fancy word for being inattentive/ overactive/impulsive due to just plain boredom or being baffled. "Information overload stress" should be considered as causing inattention/overactivity/impulsivity only after confirmation that the individual does not have ADD or ADHD. ADD/ADHD is a newcomer, popular diagnosis. ADD/ADHD diagnosis is barely a generation old, meaning that some adults may have ADD/ADHD (6%); but properly harnessed, these people can be the chomping-at-the-bit race horses of society, taking risks most people would not. But then again, the untreated ADD/ADHD "absent-minded professor" is humorous, but the absent-minded surgeon or pilot is not funny at all. Check with your local ADD/ADHD support group for information or support.
- An individual may just have ABB (Always bored or baffled) because the environment is not interesting enough or is too challenging. The average classroom teacher has to accommodate about a six-grade-level spread of skills. (In a third grade classroom there may be a gifted child capable of sixth grade work, or a child may be delayed to the pre-first grade skill level.)
- Treating an anxiety disorder with ADHD prescriptions will make an anxiety (stress) disorder worse! Emotional disorders are much more frequent than ADD/ADHD. Seek qualified professional assessment, usually an M.D. or clinical psychologist. (It is beyond the scope of this work to go into the combinations of ADD/ADHD/emotional disorders.)
- Some tips that may be useful whether the individual has ADD/ADD or just plain ABB (Always bored or baffled) include: Time management, Stress management, Desk management, Exercise, Communication skills, Memory boosters [Chapter 17]). See below for additional brain-training activities.

ONE-MINUTE ANTI-STRESS SKILL-BUILDERS ©

Dr. Ronald L. Rubenzer, 2003

From: *How the Best Handle Stress*

This educational material is not intended in any way to be a substitute for professional treatment (psychological, counseling, medical) and should be used in addition to prescribed regimens.

Chapter Three
Topic: ADD, ADHD OR JUST ABB: Always bored/baffled

Tips to improve work/study skills

SUGGESTIONS TO HELP INDIVIDUALS DEVELOP CONCENTRATION/ STUDY SKILLS (DIAGNOSED OR SUSPECTED ADHD)

- Increase individual's concentration time. Encouragement will be needed to build up the amount of time individuals can concentrate without a break. Even setting a timer inside a drawer (so he can hear it go off without hearing it ticking) would be helpful. Fifty minutes is the average adult attention span.
- Develop a work/study routine for individual. Have individual pick a set time and place to study on a daily schedule.
- Keep individual's work/study environment relatively quiet to help him improve his concentration. Individual may benefit from soft background music. During individual's work time, reduce interruptions by taking messages if needed, and keeping others from disturbing individual.
- Have individual keep all his work assignments in one folder.
- Have individual use a proven study system. Try having individual underline important material, or information he does not understand. Use the **SQ3R®** method, which stands for **S**can the reading assignment (looking at headings, graphs, summaries); **Q**uestion, that is, make up a question to keep in mind as individual reads; **R**ead, to answer the questions individual made up, then **R**ecite the answers without looking at the assignment, and finally **R**eview the material to be certain individual's notes are organized and the major ideas are understood.
- Teach individual how to plan ahead. Have individual write down, on a large planning calendar, major tasks or assignments that are due and tests/reviews that are coming up. Determine how much time each day, for how many days/weeks will be needed to get in the appropriate study time. Six hours a day is considered the maximum learning time most adults can tolerate.
- Have individual set his own goals. Individual should write down what grade or goal he wants to shoot for and how much time it would take to do well on the project or test. Individual's supervisor/teacher would be best at determining how much time it would take to accomplish a certain grade or project.

- Reward individual for achieving steps. Congratulate individual for keeping up with his planning calendar and sticking to his schedule. Provide snacks; allow him to call his friends, etc., to reward his efforts and success in developing and sticking to his study schedule.
- If you have access to a computer, use the built-in calendar program (e.g., Outlook) which provides a convenient way to plan daily, monthly and yearly. The program provides gentle reminders of tasks to be completed without nagging.

ONE-MINUTE ANTI-STRESS SKILL-BUILDERS ©
Dr. Ronald L. Rubenzer, 2003
From: *How the Best Handle Stress*

This educational material is not intended in any way to be a substitute for professional treatment (psychological, counseling, medical) and should be used in addition to prescribed regimens.

Chapter Three
Topic: ADD, ADHD OR JUST ABB: Always bored/baffled

TIPS to help students pay attention and complete tasks

To help teachers and parents help children with attentional problems. (Only a medical doctor or clinical psychologist can diagnose ADHD.) (From Harvard Medical School: *Harvard Mental Health Letter,* p. 2, Sept. 2000.)

The use of any of these tips is completely up to the discretion of educational personnel.

- Place individual in front of the classroom, near the teacher.
- Provide individual with:

  Close monitoring,

  Predictable schedules,

  Constant feedback,

  Tangible rewards and reprimands,

  Posted rules,

  Brief study periods,

  Repeated directions.
- Spare individual from having to take timed tests as much as possible.
- Flashcards, outlines, and underlining text may help individual.
- Individual should be encouraged to notice and record when he has not been paying attention.

What adults can do to help individual

- Provide clear rules for individual.
- Have a clear division of responsibility between parents (legal guardians) who should present a united front.
- Write out complaints about individual's behavior but praise good behavior immediately.
- Know the signs that individual is going to lose self-control.
- Try to balance their attention among children in the family.

SHORT-TERM MEMORY

- Make material to be remembered emotional and meaningful.
- Hold seven units of memory in short-term. Teach him to chunk information.
- Teach student to relax when listening (relaxation increases short-term memory).
- Teach mnemonics (USA stands for United States of America, etc.).
- Have pupil repeat directions back to teacher.
- Make eye contact.
- Repeat directions to individual students as needed.

Teaching tips for anti-boredom "whole-brain" approach to curriculum, (From *Educating the Other Half:* Rubenzer & Rubenzer, 1981) — See p. 207 in text.

ONE-MINUTE ANTI-STRESS SKILL-BUILDERS ©

Dr. Ronald L. Rubenzer, 2003

From: *How the Best Handle Stress*

This educational material is not intended in any way to be a substitute for professional treatment (psychological, counseling, medical) and should be used in addition to prescribed regimens.

Chapter Four
Topic: WHY INDUSTRIAL-STRENGTH STRESS CONTROL?

Are you part of the solution, or part of the problem?

EFFECTIVE JOB-STRESS MANAGEMENT HABITS CHECKLIST

Do you consistently?

1. Foster a "we attitude" rather than a "me attitude." [YES] [NO]
2. Know/do what your supervisor wants. [YES] [NO]
3. Encourage communication/trust. [YES] [NO]
4. Practice clutter management. [YES] [NO]
5. Employ consistent (daily, weekly) time management. [YES] [NO]
6. Walk at break/take legitimate breaks. [YES] [NO]
7. Use a relaxation technique (Wall Street Business professionals use relaxation breathing).* [YES] [NO]
8. Deal with difficult people/conflict effectively. [YES] [NO]
9. Use problem solving/conflict resolution. [YES] [NO]
10. Engage in professional development. [YES] [NO]

GRADE YOURSELF (SIMPLY ADD UP YOUR YES SCORES)

9-10 GRADE = A - Model employee, leader

7-8 GRADE = B - Keep up the good work

5-6 GRADE = C - Need improvement

3-4 GRADE = D - Re-examine priorities

0-2 GRADE = F - Retrain, get help

*On February 7, 2001, CNN, with an audience of 22 million, recognized the *Freeze-Framer*™ program by HEARTMATH as so effective it significantly reduces stress in teachers, students, and even policemen. Call Heartmath, 1-800-372-3100 or email: <info@heartmath.com>. This enjoyable, but highly accurate and effective biofeedback product makes relaxation training fun and fast in almost any setting, business, school, counseling setting or home.)

ATTACKING ANXIETY has been used by over 500,000 people over 17 years. It has been recently proven to clinically reduce anxiety, according to January, 2000 issue of the *Journal of Clinical Psychology,* Vol. 56 (1), 11-21, 2000, Call 1-800-944-9428. This is a cognitive-behavioral management program. In some cases, individual insurance companies, EAP's and even workers' compensation have paid for the program. Contact <www.stresscenter.com>. Always see your doctor before beginning any anxiety management program.

ONE-MINUTE ANTI-STRESS FACT SHEET ©

Dr. Ronald L. Rubenzer, 2003

From: *How the Best Handle Stress*

This educational material is not intended in any way to be a substitute for professional treatment (psychological, counseling, medical) and should be used in addition to prescribed regimens.

Chapter Four
Topic: WHY INDUSTRIAL-STRENGTH STRESS CONTROL?

- Many would rather quit than fight: 79% have been treated rudely: 42% verbally abused; 29% screaming mad; 23% brought to tears; 10% witnessed physical violence.
- Staff infections — how negative emotional contagion infects the whole staff.
- Excess stress reduces performance.
- The mean shall inherit the earth: Welcome to Business 101.
- Effective job-stress management habits — rate yourself (See Skill-Builders, Chapter 4).

ONE-MINUTE ANTI-STRESS FACT SHEET ©

Dr. Ronald L. Rubenzer, 2003

From: *How the Best Handle Stress*

This educational material is not intended in any way to be a substitute for professional treatment (psychological, counseling, medical) and should be used in addition to prescribed regimens.

Chapter Five
Topic: JOB-STRESS PRESCRIPTIONS: "When upset hit reset"

Don't let anyone push your buttons, especially your panic button. When they hit your panic button, hit your "reset button."

How to prevent "job rust out"

Relaxation and "working smart" provide the oil to prevent your "RUSTING OUT" on the job.

- Practice real PR (patience and relaxation) when faced with impatience from yourself or others. Remember, "Easy always does it."
- Try to do one thing at a time, "This one thing I do." You won't feel as overwhelmed and what you do will be done better.
- "Knowledge is power" over your job. Know your job, what is expected, when and how you will be evaluated.
- Seek positive co-workers. It only takes a QUARTER (25%) of a group to bring DOWN (infect) the entire job place with a negative attitude, so beware of the QUARTER DOWNER principle.
- Write it down. Trying to remember many important details creates stress. Remember: "The palest ink is better than the best memory."
- Schedule your work, work your schedule, to avoid getting swamped with unfinished work.
- DeRail unpleasant people by being *relaxed, assertive* and an *intensive listener.*
- Limit or even eliminate "pity parties." If you must have a gripe session, make it brief and try to come up with at least one possible solution.
- Take your breaks.
- Expect delays and have projects you can do while waiting.
- Do it now. Procrastination consists of excessive perfectionism, "I need just one more day," and lack of planning.
- Keep your eyes on the prize. Have pictures/reminders of past vacations, future trips, loved ones, etc., to help bring about peaceful moods.
- **REMEMBER: DON'T WORRY — WORK.**

ONE-MINUTE ANTI-STRESS FACT SHEET ©

Dr. Ronald L. Rubenzer, 2003

From: *How the Best Handle Stress*

This educational material is not intended in any way to be a substitute for professional treatment (psychological, counseling, medical) and should be used in addition to prescribed regimens.

Chapter Five
Topic: TIPS TO REDUCE JOB-STRESS: "Goal Setting"

Check each activity you do now. Unchecked items are your new goals.

PREPARATION (At home)

- Sleep about seven hours nightly.
- Use a "friendly" alarm clock (No cannons!).
- Eat a good breakfast (Low blood sugar causes stress).
- Make optimism your breakfast of champions.
- Exercise three times weekly vigorously (e.g., walk) with a responsible "motivated partner."
- Limit daily caffeine to two cups of coffee or two cans of soda.
- Maintain normal weight.
- Manage your time and budget.
- Do something fun (hobby) you have complete control over.
- Express affection with "loved ones"/socialize with friends/enjoy your pets.
- Hold a brief, informal family meeting weekly to discuss plans, victories, etc.
- Vent problems/complaints with focus on solutions.
- Get outside daily (Sunlight puts people in better moods). Allow as much sun in the house as possible.
- Home "work" should "contrast" job "work" (e.g., yard work vs. sedentary mental work).
- Take warm baths/get massaged.
- Prepare for work the night before (clothes, keys, breakfast).
- Celebrate life's "little pleasures."

CONTACT (!) (At work)

- Arrive early.
- Do the most difficult tasks first (if possible).
- Reduce "brainstrain" by writing things down.
- Focus on doing one thing well at a time.
- Smile/laugh when you can (Laughter releases the brain's natural tranquilizer).
- Challenge yourself to continually improve your job skills, job relations and assertiveness skills (if needed).

REWARD and RECORD

- Keep your eyes on the prize (tangible rewards with specific dates for meeting goals).
- Take one day at a time.
- Count up "unchecked" activities. Practice one new one per week. Check off when a habit is learned.

Daily REWARD YOURSELF.

- Maximize your physical comfort within company policy (comfortable shoes, ties, extra seat support if needed)
- Stretch for ten seconds every two hours. Focus your eyes at far distance hourly.
- Manage time, clutter and difficult people before they manage you.
- Make your work area "homey" (pictures, trophies, music).
- Practice one-minute relaxer.
- Develop trusted friends.
- Change what you can, accept what you need to, but know the difference.
- At day's end, write down tomorrow's priority plan; next day, follow the plan.
- Take breaks with positive people.
- Walk (outside) at lunch if you can.
- REMEMBER TGIE (Thank goodness I'm employed). Job hunting is very stressful.
- Listen to positive motivational tapes while driving or at home.

"STRESS BAGGAGE" — DO LEAVE HOME WITHOUT IT!

Dealing with Mondays: Hardly a fun day but ...

Mondays are rough on the nerves because you are using your "right brain at the wrong time." Try these "foods that soothe" on Monday to counteract "weekend treat withdrawal."

- A banana with Monday morning breakfast (It lowers blood pressure).
- Carbohydrate/protein-rich cereal (commercially-available cereals) with milk.
- Fruit juice or vegetable drink mixture.
- Extra fluids while at work.

Monday as a fun day? Hardly, but you can make it easier by:

- Writing your Monday "To-Do" list on Friday so you can forget about work and you don't fumble around confused on Monday.
- Taking a shower before you leave for work.
- Leaving home five minutes earlier.

- While commuting to work, sharpen your left brain focus by doing 10 to 1 countdowns (silently) by ones, then by two's (10, 8, 6, 4, 2, 0).
- Break your day into manageable chunks and take your breaks.
- Plan and enjoy some type of "Monday-night delight," a ball game, etc. for holding it together on Monday.

Useful reference:

Waitely, D., & Reni, L.W., (1985). *Joy of working, The 30 day system to success, wealth & happiness on the job.* New York, NY: Dodd Mead.

ONE-MINUTE ANTI-STRESS SKILL-BUILDERS ©

Dr. Ronald L. Rubenzer, 2003

From: *How the Best Handle Stress*

This educational material is not intended in any way to be a substitute for professional treatment (psychological, counseling, medical) and should be used in addition to prescribed regimens.

Chapter Six
Topic: ADJUSTING YOUR ATTITUDE: "Power" Attitudes

"SMALL THOUGHTS" VACCINE (next page)

Advice from the world's "smartest" person on the power of attitudes

- Marilyn vos Savant, who has the highest-measured IQ (230) in the world, states, "Thoughts generate emotions. You may not necessarily choose your emotions, but you control the thoughts that produce them."
- Your stress begins and ends with strong attitudes. Perceptions are real, whether they are really right or not. Use **CPR** (I'm **C**alm, **P**eaceful, **R**elaxed) before you need real CPR.
- If you work at it, you can maintain positive attitudes 90 to 95% of the time.
- Scott Ventrella in his new book, *The Power of Positive Thinking in Business, The Ten Traits for Maximum Results* (The Free Press, 2001), defines ten positive attitudes that are considered the keys to success.

SMALL THOUGHTS	"SMALL THOUGHTS VACCINE"
This job is a drag; there is too much change; these computers are driving me nuts!	Work is fun, change is good: A poor workman argues with his tools, so get back in the loop, the 21st century program!
I have to.	I want to. If I do what I have to now, I can do what I really want to, later.
I think I can't (change).	I think I can.
You are told: You will never have a perfect "score" (grade)!	No monument was ever dedicated to a critic.
This job is too stressful. I can't take the stress of these computer courses.	Job-stress is better than Jobless-stress. Choose to convert temporary stress into long-term satisfaction (e.g., taking those computer courses now for a better job life later).
The only person who likes change is a wet baby.	Change is the only sure thing in life. You couldn't even eat if food didn't change form.
Why am I in this job (course, etc.)?	What are my LFT's, "Look forward to's"?
She is impossible to get along with.	I'll try the JLU, "Just like us," approach, by finding something in common with her (dress, food, hobbies, interests).
I give up.	It is better to light a candle than to curse the darkness.
The glass is half empty.	The glass is both half empty and half full. There is some balance between good and evil.

ONE-MINUTE ANTI-STRESS FACT SHEET ©

Dr. Ronald L. Rubenzer, 2003

From: *How the Best Handle Stress*

This educational material is not intended in any way to be a substitute for professional treatment (psychological, counseling, medical) and should be used in addition to prescribed regimens.

Chapter Seven
Topic: BREATHING EASIER

Try the following RELAXATION BREATHING exercise lying down.

- Notice the rising of your stomach, then your chest as you slowly inhale. Your goal is "belly breathing" in which the belly fills with air before the upper lungs do. Notice your chest falling and then your stomach flattening as you slowly exhale. Putting your hand on your stomach will help you feel whether you are belly breathing. Practice this belly breathing at bedtime for a few weeks until it is a habit. — Try the FDA approved device RESPeRATE™.
- BREATHING BY THE NUMBERS (Do this sitting up). Breathe in on odd numbers; breathe out on even numbers up to the count of ten. For example, breathe in on the count of one, breathe out on the count of two, breathe in on the count of three, and breathe out on the count of four. Five in, six out, seven in, eight out, nine in, ten out. Practice "breathing by the numbers" several times a day until you can breathe to the count of ten some of the time without thoughts interrupting (e.g., Why am I doing this?).
- BREATHE WITH "MEANING." Once you can breath-count to ten, substitute a single word or short phrase for the numbers. For example, say silently to yourself on your inhalation, "In relaxation," then as you exhale, say "Out tension," or try, "I am — relaxed." You may want to try saying to yourself more (on the inhalation) relaxed (on the exhalation). Some self-calmers are "Just for now — I'll relax," or religious, "This too — shall pass," "The peace that passes all understanding."
- If you are trying to doze off to sleep, say as you inhale, "Deep," and as you exhale, "Sleep."
- Learn from the experts* and get group support. Relaxation breathing is simple but not easy. We have flash-bulb short-attention spans. Build up your attention span minute by minute.

*ATTACKING ANXIETY has been used by over 500,000 people over 17 years. It has been recently proven to clinically reduce anxiety, according to Jan. 2000, issue of the *Journal of Clinical Psychology,* Vol. 56 (1), 11-21, 2000, Call 1-800-944-9428. This is a cognitive-behavioral management program. In some cases, individual insurance companies, EAP's and even workers' compensation have paid for the program. Contact <www.stresscenter.com>. Always see your doctor before beginning any anxiety management program.

ONE-MINUTE ANTI-STRESS FACT SHEET ©

Dr. Ronald L. Rubenzer, 2003

From: *How the Best Handle Stress*

This educational material is not intended in any way to be a substitute for professional treatment (psychological, counseling, medical) and should be used in addition to prescribed regimens.

Chapter Seven
Topic: BREATHING EASIER

- The key to stress management is right under your nose!
- If controlled breathing calms during childbirth, it will work on the job.
- Excellent sensory perception (better attention) through deep breathing.
- Fill in the blank of boredom with breathing.
- The WHO (World Health Organization) has approved relaxation response as part of the treatment for high blood pressure. Relaxation exercises, however, are no substitute for medication and diet.
- Duke University anger research proves that if you can delay overreacting to an "incoming" stressor for 20 seconds, you are more likely to think rather than get upset. Breathing by the numbers (inhaling on odd numbers, exhaling on even) to the count of ten will give you about a 20-second stress buffer.
- Relaxation breathing is now standard preoperative procedure for hospitals.
- The FDA has just approved RESPeRATE™, a biofeedback breathing device, to reduce blood pressure, (call 1-800-509-2389 or <www.resperate.com> for more information). It should be used in addition to medication and costs $299.00.

ONE-MINUTE ANTI-STRESS FACT SHEET ©
Dr. Ronald L. Rubenzer, 2003
From: *How the Best Handle Stress*

This educational material is not intended in any way to be a substitute for professional treatment (psychological, counseling, medical) and should be used in addition to prescribed regimens.

Chapter Eight
Topic: WIN/LOSE — YOU CHOOSE: Freedom to choose
(Presented in Switzerland, World Congress on Stress, 1997)

Choice is the C in the ABC's of Industrial-Strength Stress Control. (The Attitude and Breathing components of the ABC's were discussed previously.) No one can take your freedom of choice from you. Choice empowers you to effectively handle life's struggles. Four wise choices are contained in your workplace C.A.R.E. package. Effectively taking C.A.R.E. of business involves choosing to:

C ONTROL — YOUR WORK,
A CCEPT — WHAT YOU CAN'T CONTROL,
R EST — WHEN YOU CAN,
E NJOY — MOST ASPECTS OF YOUR LIFE.

Most of your effort should go into choosing to get control over your work. Three key ways of getting control over your work are:

1. Increase your knowledge. Find a need and fill it;
2. Play by the company rules;
3. Plan and pace yourself with time management.

Two other concerns directly related to the job-stress environment

- Human relations: JLU, "Just like us," principle — key to getting and keeping a job. Trying to find something in common with your co-workers.
- Diversity and harassment on the job. Is the impact of your message the same as the intent of what you meant to say?

ONE-MINUTE ANTI-STRESS FACT SHEET ©

Dr. Ronald L. Rubenzer, 2003

From: *How the Best Handle Stress*

This educational material is not intended in any way to be a substitute for professional treatment (psychological, counseling, medical) and should be used in addition to prescribed regimens.

Chapter Eight
Topic: PASSING THE TEST OF TIME: TIME MANAGEMENT

In 1932, Albert Einstein said: "*For us . . . the distinction between the past, present and future is only an illusion, albeit a stubborn one.*"

Henry David Thoreau, in *Walden Pond,* emphasized the importance and difficulty of improving the "here and now." Thoreau said we have to put all our effort into improving the "nick of time," although we stand at the crossroads of two eternities, the past and the future.

---

1. Two critical reasons why time management is so important.

A. Time management frees you to enjoy what you want to by organizing you to do the things you have to (more easily).

B. Job security is helped or hindered by your attendance record. Friends or foes can point to your punctuality to keep you or fire you. It has been said that getting to work is about 80% of the battle. Once you get there, your habits and support systems take over and before you know it, you are "in the groove." It actually would not hurt to arrive a few minutes early.

---

2. Why time management is so stressful: It's unnatural.

Our minds are in a taffy pull! We are pulled in a tug of war between the past and the future, resulting in a kind of double vision. Time-management experts suggest 90% of your time be focused on the "here and now."

Time is relative. How long is a minute? It depends on which side of the restroom door you are on when "nature calls urgently."

---

3. How to know if you really need time management.

You really need time management IF:

- You are continually apologizing for showing up late (Then for a month, start earlier, enjoy conversation or a warm drink with your spare time);
- You just "have to" do everything yourself because nobody else gets it quite right (Then take baby-steps in assigning tasks to others, enjoy trusting others);
- You are always misplacing your door keys, glasses, handbag or briefcase (Then always put your keys on your key rack at home);
- You have piles of unread newspapers and magazines (Then sit with each day's

deliveries, and sort into trash, A-1 important, and bottom of bird cage when finished reading);

- You always need to search even for those kitchen items you use all the time (Then take one junk drawer at a time [15 minutes daily], organize it, and even label it until everyone gets the hang of the new system);
- You often feel exhausted because there seems to be so much to do and no time for you (Then for one month, have a daily "To-Do" list or system, to reach weekly activities that reflect longer-term goals, go to a movie at week's end).

---

4. How are time management and stress management, ADHD, Type A connected? Improving your quality of life on the job and at home. Giving you a sense of control and predictability.

Time management is a critical factor in helping Type A's, Type T's (thrill-seekers), ADHD or ADD individuals gain control of their environment. A high-energy person without control is like a racecar with no steering wheel; both will crash and burn. Time management gives you a sense of control and predictability, reducing your anxiety. It is considered one of the top ways to manage job-stress. Time management is a most critical key factor in helping Type A's, Type T's (thrill-seekers) and ADHD or ADD individuals gain control of their environment.

Fire-ready-aim

The opposite of managing your time well is captured by the uncomplimentary phrase fire-ready-aim. You shoot for your target impulsively, without getting ready and then aiming. You may say or do things without taking a few seconds to think first.

If you don't know where you are going, any road will get you there!

More freedom of choice

If you don't take control of your calendar first, someone else will. Block out time in advance for projects, rests, etc. Lack of control is the number one source of job-stress.

The opposite of this is that your tasks will take as long as you plan for them to take, if you don't have weekly goals.

Remember, we always make time for real priorities (e.g., dating, sleeping, eating, going to movies, etc.).

Doing well on tests because of more "time on tasks"

A multimillion-dollar study at Columbia University revealed that "time on task" is the best way to improve any type of skill. Sadly, most college dropouts quit after their junior year (of four).

Don't wish for things to be over, because some day they will be forevermore.

ONE-MINUTE ANTI-STRESS SKILL-BUILDERS ©
Dr. Ronald L. Rubenzer, 2003
From: *How the Best Handle Stress*

This educational material is not intended in any way to be a substitute for professional treatment (psychological, counseling, medical) and should be used in addition to prescribed regimens.

Chapter Eight
Topic: TIME MANAGEMENT AND OVERCOMING PROCRASTINATION

1. What to do on Monday? Basic steps in time management.

Keeping time "the old-fashioned way," the "To-Do" list

Time management is simple, but not easy. Keeping up your SINGLE daily "To-Do" list is the heart of effective time management.

1. Write down your thoughts. This will help you organize and remember. "The palest ink is better than the best memory." The best handwritten organizational system for time-management is Day-Timer. Call toll free 1-866-654-9797 or <ordersupplies.com> for calendars.

2. List your important goals. These should be your major lifetime goals, work goals, etc. For example, lifetime goals: to retire early at the beach and/or mountains, go to Tahiti, write an article. Work goal: develop systems to manage information more effectively.

3. Prioritize all your goals. For example, going to Tahiti might be more important than retiring early at the beach. Organizing your files might be more important, right now, than something else. An excellent book to help you learn how to prioritize is *First-things-first,* by Dr. Stephen Covey.

4. For each goal, list weekly activities that will help you meet your goal. Remember, everything takes twice as long as it does (If you think something will take a week, it usually takes two).

Remember the simple, but effective formula TOT = TOT (Time on Tasks = Tasks on Time). The old saying, "If you fail to plan, you plan to fail," may have some truth.

For stress relief when you are "off the clock" make time to waste time. Don't wear your watch, pager or cell phone unless, of course, you are an emergency-room physician on whom lives actually depend. You might put on your "To-Do" list at home (if you are checklist-addicted). Have fun.

You can accomplish almost any goal if you are persistent enough. People have tunneled their way out of concentration camps digging only with a spoon.

5. Now prioritize your activities to meet the goals. Assign the value A-1 to your top activity; A-2 to the second activity.

6. Get a legal pad, at the top write the words, "To-Do," with today's date. What you don't get done today, carry over to the "To-Do" list you have for tomorrow. Duplicate a month's worth of "To-Do" lists and staple them together. Stick to using a single "To-Do" list.

7. Schedule your prime time. Do the worst work first. Most people are mentally sharper in the morning, but fade mid-afternoon. Try to coordinate your schedule around other people's prime time if you need to meet them (e.g., Check to see if the dentist works on Friday afternoon).

8. Be flexible to shift goals. Give yourself weekly deadlines, not daily deadlines, if possible. The crumbs out of your pantry may be a level C goal in September, but will quickly become an A-1 goal when mice start munching on those crumbs in October.

9. Periodically review progress on your goals and, if necessary, revise your goals and activities accordingly. If you are NEVER completing any of your weekly goals, you probably are not planning properly. Remember, you can only have one A-1 priority. Again, time management is simple but not easy. Especially when it comes to procrastination, the material used to pave the road to Hades.

Don't wait for perfect timing. "When I graduate I'll . . .; When the kids stop fighting I'll improve my. . .; I'll finish that report when my desk is cleared, all my papers are filed AND all my pencils are sharpened . . . ; I'll go to Tahiti when I can afford it. . .; I'll improve my love life when I lose more weight; We'll leave for vacation when the house is spotless and could pass "the Martha Stewart" inspection.

10. Reward yourself for accomplishing. Always ask yourself: Am I making the best use of my time, right now? Use the simple if-then proposition or grandma's law (e.g., if you eat your peas, you can have dessert). If you review your "To-Do" list, reward yourself with a break.

---

2. Procrastination: seeds of failure! Eight tips to pull out these weeds before they choke you.

Procrastination is a siamese twin to poor time management. We are giving into stress when we avoid doing something we think is unpleasant, or meaningless.

1. Remember the COSTS of procrastination (what important others will think; the reputation you may be creating; the bad habit you are strengthening). Remember the rewards of completing tasks on time.

2. Use the SWISS CHEESE (Lakein, 1974) method of getting started on difficult tasks or making real molehills out of imaginary mountains.

3. List instant tasks that are easy and take no longer than five minutes (e.g., new information management system – look up phone number of administrator who will approve your project).

4. Start your instant task. Use an egg timer and set it for five minutes. You may find that you actually are involved in the task. If you feel motivated to continue after five minutes, do so. You can do anything for five minutes. Stretch your frustration tolerance to fifteen minutes. In a few months you may be able to tolerate fifty minutes of unpleasantness, without it ruining your whole day. (Fifty minutes is considered the peak performance attention span for an adult.)

5. Build in a quota of instant tasks you will accomplish each week. After a dozen or so instant tasks, you will have taken a significant number of holes out of the chunk of cheese that seemed overwhelming in the beginning.

6. Gather information about the task. This may create interest. Talk to others about the task. They may have insight on how to better approach the task.

7. Arrange yourself physically to get yourself going. If you have to write something, sharpen your pencil. Keeping the A-1 project information in a place of prominence on your desk will help. If you need to type something, sit down at the computer and turn it on.

8. Reward yourself for meeting weekly instant task quotas and for completing the goal itself.

Remember: You always have time to do those things that are truly important to you. You certainly managed the time to date as a youth, no matter how many clubs, courses, errands you had. Time management helps you decide what is important to you and when you will do it. You can even learn to make time to waste time.

ONE-MINUTE ANTI-STRESS SKILL-BUILDERS ©

Dr. Ronald L. Rubenzer, 2003

From: *How the Best Handle Stress*

This educational material is not intended in any way to be a substitute for professional treatment (psychological, counseling, medical) and should be used in addition to prescribed regimens.

Chapter Nine
Topic: COMPUTER STRESS MANAGEMENT

Adopt a humorous sense of perspective, even for those of you suffering from CSA, Computer-separation-anxiety. Fifty-five-million obsolete computers will have to be separated from computer addicts before 2003.

- Remember, you can always pull the plug. Display your sense of humor with cartoons taped on your computer or workstation area.
- Read the *Consumer Reports* article, "This @!*# Computer. How to Handle Ten Common Gripes." (March 2001, p. 65).
- Scientifically learn muscle tension awareness/relaxation with biofeedback.
- Rest your hands on your desktop or in your lap whenever possible.
- Blink. Staring at a screen can dry your eyes. Also a tip from an Emmy award-winner to reduce eyestrain – At home, light a candle to safely enjoy. Blow out candle whenever you are not in the room.
- Look away.
- Take a mini one-minute break every 15 to 30 minutes.
- Breathe slowly and deeply for a few breaths as you sit down in front of your computer.
- Get an entertaining screen saver.
- Consider learning computers like learning a foreign language. Just do it.
- Get a personal trainer. Link up with a computer store or find an expert who makes you feel comfortable.
- Make friends with a child who knows computers (and what child doesn't?). Get back with your significant other if he or she has become a web widow because you suffer from CSA, Computer-separation-anxiety (You get anxious when you aren't with your computer).

ONE-MINUTE ANTI-STRESS SKILL-BUILDERS ©

Dr. Ronald L. Rubenzer, 2003

From: *How the Best Handle Stress*

This educational material is not intended in any way to be a substitute for professional treatment (psychological, counseling, medical) and should be used in addition to prescribed regimens.

Chapter Nine
Topic: COMPUTER STRESS MANAGEMENT

Your PC contains more programming capacity than the first manned space flight on board computer.

- Half of adults avoid computers.
- Watch your language, your computer's language, that is. Is fatal really fatal?
- Excessive computer use leads to depression.
- Existence of web widows.
- When your computer has a lobotomy (hard drive crash) or why computers may be stressful.
- Being tested by computers — the future is here.
- Those with CSA, Computer-separation-anxiety, will need to be weaned from their obsolete computers as 55-million computers will be outdated shortly. Some folks afflicted with CSA would rather spend time with their computer than with their friends. CSA is a humorous acronym used to coin the symptoms (worry, sweating palms) that accompany separation of owners from their computers.

ONE-MINUTE ANTI-STRESS SKILL-BUILDERS ©

Dr. Ronald L. Rubenzer, 2003

From: *How the Best Handle Stress*

This educational material is not intended in any way to be a substitute for professional treatment (psychological, counseling, medical) and should be used in addition to prescribed regimens.

Chapter Ten

Topic: JOB-STRESS MANAGEMENT: Freedom of Choices

(Presented in Switzerland, World Congress on Stress, 1997)

Taking C.A.R.E. of Business

- **C**ONTROLLING: Find a need and fill it. Read Jason Carter's, *Nasty People: How to Stop Being Hurt by Them Without Becoming One of Them.*
- **A**CCEPTING: "God grant me the serenity to accept the things I cannot change, the courage to change the things I can, and the wisdom to know the difference." - Reinhold Niebuhr. No one was ever fired for listening.
- **R**ESTING: No one has ever been too tired to leave work and go home. Rest is absolutely important, but some of the fatigue we feel at work is in our heads, and that is job-stress. A 20-minute power-nap recharges the most powerful man on Earth — the President. Twenty minutes of rest will reset your brain back to optimal performance. You will improve your memory, sharpen your alertness and reduce fatigue. (Do at home!)
- **E**NJOYING: "No pain — no gain" makes about as much sense as "Spare the rod — spoil the child." Both principles are wrong and abusive. Pleasure-starved people are often irritable, inefficient and unfriendly. These people brighten the room by leaving it.

Whenever you are having fun, you are healing from the effects of stress

- Make and review a list of your "look forward to's."
- Try to humor yourself when you can.
- Keep your eyes on the prize. Look for "pleasure islands" to calmly escape momentarily.
- Enjoy eye candy, something you look at which is pleasing to the eye. Read Diane Ackerman's, *Cultivating Delight: A Natural History of My Garden.*
- Practice your "eye-robics" by feasting your eyes on beauty in motion. Gaze upon a flock of geese in flight, rolling ocean waves, a hummingbird suspended in flight, a horse running in a pasture.
- Conduct a "pleasure hunt" at work, to look for the most pleasant elements of your job you can enjoy daily. Pride in what you do is a close relative of pleasure, so take honest pride in what you can.
- Remember "reward revenge" is also a way to get even with life's hassles. The phrase, "I deserve this _______ (dinner, movie, sports event, book)," will help you enjoy the hard-earned fruits of your labor.

ONE-MINUTE ANTI-STRESS SKILL-BUILDERS ©
Dr. Ronald L. Rubenzer, 2003
From: *How the Best Handle Stress*

This educational material is not intended in any way to be a substitute for professional treatment (psychological, counseling, medical) and should be used in addition to prescribed regimens.

Chapter Eleven
Topic: BOOSTING YOUR WILL POWER, (The REDS program)

Sometimes our own mind "won't mind" us

For example, you've made up your mind to drop a habit, but your mind stubbornly resists (overeating, whining, etc.).

- **R**elax: It's impossible to have deeply relaxed muscles and feel nervous at the same time. Tapes are available to learn how to do "progressive deep muscle relaxation."
- **E**xercise: This is very important in stress management. Exercise changes your blood chemistry by metabolizing (neutralizing) stress hormones and introducing the brain's natural tranquilizers (enkephalins, endorphins). Always check with your doctor before beginning any exercise or diet program. Exercise also gets you away from your problems. Walking three times weekly (30 minutes) at a brisk pace is sufficient. You will be in "good" walking shape in about eight weeks. Change your routine to counteract boredom. The feeling of relaxation will be with you for about six hours. Exercise no later than two hours before bedtime. Exercising Sunday evening will ease you back into work on Monday. A 2001, Duke study showed that exercise can be more effective than zoloft in elevating moods. Exercise can reduce fatal heart attack risk by 70% according to Harvard, *Men's Health Watch* (December, 2001, p. 3). The article lists 22 ways to get exercise as recommended by the Surgeon General.

  Exercise at least three days/week (Tuesday, Thursday, Saturday).

  Move to a movie. Rent or record a movie. Set up the movie, and take the remote control with you on your exercise machine. Watch a portion (30 minutes) of the movie while you workout on the treadmill or exercise bike. You will have enjoyed a full-length motion picture in about three or four exercise periods. Try to obtain a fast-moving movie. Another good alternative is to watch your favorite TV program while you exercise. Before you know it, you will have your exercise quotient in and will have actually enjoyed your workout. Maybe your exercise time won't fly by, but at least it won't crawl by.
- **D**iet: Caffeine is a "stress amplifier." About two cups/servings of caffeinated beverage will not contribute to feelings of stress for most people. Three or more servings may result in a caffeine addiction and feelings of stress. If you are trying to cut back, taper off slowly. Don't cut back on the amount of

liquid you are drinking, but on the amount of caffeine in the drinks. Making a half/half mixture (half-caffeinated, half-decaffeinated) might be useful. Try green tea. Caffeine stays in your system about six hours. If you have difficulty sleeping, you may want to skip caffeine at the evening meal. Of course, chocolate and many headache remedies contain caffeine. Milk contains a natural tranquilizer and has a calming effect on some people.

Fruit of the vine: No wine until it's time. The rule of two for alcohol (two drinks for men or one for women) appears to have some possible overall health benefits. However, it is not recommended that you start drinking if you don't, and it is recommended that you take a vacation from alcohol weekly.

Natural remedies: "Not everything that is natural is good for you." (e.g., snake venom). There may be some calming benefit to the natural homeopathic remedy called kava. Always check with your physician for possible interactions with so-called natural remedies. Some natural remedies can do more harm than good. National Public Radio offers, "The People's Pharmacy," which is a legitimate source of information on the use and abuse of natural remedies.

- Sleep: Get about seven hours. Keep the bedroom "off limits" for business (money) or other important matters. Don't make your bedroom your boardroom. If you can't get a problem off your mind, get up; write a note about it, and go to another room to try to fall to sleep. Using a relaxation tape right before bed will aid in sleeping. Take a warm bath prior to going to bed. Use a sound soother. Install room-darkening shades. Your body reacts to sunlight as a signal to wake-up.

ONE-MINUTE ANTI-STRESS FACT SHEET ©

Dr. Ronald L. Rubenzer, 2003

From: *How the Best Handle Stress*

This educational material is not intended in any way to be a substitute for professional treatment (psychological, counseling, medical) and should be used in addition to prescribed regimens.

Chapter Eleven
Topic: BOOSTING YOUR WILL POWER

- Let's "get physical" about stress.
- Why "get physical" about stress? Because what starts off in your mind is expressed through your body. Stress generated by your mind produces physical hormones (adrenaline, cortisol and also testosterone for men). Your thoughts become things (hormones), which are measurable and can't be thought away. You have to do something physical to counteract these stress hormones. You can no more effectively "think away" stress hormones than you can "think away" coffee jitters (let's say four cups of coffee). It is now theorized that exercise neutralizes the heart-harmful effects of cortisol and adrenaline, the culprits in the "fight-or-flight" response. Exercise also produces endorphins, the brain's natural tranquilizer.
- Using the simple REDS program described below will close the gap between knowing and doing what's right for you by increasing your will power. Using the REDS program works on the body-mind aspect of stress, producing ONE-MINUTE ANTI-STRESS hormones (endorphins, enkephalins) to influence your mind.
- ALWAYS CONSULT YOUR DOCTOR BEFORE ENGAGING IN ANY TYPE OF EXERCISE PROGRAM. Being fit will help you feel somewhat more like getting back to work rather than getting back to bed. Give yourself at least a month on the exercise component of the REDS program.
- The four components of the REDS program are described below. You are probably already doing some of these.

  Relaxation

  Exercise

  Diet

  Sleep

See previous Chapter Eleven (p. 317), Skill-Builder Sheet for more specifics on the REDS program.

ONE-MINUTE ANTI-STRESS SKILL-BUILDERS ©

Dr. Ronald L. Rubenzer, 2003

From: *How the Best Handle Stress*

This educational material is not intended in any way to be a substitute for professional treatment (psychological, counseling, medical) and should be used in addition to prescribed regimens.

Chapter Twelve
Topic: CRITICAL INCIDENCE RECOVERY: Refuse to Lose (Your Mind)

Don't let stress squelch your success.

HOW TO TURN FAILURE INTO SUCCESS

- Retreat, rest, momentarily. See your doctor if you cannot sleep.
- Like former President Clinton, be a "comeback kid" — but with good judgment.
- Set reasonable goals that may be out of reach, but not out of sight.
- Have a plan B with tangible goals and progress markers.
- Confidently brace yourself for bumpy roads.
- Know yourself realistically. Brainstorm resumé/items.
- Read about heroic "successful failures."
- Truly believe in yourself (It is contagious).
- Keep your resumé up to date.
- Contact Professionals in Transition for job-search support.
- Try to maintain activities of daily living (ADL) as much as possible.

ONE-MINUTE ANTI-STRESS FACT SHEET ©

Dr. Ronald L. Rubenzer, 2003

From: *How the Best Handle Stress*

This educational material is not intended in any way to be a substitute for professional treatment (psychological, counseling, medical) and should be used in addition to prescribed regimens.

Chapter Twelve
Topic: CRITICAL INCIDENCE RECOVERY: Refuse to Lose (Your Mind)

If it doesn't destroy me it makes me stronger.
- Arthur Schopenhauer (German philosopher; b. 1788 d. 1860)

- Sooner or later everyone is "rocked" by a level 10 earthquake on the stress Richter Scale, such as the 9/11 World Trade Center suicide bombings.
- When under extreme stress, try to remember that the quick cure is sometimes worse than the disease. Giving up, extreme overindulgence, revenge or withdrawal may be some of the cures that are worse than the disease (job loss, death of a loved one, divorce, etc.).
- No matter how much it hurts, your true north emotional "compass heading" is something like, "It's better to light a candle than to curse the darkness." You have lost your direction if your main goal in life is to get even or get out of the race. Check your "compass heading" during these terrible storms when you can't see the light. Watch for your emotional lighthouses in loved ones and friends.
- Also, take advantage of professional therapy (counseling) that is usually offered by corporations. Eventually take advantage of outplacement services by your employer, whereby you will be provided with professional leads and job-interview advice. A "life raft" may be almost within reach. Don't give up!

ONE-MINUTE ANTI-STRESS SKILL-BUILDERS ©

Dr. Ronald L. Rubenzer, 2003

From: *How the Best Handle Stress*

This educational material is not intended in any way to be a substitute for professional treatment (psychological, counseling, medical) and should be used in addition to prescribed regimens.

Chapter Thirteen
Topic: HUMOR: Your Sixth Sense of Survival

*"I took an IQ test and the results were negative."**

- Anonymous

- Know yourself. Find your "sore spots" and apply humor as you would a soothing salve. For example, if your daily encounter with a computer makes you sore, find cartoons that make fun of computers.
- Go on a "humor diet." Try *Interfax Daily*. Call (336) 397-0000 for a Free-Daily humor fax. Optimism is the breakfast of champions. Instead of waking up to "doom and gloom" news, listen to upbeat radio stations. Find a radio station that emphasizes humor. Calendars are available which feature a daily cartoon or joke. When reading the newspaper, focus on the "funnies" first before finding out all the negative things thousands of people have done lately. Watch movies, listen to tapes or read books that are humorous.
- Develop your sense of humor. Often people feel worse after listening to everyone's complaints during breaks, so choose to be around more uplifting people.
- Watch the company you keep. Avoid "pity parties." Fly with eagles . . . don't flounder with turkeys. Seek out and be around people known for their uplifting jokes and/or sense of humor.
- "Lock it in." Treat yourself to a humor treatment on a regular basis. Don't let a day pass without some exposure to humor.
- Remember: Your sense of humor is your sense of balance. People who need humor the most, seek it the least. When you feel you no longer have the time or mood for humor, perhaps you should slow down, relax, and smile.

**Used by permission. As seen in InterFax Daily.*

ONE-MINUTE ANTI-STRESS FACT SHEET ©

Dr. Ronald L. Rubenzer, 2003

From: *How the Best Handle Stress*

This educational material is not intended in any way to be a substitute for professional treatment (psychological, counseling, medical) and should be used in addition to prescribed regimens.

Chapter Thirteen
Topic: HUMOR: Your Sixth Sense of Survival

- He who laughs… lasts. Although leading a humorless life is not fatal, it can be unhealthy psychologically. Humor serves as a balancing pole on the tightrope of life. Humor is a powerful force in releasing stress's stranglehold. In fact, humor is such a powerful antidote to stress that many corporations hire humor consultants to "lighten up" office environments.
- Laughter is a natural mood elevator and, according to a Cornell University study, also increases creativity and flexibility of thought. Humor gives a more balanced sense of perspective. Appropriately timed humor has even been found to be useful in alleviating the pain of injections as well as post-operative pain.
- Three important benefits to humor at work. Humor can: motivate, strengthen bonds between workers, and reduce stress.
- Humor can enhance your career up the ladder. One CEO says, "Competent people with a sense of humor are more likely to be promoted." People are more likely to want to work for someone who has a sense of humor.
- The key attribute of humor in the workplace is to motivate and create team spirit without wasting time.
- Humor should be used like a spice, to enhance your career. Overusing humor is like ruining a dish with too much flavoring. You should use the right amount of humor at the right time.
- IBM executives have attained a 30% increase in sales by injecting fun and humor into a very competitive, intense office.
- The main mechanism of humor or laughter appears to be the release of endorphins or the brain's natural tranquilizer into the system. Laughing results in an "endorphin high." Furthermore, laughter stimulates internal organs, making them work better through the increase of circulation that follows the vibrating massage that accompanies it and heightens resistive vitality against disease. We smile because we are happy. Interestingly, it has been discovered that our smile also causes our feelings of happiness. That is, the act of smiling elevates moods.

ONE-MINUTE ANTI-STRESS SKILL-BUILDERS ©
Dr. Ronald L. Rubenzer, 2003
From: *How the Best Handle Stress*

This educational material is not intended in any way to be a substitute for professional treatment (psychological, counseling, medical) and should be used in addition to prescribed regimens.

Chapter Fourteen
Topic: PUBLIC SPEAKING: A step-by-step guide

Lady luck favors the prepared.

- Don't sweat (while presenting). Sweat while preparing. A ten to one ratio of preparation to presentation time is typical. (It takes ten hours of preparation for an hour of good presentation.) This includes needs assessment, product development and practice.
- Attitude affirmation. Repeat to yourself. "I know — that I know" to build your confidence. You will always know a little more than your audience (at least new jokes).
  Smile and say to yourself and then to your audience, "I'm glad to be here," (Whether you are or not, fake it till you make it). Find one friendly face in the audience.
- Practice makes permanent. Use the rule of 7 – go through your talk at least seven times. Practice once to a live audience (of one) sitting at the back of the room or tape-record your speech. Make sure your practice audience feigns boredom and distraction so you are not upset when it happens in real life. Have your "guinea pig" audience sit at least twenty feet away from you so you learn to project your voice.
- Double the amount of enthusiasm you speak with normally and slow down your pace.
- Practice the main points of your speech right before you go to sleep. This will solidify it in your memory.
- Drink a warm (decaffeinated) drink right before you talk. It will relax you and your voice. Take three or four slow deep breaths, belly breathing if you can.
- Use cue cards and technology but don't depend on them entirely. Have your major points memorized. Probably a twenty-point font size type would be helpful. Also, you can even put breathing/pause marks in your notes so you don't talk too fast under stress.

ONE-MINUTE ANTI-STRESS FACT SHEET ©

Dr. Ronald L. Rubenzer, 2003

From: *How the Best Handle Stress*

This educational material is not intended in any way to be a substitute for professional treatment (psychological, counseling, medical) and should be used in addition to prescribed regimens.

Chapter Fourteen
Topic: PUBLIC SPEAKING

Private & Public speaking are basically the same, you just need more "wind" for the latter.

- You just need more "wind" for public speaking. Most people will eventually overcome this stressor; public speaking. Probably the main reason public speaking is stressful is that we cut off our own air supply. We squeeze our own wind pipes with stress.
- When we are not used to projecting our voices, we tend to breathe shallowly and quickly, almost hyperventilating. Of course, oxygen deprivation will set off all kinds of alarms in your brain, even leading to panic attacks.
- Seasoned actors know the importance of deep breathing to speak well and even feel well during performances.
- Mastering public speaking is an art. How you react to the stress of public speaking is up to you. Many consider pre-speaking jitters as a sign of respect for your audience.
- Stress is simply energy, and stress management is simply energy conservation. Choose to use stress as an energy source. If you interpret the butterflies in your stomach as excitement, you are converting negative stress (distress) into positive stress (eustress).
- To disarm the number one stressor on the job, a step-by-step guide has been provided in the Chapter Fourteen Skill-Builders based on information gleaned from the American Society of Training and Development. (See previous page.)

ONE-MINUTE ANTI-STRESS SKILL-BUILDERS ©

This educational material is not intended in any way to be a substitute for professional treatment (psychological, counseling, medical) and should be used in addition to prescribed regimens.

Chapter Fifteen
Topic: CHILDREN: Stress Cures at Home

Listen to your child and take a real recess.

- Watch out for excessive preschool competition, TV violence, and family discord.
- Listen to your child.
- Get help with schoolwork. Call the Homework Hotline. Get your high school child classic reference books, (e.g., Strunk's and White's fourth edition of *The Elements of Style,* 2000, Allyn & Bacon). Use the ISP WorldCat for references, by simply calling your librarian. It searches the world's catalogues.
- Join the PTA.
- Tackle test anxiety.
- Have a real twenty-minute recess with your child.
- Try not to "club your child" to stress with excessive clubs and after-school activities.
- Encourage a stress-reducing diet.
- Use sports as a way to "blow-off" steam.
- Make certain your child gets enough rest.
- Provide a quiet environment.
- Pet your pet.
- Be tough minded but tenderhearted.
- MOST IMPORTANTLY: Be a "good example." You can't give what you don't have.

ONE-MINUTE ANTI-STRESS FACT SHEET ©

Dr. Ronald L. Rubenzer, 2003

From: *How the Best Handle Stress*

This educational material is not intended in any way to be a substitute for professional treatment (psychological, counseling, medical) and should be used in addition to prescribed regimens.

Chapter Fifteen

Topic: CHILDREN: Stress Cures at Home

- Children have never been under more stress and this stress is predicted to mount. The reasons cited for this increased stress are the pressure youngsters are under to deal with academic demands and other tasks for which they are not developmentally ready.
- Trying to artificially pump-up IQ's in the very young may also lead to increased stress in kids, because the parents' anxiety tends to rub off. As early as four years of age the brains of stressed kids look similar to brains of stressed adults, being flooded with "fight-or-flight" response hormones. If the brain is kept on edge long enough, the changes become more or less permanent, and as these stressed-out kids get older, learning becomes harder.

Five benefits resulting from stress management in children include

- Enjoying better physical health.
- Increased resistance to negative peer pressure.
- Less fighting.
- Preventing and controlling emotional problems.
- Opening lines of communication: Highly-anxious children may be afraid to displease their parents, and may even tend to hide problems. Unrelieved stress from a child's problems will eventually erupt.

TEN WARNING SIGNS OF EXCESSIVE STRESS

1. Sudden, dramatic increase or decrease in effort at school.
2. Major change in attitude/temperament (irritability, lack of enthusiasm, carelessness).
3. Withdrawal or outbursts.
4. Nervous tics, fidgeting, jumping from task to task, difficulty concentrating. Pulling eyebrows, twirling hair, bouncing knees, frequent unnecessary trips to the bathroom can be forms of nervous energy overflow.
5. Complaints of fatigue and vague illnesses.
6. Difficulty sleeping.
7. Stomachaches, headaches.
8. Drug abuse.
9. Increase in allergic/asthmatic attacks.
10. Avoidance of school or testing situations by direct refusal or convenient illnesses. Frequent visits to the school nurse's office for no diagnosable cause.

ONE-MINUTE ANTI-STRESS SKILL-BUILDERS ©

Dr. Ronald L. Rubenzer, 2003

From: *How the Best Handle Stress*

This educational material is not intended in any way to be a substitute for professional treatment (psychological, counseling, medical) and should be used in addition to prescribed regimens.

Chapter Sixteen
Topic: STUDENT STRESS MANAGEMENT

MODEL "GRACE UNDER PRESSURE"

- You can telegraph relaxation by smiling, talking and moving calmly but enthusiastically.
- Try the W.A.L.K.E.R. program: Students can exit the "stress express" through following this 6-step WALKER program. Encourage:

  Walking (briskly 20-minutes, three times weekly to burn-off stress);

  Attitude (of positive organized persistence - POP);

  Laughter (Use a humor board for students' cartoons);

  Keeping up (with homework, studying, test preparation);

  Expressing stress (through writing, art, music, sports, counseling);

  Rewarding (Teach students to keep their "eyes on the prize" — earn praise, privileges, pride, support cards along with report cards).
- Offer specific skills training in test-taking, homework management and dealing with conflict/criticism.
- Post relaxation reminders. Motivation posters can serve as relaxation reminders.
- Make relaxation the fourth "R" in education. The classroom may be the only place where achievement-stressed students learn to identify and control stress. The turn-of-the-century curriculum needs to incorporate relaxation as the fourth "R" to maximize our students' success and satisfaction when challenges rise on the horizon.
- ASSURE THE CHILDREN THAT THE U.S. IS STILL SAFE even after 9-11-01. Explain "lessons to be learned," as detailed in Dr. Arthur Levine's 9-18-01 Columbia University letter to teachers. (See Chapter 16.)

ONE-MINUTE ANTI-STRESS FACT SHEET ©
Dr. Ronald L. Rubenzer, 2003
From: *How the Best Handle Stress*

This educational material is not intended in any way to be a substitute for professional treatment (psychological, counseling, medical) and should be used in addition to prescribed regimens.

Chapter Sixteen
Topic: STUDENT STRESS MANAGEMENT

- Stress impairs performance: Millions of students suffer from test anxiety. Decades of research have proven that test anxiety lowers test performance. According to learning researcher, Eric Jensen, stress may be the leading contributing factor to student underachievement (e.g., poor test scores).
- Thirty percent of 8,000 high-schoolers reported they were under great stress.
- Stress increases absenteeism: About one in six students misses an average of a week of school from stress-induced severe stomach pains.
- Stress leads to unhealthy Type A development: As early as three years of age, Type A habits are being crystallized. Untreated, these habits solidify into Type A personalities by fourth grade. Type A students are often inappropriately perfectionistic, competitive, urgent, overreactive and/or anger-prone.
- Stress causes obesity due to stress-relieving eating. Stress, along with food choices and eating habits, is something we can control. Sadly, when children are most sensitive about their appearance, the temptation to stress-relief eat is great.

Benefits of student stress management

- "Taking off the edge" Gives children "the edge" on tests.
- More teachable moments: Excess stress is a nonconductor of learning.
- Curbing school violence: "To curb violence, it's essential to establish a relaxed, positive climate in school," says Cohn Greer, author of *"How Safe is Your Child's School?"*.
- Males under stress, aggress. Male children are more likely to need stress management.
- Males are particularly prone to react to tension with hostility and aggression because their bodies are flushed with testosterone (aggression hormone). This testosterone flushing does not occur in females, who try to befriend potentially stress-producing people.
- Reducing drug abuse: The local D.A.R.E. (Drug Abuse Resistance Education) program points to stress as one reason people use drugs. Reducing stress reduces the risk of drug use for some.
- Need for reduction in extreme stress-reaction behaviors, including copy-cat shootings and suicidal bombings. (On January 6, 2002, fifteen-year-old high school freshman killed himself by flying a private plane into a building.)

ONE-MINUTE ANTI-STRESS FACT SHEET ©

Dr. Ronald L. Rubenzer, 2003

From: *How the Best Handle Stress*

This educational material is not intended in any way to be a substitute for professional treatment (psychological, counseling, medical) and should be used in addition to prescribed regimens.

Chapter Seventeen
Topic: TEST-TAKING SKILLS

GENERAL TIPS FOR HELPING STUDENTS TO BECOME "FACT SMART" (Left brain)

- Make these tips part of each student's study habits by introducing them at the beginning.
- Get the "big picture" (Overview first, read end of chapter questions next).
- "Seeing is believing" for most students. "Teach smart" (Visually).
- Make meaningful memories.
- Teach memory mechanics. (Repeat information at least seven times.)
- Students develop flashcards. Submit flashcards as an assignment immediately before the test.
- Encourage note-taking while students are reading or listening.
- Divide and conquer information (more frequent, shorter study periods spread over time).
- If appropriate, provide a test-specific diagnostic survey.
- As a reward, have students play "not-so-trivial pursuit" by making up their own questions about material and having a rival team answer the questions under a time limit.
- Celebrate "sticking to their test-prep schedule."

TIPS FOR IMPROVING "TEST-SMARTNESS" (Left and right brain)

- Answer the questions (Multiple-choice tests are not multiple-guess tests, but use creative problem solving, if needed).
- Be clerically correct.
- Provide practice sessions (with time limits) if appropriate. Check out "test-prep" services. SAT scores can increase up to 300 points with expert coaching.

BUILDING "STRESS-SMARTNESS" (Primarily a right brain skill) Weeks before the test

- Conduct a "reality checklist" of what the student can expect to avoid shock on test day.

- Prior to the testing situation, provide a "relaxed exposure" to these "test reality conditions."
- Positive attitude: Expect the best but respect the test. The test is the reward to prove your knowledge. "Inch by inch, anything's a cinch, yard by yard, life is hard."
- Use positive peer pressure: Bring in cartoons about testing stress — (e.g., I took an IQ test and the results were negative).
- Good modeling by all adults.
- Start an exercise program at least a month before the big event. This can consist of simply walking briskly for thirty minutes, three times a week. Exercise improves memory and the ability to juggle mental tasks better according to Duke University research (2001).
- Food for thought — natural sugars. Honey on toast will give your brain a natural boost. Any sweet fruit (peaches, oranges, melons) followed by a glass of water will provide your brain with a natural power boost.
- Caffeine is at best a double-edged sword. While it can sharpen your thinking (no more than two cups of coffee), you pay for it with caffeine jitters. If you don't use caffeine, don't start.

ONE-MINUTE ANTI-STRESS FACT SHEET ©
Dr. Ronald L. Rubenzer, 2003
From: *How the Best Handle Stress*

This educational material is not intended in any way to be a substitute for professional treatment (psychological, counseling, medical) and should be used in addition to prescribed regimens.

Chapter Seventeen
Topic: TEST-TAKING SKILLS

If stress is sand in the machinery of thought, then relaxation is the oil.

Why do well on tests?

- Testing in math and reading has been federally mandated for grades 3-8 (June 14, 2001).
- Tests are here to stay.

  One-hundred-million standardized tests are administered for elementary and middle school children yearly. Since tests (which are better than guessing what a person might know) are obviously here to stay, we might as well learn how to master them.
- Enjoying a successful twelve-year career. Tests are "success benchmarks" during everyone's twelve-year academic career. Used correctly, tests actually serve as "success stepping-stones" rather than stumbling blocks. Triumphing over fear of failure.
- Fifteen-percentile point test-score increase, or a whole letter-grade improvement results from learning test-taking skills for students. A fifteen-percentile point increase is the difference between your child's functioning in the high average range, to performing in the superior (gifted) range and possibly being considered for advanced learner programming. It's the difference between being on the B honor roll and A honor roll. This could make the difference between your child winning a scholarship or her being on a "parentship," where you pay all college tuition costs. (Scruggs & Mastropieri, Purdue University, 1992).
- Fear of academic failure was the leading "most difficult problem" American teenagers face according to a 1994 Gallup Poll. Equipping students with proven "test-taking tools" results in real success experiences to triumph over imaginary fears.
- Proving your knowledge is power to succeed. The ladder of success is built with small but measurable steps. Tests can help measure readiness for the next step toward goals.

- Why reduce test anxiety? It is even "front-page" news. The "front-page" news item read, "Pretest jitters will try to be soothed by schools."
- The $64,000 question: Why should my child take a test-prep course? Score gains from 140 to 300 points on SAT (Spelled $AT). Talented test-takers (95% and above) coach students. Testimonials by Princeton Review students having taken a course revealed score gains of 190 to 300 points. They received admission to schools of their top choice. Tell yourself as a parent that you could spell SAT as $AT. Your child can win thousands of dollars in scholarships by doing well (High SAT students improve a university's standing). Don't tell your child ahead of time about the $AT angle, it may create additional, unneeded pressure, which will actually decrease your child's score.
- Aim high: An SAT Score of 1394 (693 verbal/710 math) may win a scholarship at Columbia University, the most expensive university in the nation, at $29,000 per year for tuition only (2000). Columbia has been ranked the number one university in the country at least twice in the last decade (America's Best Graduate Schools – Exclusive Rankings, *U.S. News & World Report,* March 18, 1996).

ONE-MINUTE ANTI-STRESS SKILL-BUILDERS ©

Dr. Ronald L. Rubenzer, 2003

From: *How the Best Handle Stress*

This educational material is not intended in any way to be a substitute for professional treatment (psychological, counseling, medical) and should be used in addition to prescribed regimens.

Chapter Seventeen
Topic: MEMORY BOOSTERS

GENERAL TIPS FOR HELPING TO HAVE A RAZOR SHARP MEMORY (Left brain)

- A normal memory problem is when you can't remember where you put your car. A serious memory problem is when you can't recall how to drive home. In either case, you should go see your doctor.

Simple memory boosters include

- "The palest ink is better than the best memory," so put it in writing. Write notes to yourself. If you have to, use hyper notes (those small, yellow sticky notes that allow you to cover an entire desk top or refrigerator with reminders). Leave messages to yourself on your answering machine. Like location, location, location, remember, "repetition, repetition, repetition."
- Play with your brain, that is, keep your brain in tune by playing games.
- Bridge the gap. (One of the brightest people this author knows plays bridge youthfully and expertly and technically qualifies for AARP membership.) *Games* magazine, which emphasizes word play, is great. Maybe the *New York Times* crossword puzzle is not your style, but any crossword puzzle will do. You can even get crossword puzzles that deal with a hobby interest of yours. Even playing checkers exercises your brain better than playing your TV remote.
- Remember the old saying, "A place (and time) for everything and everything in its place." It may be boring, but learn to routinely put your keys (wallet, etc.) in one place. That will be one less thing you have to remember. It takes about three weeks to a month for your brain to reroute to a new routine. So remind and reward yourself for the first month in retraining your brain.
- Tell jokes (to tested audiences, like your best friends). This requires timing and remembering the punch line. If you can't remember punch lines, write them down.
- Communicate. If you are not computer phobic, join a chat room (There are even chat rooms devoted exclusively to standard poodle lovers). Get on the Internet, or if nothing else, write a letter to your friends, using snail mail.

- Take up a course that has nothing to do with what you have to do, but something you want to do (painting, coin collecting). You probably don't need the extra credit but it will give you something to look forward to. Even your classmates can keep you young.
- Exercise by taking a brisk thirty-minute walk, three times weekly (Always get your doctor's permission first). Mental decline over age is blamed to a degree on decreased circulation to key parts of the brain. Exercise supplies these deprived key areas with freshly oxygenated blood (Duke University study, 2001).
- If older, try ginkgo, only after consulting your doctor. It is the only clinically-proven (but not FDA approved) herbal remedy that shows promise for improving memory.

ONE-MINUTE ANTI-STRESS SKILL-BUILDERS ©

Dr. Ronald L. Rubenzer, 2003

From: *How the Best Handle Stress*

This educational material is not intended in any way to be a substitute for professional treatment (psychological, counseling, medical) and should be used in addition to prescribed regimens.

Chapter Eighteen
Topic: RELAXATION FOR TEACHERS

How to Have Less-Stress, Tomorrow: A Checklist

THE PRRICE APPROACH

- **P**REVENT the causes of stress.
- **R**ELAX your jaws, neck muscles, hands and breathing.
- **R**EDUCE the impact of remaining stressors.
- **I**GNORE unimportant irritations.
- **C**OMMUNICATE, COPE, AND HOPE.
- **E**SCAPE.

LOUNGE TIPS

- Offer decaf coffee or tea.
- Drink something warm.
- Have a humor board with cartoons and jokes.
- Put a TGIE poster up (Thank goodness I'm employed).
- Provide pleasant music.
- Make sure your lounge doesn't become "whine country" where people actually compete to see who can whine the most.

BREAK TIPS

- Take your breaks. Be around pleasant adults if at all possible.
- Walk outside during lunch if possible.
- Avoid "pity parties."

BUILD IN STRESS BUFFERS

- Cultivate strong work-related friendships.
- Have your "pleasure islands" at work.
- Have a fish tank in your classroom.
- Posters of nature scenes soothe nerves also.

ONE-MINUTE ANTI-STRESS FACT SHEET ©

Dr. Ronald L. Rubenzer, 2003

From: *How the Best Handle Stress*

This educational material is not intended in any way to be a substitute for professional treatment (psychological, counseling, medical) and should be used in addition to prescribed regimens.

Chapter Eighteen
Topic: RELAXATION FOR TEACHERS

"Without teachers I would not, could not, have become an astronaut. How else do you think I got here?"

- Astronaut addressing the North Carolina Association for Gifted and Talented Conference, Wilmington, North Carolina

- Currently there are 3,071,000 public- and private-school teachers. As stress builds throughout the school year, so does the volume of teachers' voices. The noble profession of teaching is becoming less attractive to young people because of the high degree of stress from behavioral problems and ever-escalating accountability from test results. It's hard to be dedicated when you feel battle-fatigued at the end of each day.
- Stress is blamed for the 30% new teacher dropout rate. The rate is much higher in poorer urban areas.
- Every school day across America, 52-million children are greeted by about 3-million teachers. Many teachers and pupils pass through metal detectors to get to their rooms. Most are under intense test-score improvement pressure.
- Landmark legislation passed by the U.S. Senate on June 14, 2001, requires math and reading testing of **all** 3rd through 8th graders. If students do not do well on tests they have the option to leave the school and/or get tutoring at taxpayer's expense. It's the law. Hopefully this won't be the last straw for many conscientious teachers who are pouring their lives into helping disadvantaged students to do well on standardized tests. Unfortunately, teachers are evaluated on the class's performance, just as a coach is judged on his team's performance.
- Job-stress topped the list of teacher-stressors in an international study conducted by this author. School can be stressful, but it doesn't have to be.
- Stress makes you fat, according to Harvard researchers.
- Test scores rise as performance anxiety falls. Students will catch your stress.
- Crossing the won't/can't let go line. Stress is not a neutral force. If you won't let go of stress, eventually you can't let go of stress (headaches, insomnia, high blood pressure, irritability, stomach problems).

ONE-MINUTE ANTI-STRESS SKILL-BUILDERS ©

Dr. Ronald L. Rubenzer, 2003

From: *How the Best Handle Stress*

This educational material is not intended in any way to be a substitute for professional treatment (psychological, counseling, medical) and should be used in addition to prescribed regimens.

Chapter Nineteen

Topic: THE 21st CENTURY "RULES FOR THE SEXES." Improving communication between males and females: You don't bring me compliments any more

- To narrow the communication gap and reduce the stress between sexes when communicating, simplify the number and details of the messages, and have the receiver rephrase the message to make sure it just didn't go in only one brain, and out the other.
- Since the right side of the brain, which women also use to communicate, is more sensitive to the tone of voice, make sure your tone of voice matches the intent of your message. The right brain is also responsible for reading facial expressions, so once again, try to make your facial expression match your verbal expression.
- On the home front, remember it is better to be happy than right.
- Seeing eye-to-eye may require holding back on what seems natural. Of course, until we know better, we think everyone thinks as we do. Nothing could be further from the truth. Trusting the value of the other person's thinking style (he or she did make it this far using that style), it may be necessary to show a little respect, back off and listen to the other person. This may reduce a lot of stress from unchangeable brain-based communication gaps.
- Surprise your mate with an unexpected, but "on-target" gifts.
- Correctivitis (overly correctness) is the obsession with being right, having the last word and dominating. This common malady is highly stressful to surrounding people. Being a target of someone with correctivitis is like driving over jarring and unnecessary speed bumps when you are trying to talk. People with correctivitis are always interrupting and correcting you, whether they know what they're talking about or not. They look for any loophole to unravel your thread of thought until you completely lose your train of thought.
- This is a good time to try the "In one ear out the other" technique if you can.
- Smile if you can manage it.
- Do take notes if it's appropriate to review later. Even better, have them write down their suggestions.

The 21st century "Rules for the sexes." Important Rules for partners

Rules for Men

- Apologize — even though you don't know what you've done wrong.*
- Don't count her shoes. Pointy toes, square toes, round toes, no toes. It will never make sense to you.
- Don't burp and then laugh about it. Only men and their sons think that burping is funny.
- Don't make fun of Oprah.

Rules for Women

- No trick, "Am I fat?" questions.
- Beer is to men what flowers are to women.

*Thanks to top radio personality, Mr. Bill Flynn, of North Carolina, for publicizing the books, *The Rules for husbands;* Sarah Andrews and Jim Dale, and The *Rules for wives*; Jim Dale and Ellen Small, 2001. See Chapter 19 for more details.

ONE-MINUTE ANTI-STRESS FACT SHEET ©
Dr. Ronald L. Rubenzer, 2003
From: *How the Best Handle Stress*

This educational material is not intended in any way to be a substitute for professional treatment (psychological, counseling, medical) and should be used in addition to prescribed regimens.

Chapter Nineteen
Topic: "RULES FOR THE SEXES:" Improving Communication between Males and Females

"At home it is better to be happy than right;
At work it is better to be right than happy."
- Dr. Ron Rubenzer, 2003

Change your mind to change your life. (See the "Rules for the sexes" on previous page.)

- The only adult's mind you can really change is your own. If you are constantly in a state of agitation because everyone else seems scatterbrained, you might consider consciously trying to change your mind.

Male aggression—female expression: Possibly different brain styles

- Seeing eye-to-eye is difficult.
- There is some research that suggests that the male brain is more designed for aggression. The female brain may be better designed for expression. One brain style wants to aggressively get to the bottom line, the other wants to talk in a free-flowing stream of words. For example, Delia presents a problem. Bob poses a solution. Delia actually only wants to express her frustration, not necessarily solve the problem. Bob aggressively tries to get to the "heart of the matter" by taking care of business and solving the problem. To Delia, expressing herself about the problem is part of the solution and not just describing the facts of the matter.

Brain-based communication gaps. Won't versus can't remember

- You never listen to me! "It seems like you are only half-paying attention to whatever I say," said Delia, as Bob once again forgot half the items on the "mental" shopping list he made. "Furthermore you completely forgot about that dinner we set up with the Epicures."
- Men may only be "half-listening" when women are trying to communicate. A November 2000, brain study conducted at the Indiana University School of Medicine shows that men may only be half-brained listeners. When listening to a story, men used only the left side of their brain, whereas women used the left side and the right side of the brain (associated with more abstract reasoning). There seems to be a biological brain-based difference between the sexes in information processing.

- Women are better at listening to two conversations at once, which may be overwhelming for men. In phone conversations, it would probably be annoying to most males if you try to talk to them while they're talking on the phone, since they devote one brain to one conversation at a time.
- It is not that the opposite sex won't think like you do, it's that they can't think like you do.
- Learn the thirty-second secret-insights to the "Rules for the sexes," to save thirty years of stress. (See previous pages).

Get a Brain Scan! Take the five-minute, paper/pencil Brain Scan (next page). We can all improve by exercising our weaker side of thinking.

BRAIN SCAN

Some of the characteristics that correspond to left-right brain thinking styles are listed below. (Of course, we always use more than "half a brain" when thinking, just as we actually use more than one hand [even back muscles] when we pick up a soda to drink. For the overly left brained, a set of serious resources is provided in the text for follow-up).

How to do your own Brain Scan

- Casually read each left brain/right brain style choice on the following page (they are not prioritized).
- Circle the one that seems more like you.
- It is all right to circle corresponding opposites if both describe you.
- Add the column totals (Write L= [for left brain column total]; R = [right brain]).
- The column (left or right) with more items circled suggests your tendency or thinking style (left or right brain).
- Have your partner (child, etc.) take the Brain Scan.
- See if you are on the same "brain-wave" length. If you have all L's and your partner has all R's this could create stress. Opposites may attract, but may also result in thinking the other person is only using half their mind.
- Learn to compromise and use both your brains.

LEFT BRAIN	RIGHT BRAIN
Early bird	Night owl
Analytical (breaks things down)	Analogical (makes connections)
Prefer clarity	Prefer vagueness
Prefer correct answer	Seek alternative responses
Doer	Dreamer
Exactness and precision desired	Tend to exaggerate
Structured, forced	Unstructured, free
Intellectual	Artistic
Test ideas	Make ideas
Serious	Jokester
Logical	Intuitive
Motivated by external rewards	Motivated by satisfaction
Focused, narrow	Nebulous, diffuse
Makes Order out of Chaos	Makes Chaos out of Order
Opinionated	Open-minded
Planned	Directionless
Ask factual questions (what, when, who)	Ask speculative questions (what if, why not)
Rule maker	Rule breaker/bender
Interested in science fact	Interested in science fiction
By the clock, (e.g., lunch is always at noon)	Timeless (lunch is "whenever" you are hungry)
Uptight	Uninhibited
Verbal	Visual
Task oriented	Idea Oriented
Enjoy complicated	Keep it simple
Astronomy Buff	Astrology Fan
Loathes Surprises	Loves Surprises

ONE-MINUTE ANTI-STRESS SKILL-BUILDERS ©

Dr. Ronald L. Rubenzer, 2003

From: *How the Best Handle Stress*

This educational material is not intended in any way to be a substitute for professional treatment (psychological, counseling, medical) and should be used in addition to prescribed regimens.

Chapter Twenty
Topic: USING STRESS FOR YOUR SUCCESS: How the Best Handle Stress

You can learn how to have success without distress.

- Life in the fast lane may be the only way to stay ahead.
- Deadlines, lack of time, competition, difficult people, and criticism are roadblocks that are common to everyone. While these may be obstacles for some, the best actually use these stressors as stepping-stones rather than stumbling blocks to get where they want.

Those best at handling stress included

- An Emmy award-winning writer.
- A top Nielson-rated TV personality with an earned doctorate, and an international Toastmasters award for outstanding leadership.
- An Olympic pretrial competitor.
- A world leader in stress management.
- A former Special Forces Ranger, now an English professor.
- A *Sports Illustrated* photographer.
- A federal judge.
- A top radio personality.
- The director of the North Carolina Writers' Network.
- A Yale educational consultant/retired interim superintendent of a 62,000-student school system.
- A private-school teacher from Australia.

One of their personal formulas described in Chapter 20 could work for you.

ONE-MINUTE ANTI-STRESS FACT SHEET ©

Dr. Ronald L. Rubenzer, 2003

From: *How the Best Handle Stress*

This educational material is not intended in any way to be a substitute for professional treatment (psychological, counseling, medical) and should be used in addition to prescribed regimens.

Chapter Twenty
Topic: USING STRESS FOR YOUR SUCCESS: How the Best Handle Stress

You can learn how to have success without distress

- Enjoy all aspects of your life.
- "Stress management is thought management."
- It is the strength and focus of the mind that allows one to overcome fear.
- Meditate, exercise, enjoy and achieve.
- Have fun in all you do, and leave a legacy.
- Forget yourself by serving others.
- Keeping calm to help others under adversity.
- Using a proven technique.
- "Get physical" and focus on family.
- Making the right decision.
- Tips from our Australian neighbors: Meditate, exercise and dine.
- "Creating what makes one happy."
- Providing the most good for the "cause."
- Walking, massages and movies.
- Stress-management techniques unique to these high achievers.
    1. Accentuate the positive.
    2. Take pride in accomplishing goals on the way to excellence (e.g., continual self-improvement).
    3. Possess a strong "service-to-others" orientation without undue concern over immediate rewards.
    4. Reduce one's "fun-deficit" by enjoying all aspects of life (e.g., music, dining, family, work).
    5. Exercise.
    6. Practice a proven relaxation technique.

ONE-MINUTE ANTI-STRESS FACT SHEET ©

Dr. Ronald L. Rubenzer, 2003

From: *How the Best Handle Stress*

This educational material is not intended in any way to be a substitute for professional treatment (psychological, counseling, medical) and should be used in addition to prescribed regimens.

Chapter Twenty-One
Topic: CONQUERING ANGER, WORRY, HEADACHES AND SLEEPWORKING

HOW TO CONQUER ANGER

Move to a different city

- There is a strong link between hostility and death rates. Cities reporting the lowest levels of hostility enjoyed much lower mortality rates than high-hostility cities. Honolulu, having the lowest self-reported hostility level also had the lowest death rate. Mainland cities reporting low hostility rates included Seattle, Minneapolis, Denver, and Des Moines.

The American Psychological Association suggests that you

- Calm down by deep breathing and creating pleasant images.
- Change your thinking when mad (attitude).
- Plan problem solving without self-blame.
- Communicate better, apply humor.
- Improve your surroundings and schedule your time better.

Getting along with others

- We need to learn to make decisions when we get mad. We need to ask ourselves whether this irritation is worth our attention. Is our anger justified or not? If our anger is not justified, we should try to talk ourselves out of anger. If self-talk does not work, use meditation or some type of distraction. If we are justified in getting angry, we need to think of a sensible response, and deliver our message calmly and respectfully.

Fighting fair

- Do not use name-calling, do not try to psychoanalyze the other person.
- Do not fight the last thing at night or right after getting home from work.
- Both parties sit down to keep cool. Have a glass of cool water.
- Young males are at risk for learning anger, because males are flooded with testosterone (the aggression hormone), in addition to stress hormones, cortisol and adrenaline, that both sexes produce when stressed.

- Therefore anger management should be taught early. Learning to prevent or control anger impulses is what separates us from the animals. Learning to make the right choices under stress can be started even at the preschool level.

HOW TO OVERCOME WORRY

- Don't bleed until you are cut. Worrying is 97% wasted mental effort.
- Throw your worries away — write them down and trash or burn them.
- Dissect your real problems into solvable steps.
- Weave your own "psychological safety net" with those you trust.
- Use humor to whittle down your worry to size.
- Avoid "pity parties."
- Get or give help.
- Don't worry — work, (hard and smart).
- Engage yourself in physical activity.
- Learn to focus on today. (Live in daytight compartments.)

"Don't borrow sorrow" by worrying about things beyond your control.

HOW TO PREVENT HEADACHES

- Regular exercise is the best way to prevent headaches.
- Practice muscle relaxation during your breaks.
- Take a warm bath or shower.
- Get a massage from a licensed professional.
- Smile more, frown less.
- Practice deep breathing.
- Reduce eyestrain.
- Maintain good posture.
- Eat properly.

ONE-MINUTE ANTI-STRESS FACT SHEET ©

Dr. Ronald L. Rubenzer, 2003

From: *How the Best Handle Stress*

This educational material is not intended in any way to be a substitute for professional treatment (psychological, counseling, medical) and should be used in addition to prescribed regimens.

Chapter Twenty-One
Topic: CONQUERING SLEEPWORKING

(See previous pages for Conquering Anger, Worry, Headaches)

HOW TO DEAL WITH SLEEPWORKING (Insomnia due to worrying about work)

- Don't drink coffee or caffeinated drinks after lunch. Try green tea instead of coffee.
- Exercise no later than two hours before you go to bed.
- Shift into a relaxed gear about an hour before you go to sleep.
- Don't watch exciting sports shows or adrenaline-surging movies right before bed.
- Keep your room cool (about 68 degrees) and dark.
- Don't use your bedroom as a boardroom (Don't discuss money, calendars, etc.).
- If you eat before bed, eat lightly (a small bowl of cereal, graham crackers, etc.).
- Read something light and inspirational right before you go to sleep.
- Go to sleep to the sound of the beach (or running water, rainfall, etc.). Get a sound soother!
- Bore yourself to sleep. Read about something you have absolutely no interest in. Turn on the weather channel.

ONE-MINUTE ANTI-STRESS FACT SHEET ©

Dr. Ronald L. Rubenzer, 2003

From: *How the Best Handle Stress*

This educational material is not intended in any way to be a substitute for professional treatment (psychological, counseling, medical) and should be used in addition to prescribed regimens.

Chapter Twenty-One
Topic: CONQUERING ANGER, WORRY, HEADACHES AND SLEEPWORKING

"Genius is eternal patience." - Michelangelo

WHY CONTROL YOUR ANGER?
AVOIDING ANGER HANGOVERS

Anger is the worst stress-reflex because it is doubly destructive. Your anger destroys your health and your relationships. Anger hangovers are a bad way to start your day. An anger hangover is simply waking up mad from the fight you had the previous night.

"I will not let any man diminish my soul by making me hate him." - George Washington

- Anger hangovers: Waking up still angry from the fight you had the night before is an anger hangover. You start your day off on the "wrong foot" and increase your health risks.
- Holes in the block of wood. It has been said that in anger we "nail" our victims with sharp words like driving nails into a block of wood. When the heat of our anger subsides, we pull out the nails, but the holes in the wood remain. The holes in our relationship are often not worth the satisfaction we derived when we attacked our victim (Al Pecor).
- Redford Williams, M.D., Director of the Behavioral Medicine Research Center at Duke University, states that people today appear angrier than ever. A 2002 study revealed that treatment for depression has grown 500% since 1987.
- Anger, whether inner-or outer-directed, can kill you. Men with higher hostility levels were $2^1/_2$ times more likely to have evidence of developing heart disease. Postmenopausal women who were angry also had increased heart disease symptoms.
- Men are more prone to react to anxiety with anger and hostility because a surge of testosterone is added to the stress hormone cocktail (adrenaline and cortisol).
- Being socially isolated and depression are key factors linked to anger and heart disease.

- A double "whammy" would be a man who is hostile under great job-stress where he has little control and high demands.
- Too much technology, too little time, fuels the rage of anger. Too much attachment to technology leads to CSA, Computer-separation-anxiety.
- Much of today's unhappiness comes from the collision of too much technology with too little time.

WHY CONTROL WORRY? DON'T GET MAD — GET SMART

"We cannot solve problems at the same level they were created." - Albert Einstein

- To solve problems we must get above the worries that we attach to problems. Learning to relax will help us see that many of our worries are unfounded, never come true or are exaggerations.

GENERALIZED ANXIETY DISORDER

- Unchecked, a worry habit can solidify into a generalized anxiety disorder requiring professional treatment.
- Blocking your worry-urge can actually improve your physical health and emotional well-being. It may even improve your human relationship skills. "Chicken Littles" are notoriously unpopular with their constant ranting and raving, "The sky is falling."

ONE-MINUTE ANTI-STRESS FACT SHEET ©

Dr. Ronald L. Rubenzer, 2003

From: *How the Best Handle Stress*

This educational material is not intended in any way to be a substitute for professional treatment (psychological, counseling, medical) and should be used in addition to prescribed regimens.

Chapter Twenty-One
Topic: CONQUERING HEADACHES AND SLEEPWORKING

WHY PREVENT AND RELIEVE HEADACHES

- The headache is the most frequent single complaint of modern times. Most headaches are stress headaches.
- Headaches that occur at work make work even more stressful because you may anticipate getting a headache (which can actually trigger a headache).
- Headaches prevent you from concentrating well and can make the cause of your headaches (workload) increase because of errors or sick-time due to headaches.

Possible causes of tension headaches

- The exact cause of tension headaches is not clear, but the most likely culprits are: stress, muscle tension, restricted blood flow from sustained muscle tension, fatigue or too much or too little sleep.
- Other common causes of headaches include: holding a "frozen posture" for too long (e.g., looking at a computer screen too long), grinding one's teeth or even chewing gum too hard.

WHY CONTROL INSOMNIA?

Sleepworking: A common story, a highway hazard

Bob, with dark circles under his eyes and looking like he hadn't slept in days, confided in his friend during his break; "Like Hal, the uncooperative computer in the movie, *2001*, the computer side of my brain refused to shut down, working on work even though I was trying to sleep. My mind kept going over the problem like a broken record, refusing to let me sleep. I was sleepworking instead of sleepwalking."

- Sleep disorders are increasing as stress is increasing. But don't lose any sleep over that fact. If you try to practice stress management (including anger and worry management) you may improve your sleep. Always see your doctor if you are having significant problems sleeping.

What is sleepworking?

- Sleepworking is sleeplessness due to dreaming/worrying about work problems. Your sleep is invaded by unwanted thoughts. You sleepwork trying to solve problems or complete work. The problem with sleepworking is that you are only using half-a-mind. Your right brain, which functions at about a five-year-old level mentally and emotionally, dominates at night just as the stars come out at night when the sun goes down.
- Safer driving: It is common knowledge that many car accidents are caused by those asleep at the wheel.

ONE-MINUTE ANTI-STRESS SKILL-BUILDERS ©

From: *How the Best Handle Stress*

This educational material is not intended in any way to be a substitute for professional treatment (psychological, counseling, medical) and should be used in addition to prescribed regimens.

Chapter Twenty-Two
Topic: AGING GRACEFULLY

- Using it or losing it. This refers to both your mind and body.
- Use the real "fountain of youth" (sweat) to add years to your life and life to your years. (Always see your doctor before starting any type of exercise program.)
- Make today count.
- Maintain a sense of humor to maintain your sense of balance.
- Stay informed and in tune. Join AARP.
- Become knowledgeable about the many advances being made in how to improve the quality of your life.
- Expand your friendship horizons.
- If alone, get a pet, even a wet pet (fish).
- Optimism is the breakfast of champions!
- Volunteer your services and wisdom to the new generation
- The Eden Alternative: Improving quality of life in elder-care.

ONE-MINUTE ANTI-STRESS FACT SHEET ©

Dr. Ronald L. Rubenzer, 2003

From: *How the Best Handle Stress*

This educational material is not intended in any way to be a substitute for professional treatment (psychological, counseling, medical) and should be used in addition to prescribed regimens.

Chapter Twenty-Two
Topic: AGING GRACEFULLY

You will never ever be younger than you are today.
Enjoy this day.

- Seventy-six-million baby boomers have now joined the 40 to 50 year-old rank. In fact the entire baby boomer generation is rushing into the "rest of us" camp. Even Bob Dylan (a legendary singer) just turned 60 years-old (May 24, 2001).
- Ten-thousand baby boomers a day are turning fifty and entering what has been called the "second adulthood."
- One of these baby boomers was already President, sending a clear message that the "young old" are becoming establishment. Our society is aging, but gracefully.
- An individual's chances of living beyond 65 are four times greater now than they were in 1900.
- Differing concerns for men and women.
    1. Career focus. Men in their fifties often reach their professional peak, with an eager eye toward retirement. By contrast, women, after completing their child raising work, often become interested in entering the work force or improving skills.
    2. Health issues. Many women, as much as 50-85%, will experience mild menopausal symptoms. Many heart attacks surface for men in their fifties.
- Being orphaned at 55, being widowed at 75. Dealing with loss. Work with your local hospice, church, clinic or call United Way to get help. There is no reason to try to handle it on your own. It could shorten your life by years if you grieve beyond a certain point.

Several advantages that accompany aging. The elderly:

- Are less irritated by things;
- Become reflective;
- Grow wiser;
- Spend less time worrying and fighting;
- Improve mental performance especially in job-related and verbal skills;
- Report positive life satisfaction.

APPENDIX B

TIME-CAPSULE

HOW TO MANAGE TIME

More Tips on Time Management, Procrastination, Timer-Projection Devices

1. Write down your thoughts.

This will help you organize and remember. "The palest ink is better than the best memory." The best handwritten organizational system for time-management is Day-Timer. The Day-Timer Corporation even reminds you when you are running out of day timers. Give this system one-hundred days, and you will suddenly make time to waste time (like enjoying your family, improving the quality of your life, etc.). Call toll free 1-866-654-9797 or <ordersupplies.com> for calendars. But remember, having great calendars is like having a great set of weights and only looking at them. Use your calendars.

2. List your important goals.

These should be your major lifetime goals, work goals, etc. For example, lifetime goals: Retire early at the beach and/or mountains, go to Tahiti, write an article. Work goal: Develop systems to manage information more effectively.

3. Prioritize all your goals.

For example, going to Tahiti might be more important than retiring early at the beach. Organizing your files might be more important, right now, than something else. An excellent book to help you learn how to prioritize is written by Dr. Stephen Covey. In his book, *First-things-first*, he provides realistic, effective and humanistic ways to look at and organize your life.

4. For each goal, list weekly activities that will help you meet your goal.

For example, if developing an information management system is your top goal, then you will have to find out: where and if this has been done before; what materials might be the best; what methods seem to work the best; what assistance you will need to do your job well; who needs to approve your plan; and how will you measure and report progress. Remember, everything takes twice as long as it does (If you think something will take a week, it usually takes two).

Remember the simple but effective formula TOT=TOT (Time on Tasks = Tasks on Time). In your monthly planner, mark your project due date. Then mark the day before as your internal due date. If you think the project will take a week, go back two weeks for your start date. The old saying, "If you fail to plan, you plan to fail" may have some truth.

For stress relief when you are "off the clock," make time to waste time. Don't wear your watch, pager or cell phone, unless of course, you are an Emergency Room physician on whom lives actually depend. You might put on your "To-Do" list at home (if you are checklist-addicted), have fun.

You can accomplish almost any goal if you are persistent enough. People have tunneled their way out of concentration camps digging only with a spoon. One of the greatest books ever written was scratched out on bits of paper while the author, Victor Frankl, was brutalized in a concentration camp, facing certain death. No one's job is as bad as a concentration camp, and you can do great things over a long time (learn advancement skills, write books) if you are planned, patient and persistent. Sadly, most college dropouts quit after their third year.

---

5. Now prioritize your activities to meet the goals.

Assign the value A-1 to your top activity; A-2 to the second activity. For example: Goal Develop Information Management System; A-1 activity — find out who needs to approve your approach; A-2 what has already been done in this area. As mentioned above, Dr. Covey's book, *First-things-first,* is a useful guide in helping you make decisions.

---

6. Get a legal pad and at the top write the words "To Do" with today's date.

What you don't get done today, carry over to the "To-Do" list you have for tomorrow. I would duplicate a month's worth of "To-Do" lists and staple them together. It will take at least a month for the habit to kick in. Stick to using a SINGLE "TO-DO" LIST. If you must use hypernotes (little square pieces of paper that leach themselves on refrigerators, desks, etc.) at least put them in one envelope. Using a single legal pad is a much better practice. Time management is simple, but not easy. It takes discipline at first.

---

7. Schedule your prime time.

Do the worst work first. Most people are mentally sharper in the morning, but fade mid-afternoon. Morning may be best to do hard-core left brain planning, writing or calculating. Mid-afternoon might be a good time to sharpen your pencils or straighten your desk. Try to coordinate your schedule around other people's prime time if you need to meet them (e.g., Check to see if the dentist works on Friday afternoon).

---

8. Be flexible to shifting goals.

Give yourself weekly deadlines, not daily deadlines, if possible. Sweeping the crumbs out of your pantry may be a level C goal in September, but will quickly become an A-1 goal when mice start munching on those crumbs in October.

If you feel your youth has passed you by in terms of getting an education, don't despair. Four years from now you will be thirty, whether you have your degree or not. Wouldn't it be better to be thirty with a degree than regretting your not going back to school?

As previously stated, "nimble" is the key word to survival in today's business. If you have a hard time changing your routine, just put the word "nimble" on an index card and carry it with you. Then say the "nimble-jingle" you learned as a child (Jack be nimble, etc.) to yourself.

---

9. Periodically review progress on your goals and, if necessary, revise your goals and activities accordingly.

If you are NEVER completing any of your weekly goals you probably are not planning properly. Remember, you can only have one A-1 priority. Again, time management is simple but not easy, especially when it comes to procrastination, the material used to pave the road to Hades. Don't wait for perfect timing. "When I graduate I'll . . .; when the kids stop fighting I'll improve my . . .; I'll finish that report when my desk is cleared, all my papers are filed, AND all my pencils are sharpened . . .; I'll go to Tahiti when I can afford it . . .; I'll improve my romance life when I lose more weight; We'll leave for vacation when the house is spotless and could pass "the Martha Stewart" inspection.

---

10. Reward yourself for accomplishing.

Always ask yourself: Am I making the best use of my time, right now? Use the simple if-then proposition or Grandma's Law (e.g., if you eat your peas, you can have dessert). If you review your "To-Do" list, reward yourself with a break.

Timekeeper technology: transparency projector countdown

Stokes Publishing Company, out of Sunnyvale, California, offers a calculator-sized countdown timer that can be projected by a transparency projector, for a very large countdown timer image on a screen. This $52 device is excellent when you are giving timed tasks to large groups of individuals where time limits are important. It is also excellent for keeping presentations within time limits.

Procrastination: seeds of failure! Eight tips to pull out these weeds before they choke you.

PROCRASTINATION IS A SIAMESE TWIN TO POOR TIME MANAGEMENT. We are giving in to stress when we avoid doing something we think is unpleasant or meaningless. Even wild animals keep a work schedule even though it's more like flex-time. If they don't work, they starve. Yet they also have sense enough to avoid toxic situations, and will migrate if their work environment is too hostile.

---

1. Remember the COSTS of procrastination.

What important others will think; the reputation you may be creating; the bad habit you are strengthening. REMEMBER THE REWARDS OF COMPLETING TASKS ON TIME.

---

2. Use the SWISS CHEESE (Lakein, 1974) method of getting started on difficult tasks or making real molehills out of imaginary mountains.

This method also works very well for at least beginning your exercise session. Tell yourself, I'll exercise for five minutes, and then see how I feel. I'll continue exercising if I feel like it.

---

3. List instant tasks.

List tasks that are easy and take no longer than five minutes (e.g., new information management system – look up phone number of administrator who will approve your project).

---

4. Start your instant task.

Use an egg timer and set it for five minutes. You may find that you actually are involved in the task. If you feel motivated to continue after five minutes, do so. You can do anything for five minutes. Stretch your frustration tolerance to fifteen minutes. In a few months you may be able to tolerate fifty minutes of unpleasantness, without its ruining your whole day. (Fifty minutes is considered the peak performance attention span for an adult.)

---

5. Build in a quota of instant tasks you will accomplish each week.

After a dozen or so instant tasks, you will have taken a significant number of holes out of the chunk of cheese that seemed overwhelming in the beginning.

6. Gather information about the task.

This may create interest. Talk to others about the task. They may have insight on how to better approach the task. However, do not use talking to others as a pleasant escape from the task itself.

7. Arrange yourself physically to get yourself going.

If you have to write something, sharpen your pencil. Keeping the A-1 project information in the middle of your desk will help. If you need to type something, sit down at the computer and turn it on.

8. Reward yourself for meeting weekly instant task quotas and for completing the goal itself.

Remember: You always have time to do those things that are truly important to you. You certainly managed the time to date as a youth, no matter how many clubs, courses, errands you had. Time management helps you decide what is important to you and when you will do it. You can even learn to make time to waste time.

And if it is of any consolation, everyone leaves this earth with uncompleted tasks on their "To-Do" list. Chance are you will too, so don't get too "check-list" obsessed. As Ms. Loretta LaRoche advises: Have a *Don't Have To-Do* list.

BIBLIOGRAPHY

(200 Citations)

Note to the "want-to-know-more" reader. The Internet Research Engine WorldCat, provides complete information on practically every known book (including a photo of the front jacket) in the world's libraries. This service even tells you if you have this book in your local library. All you need is a library card, a password from your reference librarian.

Ackerman, Diane. (1990). *A natural history of the senses.* Random House.

ADHD and Posttraumatic Stress Disorder. (2000, October). *ADHD Report,* Vol. 8, No. 5, p. 1-7.

Allen, Catherine; O'Connor, Christopher; & Blumenthal, James A. (1993, Spring). Stress breaks silence of heart conditions. *Psychiatry at Duke, Vol. IV, Issue 1, p. 1.* Duke University Medical Center.

American Psychiatric Association. (1998, May). Practice guidelines for the treatment of patients with panic disorder. *American Journal of Psychiatry, Supplement Vol. 155, No. 5.*

Anxiety Disorders Association of America, 6000 Executive Boulevard, Suite 200, Rockville, Maryland 20852-4004. Phone (301) 231-8368. On the Web: <www.adaa.org>.

Anxiety disorders. Decade of the brain. (1994, September). *National Institute of Mental Health,* pp. 12-13. (Booklet). National Institute of Health Consumer information center. Dept. 42, Pueblo, Colorado 81009. Free 24-page booklet.

Are you hip to new workplace lingo? (1995, July 3). *Cambridge Human Resource Group.* Greensboro, NC. *News and Record,* D3.

Babyak, M., et. al., (2000, September/October). Exercise treatment for major depression: Maintenance of therapeutic benefit at ten months. *Psychosomatic Medicine,* Vol. 62, No. 5, pp. 633-638.

Barkley, Russell. (1998). *Attention-deficit hyperactivity disorder, a handbook for diagnosis and treatment.* New York: Guildford.

Benson, Herbert; Grandjean, Ann; Pelletier, Kenneth R.; Rosch, Paul J.; Winick, Myron; Gardiner, Kevin; Honda, Charlotte; Klitsner, Nancy; & McGregor, Paul. (1987). *Managing stress- from morning to night.* Alexandria, Virginia: Time-Life Books.

Benson, Herbert; Kornhaber, Arthur; Kornhaber, Carol; Le Chanu, Mila; Zuttermeister, Patricia C.; Myers, Patricia; & Friedman, Richard. (1994, Summer). Increases in positive psychological characteristics with a new relaxation response curriculum in high school students. *The Journal of Research and Development in Education, Vol. 27, No. 4,* pp. 226-231.

Biofeedback is considered to be the most effective way of stress-self-management in terms of how quickly relaxation is learned. Call Heartmath, 1-800-372-3100 or email: <info@heartmath.com>.

Blake, Lois. (1989, July/August). The stress of staying at home. *Psychology Today.*

Blank, A.S. (1994). Clinical detection, diagnosis and differential diagnosis of post-traumatic stress disorder. *Psychiatric Clinics of North America, 17,* pp. 315-383.

Blehar, Mary C.; Rosenthal, Norman; Terman, Michael; & Wehr, Thomas. (1990). Identification, assessment, and treatment of seasonality in mood disorders. *Psychopharmacology Bulletin. (New clinical drug evaluation unit issue) Volume 26, No. 1,* pp. 3-10.

Bonny, H., & McCarron, N. (1984, February). Music as an adjunct to anesthesia in operative procedures. *Journal of the American Association of Nurse Anesthetists,* pp. 55-57.

Bresnick, Jan, (1985). Fighting fatigue. Everyday health hints. (*Prevention* total health system) Rodale Press, Inc., pp. 58-61.

Bryan, T., & Bryan, J. (1991a). Positive mood and math performance. *Journal of learning disabilities,* 24, pp. 490-494.

Bryan, T., & Bryan, J. (1991a). Positive mood and vocabulary learning, reported in: *Yasutake.* (1995, June-July). The influence of affect on the achievement and behavior of students with learning disabilities. *Journal of Learning Disabilities, Volume 28, No. 6,* pp. 329-334.

Burley-Allen, Madelyn. (1995). *Managing assertively.* John Wiley & Sons, Inc.

Caffeine: what it does. (1981, October). *Consumer Reports,* pp. 595-599.

Cardiac Alert, Heart Disease Education and Prevention, Phillips Publishing, Inc., 7811 Montrose Road, Potoma, MD 20854.

Castleman, Michael. (1991, July-August). How experts cope with Stress. *Men's Health.*

Chambers, Harry. (1996, August 19). How to overcome negativity in the workplace. Greensboro, NC. *News and Record.*

Cobb, Kevin. (1992, April). Stress reduction goes mainstream. *American Health,* p. 84.

Cohen, S.; Tyrrell. D.A.; & Smith, A.P. (1993). Negative life events, perceived stress, negative affect, and susceptibility to the common cold. *Journal of Personality and Social Psychology, 64,* pp. 131-140.

Cohen, S.; Tyrrell., D.A.; & Smith, A.P. (1991). Psychological stress and susceptibility to the common cold. *New England Journal of Medicine, 325,* pp. 606-612.

Coleman, Paul. (1990). *The forgiving marriage: resolving anger and resentment and rediscovering each other.* Contemporary Books.

Condor, Bob. (1996, July 24). ABZzzz'z of sleep: The more you exercise the more you need. *Chicago Tribune* and Greensboro, NC. *News and Record.*

Controlling Anger (Brochure). American Psychological Association, 750 First Street NE, Washington, DC 20002-4242. Free brochure on controlling anger from the APA.

Cornell University Study. (1996, August 23). Executive stress highest level ever. *National Business Employment Weekly.*

Covey, Stephen R.; Merrill, Roger A.; & Merrill, Rebecca R. (1994). *First things first. To live, to love, to learn, to leave a legacy,* pp. 36-43. New York, NY: Simon & Schuster.

Craske, M. (2000). *Mastery of your anxiety and panic: therapist guide,* (3rd ed.) Academic Press.

Dannheisser, Lynn. (1996, August 19). You can neutralize negativity. Being pessimistic can prevent you from reaching your potential. Greensboro, NC. *News and Record,* B4.

Davis, Susan, & Freudenberger, Herbert. (May 30, 1995). Burnout. *Your Health,* 52-56.

Dawkins, Beth. (1995, March-April). All creatures great and small. *Arthritis Today, Vol. 9, No. 2,* pp. 29-34.

DeRoches, Brian. (1995). *Your boss is not your mother.* William Morrow and Company.

Donnelly, Kathleen. (1995, September 8). The lord of discipline. Greensboro, NC. *News and Record,* Section D.

Donovan, Priscilla. (1991). Shifting Back to left brain. *Men's Health Magazine.*

Dorian, B.J.; Garfinkel, P.E.; Keystone, E.C.; Gorcyzynki, R.; & Darby, P. (1986). Stress immunity and illness. *Psychosomatic medicine, 48,* pp. 304-305.

Dreyfack, Raymond. (1988, February). Interested in life extension? Pay attention to tension. *American Salesman, Vol. 33,* p. 20.

Dumaine, Brian. (1988, June 20). Executive life: cool cures for burnout. *Fortune magazine,* pp. 78-84.

Exercise against depression. (2001, March). *Harvard Mental Health Letter.*

Eyre, Richard. (1995). *Don't just do something, sit there.* Simon & Schuster.

Fader, Shirley Sloan. (1984, December). 25 things your boss wants you to know. *Working Woman,* pp. 112-113.

Faigel, C.H. (1988, January). An SAT pill? *Gifted children monthly,* p. 4.

Finholm, Valierie. (2001, March 11). Also roots of our rage: little annoyances, petty frustrations. The Hartford Courant, Greensboro, NC. *News & Record,* D8.

Fischman, J. (1987, February). Type A on trial. *Psychology Today,* pp. 42-50.

Flynn, J.R. (1987). Massive IQ gains in 14 nations. *Psychological Bulletin, 101,* pp. 171-191.

Forbes ranks Gates world's richest person. (1995, July 5). *Forbes Magazine, Vol. 105, No. 186.*

Frances, Allen. (1995, July 9). How to deal with difficult people. *Parade Magazine,* p. 8.

Friedman, Rodney M. (1995, August). The energizer. *The University of California at Berkeley Wellness Letter, Vol.11, Issue 11.* New York: Health Letter Associates.

Friedman, Rodney M. (1995, September). Ten minute workouts. *The University of California at Berkeley Wellness Letter, Vol. 11, Issue 12,* p. 7. New York, NY.

Friedman, Rodney M. (1995, August). Java Jolt. *The University of California at Berkeley Wellness Letter, Vol. 11, Issue 11.* Health Letter Associates.

Friend, Tim. (1990, April 2). Type A traits are risky. *USA Today.*

Gabor, Don. (1994). *How to start a conversation and make friends.* Conversation Arts Media.

Gabor, Don. (1994). *Speaking your mind in 101 difficult situations.* Stonesong Press, Inc., Fireside/Simon & Schuster, Inc.

Gibbs, Nancy. (1995, October 2). The EQ factor: New brain research suggests that emotions, not IQ may be the true measure of human intelligence. *Time Magazine*, pp. 60-68.

Gibson, James L.; Ivancevich, John M.; & Donnelly, James H., Jr. *Organizations: behavior, structure, processes,* p. 205. (5th Ed.) Plano, TX: Business Publications.

Gilner, Art. (Speaker). *Developing your sense of humor.* (Cassette Recording). Silver Spring, MD: The Humor Communication Company.

Gilroy, Diane K., Ed. (1995). *Prevention's book of home remedies and super healing foods,* p. 13. Emmaus, PA: Rodale Press, Inc.

Glaser, Ronald; et. al. (1994). *Handbook of human stress and immunity.* Academic Press, Inc. Harcourt Brace & Company. San Diego, CA.

Gold, Phillip, W. (1991). Stress implicated in Chronic Fatigue Syndrome. *American Institute of Stress* No. 8, p. 5.

Goldling, Jacqueline. (1992). *Beyond strength.* Brown and Benchmark.

Goldstein, Ross. *Fortysomething.* Jeremy Tarcher (in press).

Goleman, Daniel. (1996). *Emotional Intelligence,* pp. 82, 91-92. Bantam Books.

Gorman, J. (2000, April). Neuroanatomical Hypothesis of Panic Disorder Revised. *American Journal of Psychiatry*, Vol. 57, No. 4, pp. 493-505.

Gregory, Ted. (1994, November 6). Before Monday blues, come Sunday blahs. *Chicago Tribune* and Greensboro, NC. *News and Record,* D3.

Groppel, Jack L. (1995). *The science of success, mentally tough.* Executive Vice-President of LGE Sports Science, Inc., & Mentally Tough, Corporate Training Program. 9803 Lake Nona Rd., Orlando, FL. 32827. Phone (407) 438-9911 Fax (407) 438-6667. 1-800-LGE-PROG.

Hales, Dianne, & Hales, Robert E. (1995). *Caring for the mind: The comprehensive guide to mental health.* Bantam Books.

Hall, Nicholas R.S.; Anderson, Julie A.; & O'Grady, Maureen, P., (1994). Stress and immunity in humans modifying variable. *Handbook of human stress and immunity,* pp. 183-208. Academic Press, Inc.

Hallowell, Edward M., & Ratey, John J. (1994). *Answers to distraction.* Pantheon Books, New York.

Hallowell, Edward, Ph.D., Co-author. *Driven to distraction.* Quoted in Hales, Dianne.

Hales, Robert E. (1996, January 7). Finally I know what's wrong. *Parade Magazine,* pp. 8-11.

High stress individuals had 47% colds versus 27% colds for low stress. (1992, April, May). *New England Journal of Medicine.*

Huberty, Thomas J. (1996, March 16). *Differentiating Anxiety and Depression in Children: Assessment and Intervention,* pp. 3, 5, 8, 9. Highlights from notes and handout. National Association of School Psychologists (NASP) Convention 1996. Atlanta, GA.

Hull, Nancy R.; Hall, W. Dallas; Purcell, Julia Ann; & Payne, Yvonne. (1988). *Blood pressure control: a matter of choices.* Atlanta, GA: Pritchett & Hull Associates.

Human Synergetics: Ten year study of 10,000 managers, professionals. (1994, November 21). *Detroit News.*

Interfax Daily, Vol. WZ1V7101. (2001, March 5). Baton Rouge, LA.

Isaacson, Peggy, & O'Connell, Loraine. (1995, May 29). Learn how to handle ill-will at work. *Orlando Sentinel,* D3.

It's just a little . . . I can handle it. (1994, September). *National Institute of Mental Health.* (Booklet). Anxiety disorders. Decade of the brain. National Institute of Health. Consumer information center. Dept. 42, Pueblo, Colorado 81009. Free 24-page booklet.

Ivancevich, John M.; Matteson, Michael T.; Freedman, Sara M.; & Phillips, James S., (1990, February). Worksite stress management interventions. *American Psychologist, Vol. 45, No. 2,* pp. 252-261.

Jensen, Eric. (1998). How threats and stress affect learning. *Teaching with the Brain in Mind,* p. 52. Website: <http://www.ascd.org>; E-mail <member@ascd.org>.

Jensen, Eric. (2001), *Brain Based Learning, Brain Compatible Strategies, and Super Teaching.* Washington, DC: American Society for Curriculum and Development.

Jonson, Angela. (1997). Anger control games for grades 2-6. *Keep your cool.* Marco Products. Warminster, PA: Marco Products.

Kearney, Jay, Ph.D., (1996, June). Training Olympic athletes. *Scientific American,* pp. 52-63.

Keeping the Lid on Anger and Hostility (2001, March). *Vitality — Good News about Health, Happiness and Productivity,* p. 7.

Keller, Steven, E.; Shiflett, Samuel C.; Schleifer, Steven J.; & Bartlett, Jacqueline, A. (1994). Stress Immunity and Health. In *Handbook of human stress and immunity,* (pp. 217-244). San Diego, CA: Academic Press, Inc.

Kiecolt-Glaser, J.K.; Dura, J.R.; Speicher, C.E.; Trask, O.J.; & Glaser, R. (1991). Spousal caregivers of dementia victims: longitudinal changes in immunity and health. *Psychosomatic Medicine, 53,* pp. 345-362.

Kishline, Audrey; Marriott, Michel; Stokes, Myron; King, Patricia; & French, Rob. (1995, March 27). Moderate drinking half steps vs. 12 steps, Health: Can moderation help problem drinkers? *Newsweek,* p. 62.

Kowalski, Robin. (1995, January 1). Studies complaining – Griping researcher finds niche. *Associated Press.* Under consideration for publication in Psychological Bulletin.

Kreitner, R.; Wood, S.D.; & Friedman, G.M. (1979, August). Just how fit are your employees? *Business Horizons,* 22, pp. 39-45.

Kuczen, Barbara. (1990). *Childhood stress: How to raise a healthier, happier child.* Delta.

LaBier, Douglas. (1986). *Modern madness: The emotional fallout of success.* Reading Mass: Addison-Wesley Publishing Company.

LaLane, Jack. (1995). *Revitalize your life after fifty.*

Lancaster, Hal. (1996, May 7). Procrastinators: Mend your way before your job stalls. Managing your Career. *Wall Street Journal,* B1.

Last, C.G.; Perrin, S.; Hersen, M.; & Kazdin, A.E. (1992). DSM-III-R anxiety disorders in children: Sociodemographic and clinical characteristics. *Journal of the American Academy of Child and Adolescent Psychiatry, 31,* pp. 1070-1076.

Last, C.G.; Strauss, C.C.; & Francis, G. (1996). Comorbidity among childhood anxiety disorders. *Journal of Nervous and Mental Disease, 175,* pp. 726-730.

"Learning to Live Well With Chronic Illness." (2000, December). *Vitality,* p. 7.

Leutwyler, Kristin. (1996, August). In focus, paying attention. *Scientific American,* pp. 12 -14.

Life span doubles since George Washington's time. (1992). *Longevity Magazine.*

Lovell, James. (1995). Mission interview after successful landing. *Arts & Entertainment.*

Lowest blood pressure found for those describing faith as very important, even those who smoked. (1991). *Journal of Religion and Health, 28,* pp. 265-278.

Manley, Audrey, Acting US Surgeon General. America gets a wake-up call on exercise. As reported by Dustin, Diane. (1996, July 12). Greensboro, NC. *News and Record,* D1.

McClelland, D.C. (1989). Motivational factors in health and disease. *American Psychologist, 44,* pp. 675-683.

McGinnis, Alan Loy. (1990). *The power of optimism.* Harper & Row Publishers, San Francisco, New York.

McGrady, Angele. (1991, May). Diabetes: Tipping the scales of health. *Diabetes Care, Vol. 14, No. 5.*

Mead Johnson Pharmaceuticals. (1990). *Working through stress and anxiety.* [Brochure J-F98-6-90]. Evansville, Indiana: Bristol-Myers Squibb Company.

Mehta, Satish. (1999, November). A sick crew can't work well in space. *Odyssey, Vol. 8, Issue 8,* 2p., 1c.

Mellin, Laurel. *The solution: 6 winning ways to permanent weight loss.*

Migraine headaches reduced by hand warming biofeedback by controlling swelling of blood vessels and muscle contraction. (1995). National Headache Foundation, Chicago, IL.

Milstrey, Susan. (2000). *A delicate balance: living successfully with chronic illness.* Perseus Books. Also <www.adelicatebalance.com>.

Mind over Bunker, golf's a mental game. (1995, April 20). Greensboro, NC. *News and Record,* B1, B3.

Moran, Elizabeth J. (1990, May 5). CEO burnout: Shift priorities to manage stress. *Hospitals,* p. 67.

Moyers, Bill. (1990). *Full catastrophe living: Using the wisdom of the body and mind to face stress and pain-illness.* New York: Bantam Doubleday Dell Publishing Group, Inc.

Muriel, Solomon. (1990). *Working with difficult people.* Englewood Cliffs, NJ: Prentice Hall.

Murphy, L.R. (1984). Stress management in highway maintenance workers. *Journal of Occupational Medicine 26,* pp. 436-442.

Myers, David G., & Diener, Ed. (1996, May). The pursuit of happiness. New research uncovers some anti-intuitive insights into how many people are happy and why. *Scientific American,* pp. 70-72.

National Institute of Mental Health. (1987). *Plain talk about handling stress.* {Brochure}. DHHS Publication, No. 87-502.

National Institute of Mental Health. (1994, September). *Anxiety disorders. Decade of the brain.* [Booklet]. National Institute of Health. Consumer information center. Dept. 42, Pueblo, Colorado 81009.

Neisser, U. (1998). *The rising curve.* Washington, DC: American Psychological Association.

Noble, Elizabeth. (1983). *Childbirth with insight,* pp. 32, 33, 48. Boston, MA: Houghton Mifflin Company.

Oeschli, Matt. *Mind Power for Students.* (1996). St. Martin's Paperbacks. The Matt Oeschli Institute can be contacted at 336-273-6582.

Ornish, D. (1990). *Dr. Dean Ornish's program for reversing heart disease.* Random House.

Ornstein, Robert, & Sobel, David. (1989). Brahms valium. *Healthy Pleasures,* p. 60. Addison-Wesley Publishing Company.

Ornstein, Robert, & Sobel, David. (1989). *Healthy Pleasures,* p. 148. Addison-Wesley Publishing Company.

Ornstein, Robert, & Sobel, David. (1989). *Healthy Pleasures,* p. 240. Addison-Wesley Publishing Company.

Ornstein, Robert, & Sobel, David. (1989). *Psychology of consciousness,* p. 240. Addison-Wesley Publishing Company.

Papatheodorou, N. (1983). *Getting Started: How to handle stress.* Franklin Lakes, NJ: Becton Dickinson.

Parker, Harvey C.; Storm, George; Petti, Theodore A.; & Anthony, Virginia Q. (1991, Fall/Winter). Medical management of children with Attention Deficit Disorders commonly asked questions. *Children with Attention Deficit Disorders,* pp. 17-20. Plantation, FL.

Pearce, Kelley, Colorado Springs Gazette Telegraph (1995, December 23). US troops sent to Bosnia get help coping with stress: Mental health team will help troops deal with "psychological bullet wounds." Greensboro, NC. *News and Record,* D1.

Pennebaker, Ph.D. (1990). *Opening up: the healing power of confiding in others.* William Morrow (Publishers).

Peper, Erik; Wilson Vietta S.; Taylor, Will; Pierce, Alex; Bender, Kathy; & Tibbetts, Vicci. (1994). Repetitive Strain Injury – Prevent computer user injury with biofeedback: Assessment and Training Protocol. *Electromyography — Applications in physical therapy, Issue 9,* pp. 1-12.

Phillips, Don. (1996, March 2). Fitness tests: Because everyone has bad days. *The Washington Post,* D1-2.

Pierce, J.L., & Newstrom, J.W. (1983). The design of flexible work schedules and employee responses: Relationships and processes. *Journal of Occupational Behavior 4,* pp. 247-262.

Politzer, Brianna. (1990, December 27). Seasonal affective disorder called a common problem. Depression treated with light. *Medical tribune, Vol. 1, Number 26.*

Powell, D.; Gordon, Williams; & Powell, Don. (1991, October-November). Flaming, how to recognize when it's all too much. *Modern Maturity, Vol. 34, No. 5,* pp. 26-29.

Prepare for SAT. An excellent online resource for specific SAT preparation is located at the Web site <www.collegeboard.com>.

Relaxation techniques improve self confidence and control for competition. (1992, November). *Vitality Magazine,* p. 12.

Revicki, D.A., & May, J.H. (1989, Spring). *Behavioral medicine,* pp. 31-35.

Ritter, Malcolm. (1996, July 15). Study: Southern men hate jeers. Greensboro, NC. *News and Record,* A1, A2.

Rosch, P.J. (1993, November 19). Prolonged exposure to stress causes atrophy in the hippocampus, a region of the brain involved with learning and memory. *Newsletter of the American Institute of Stress* AIS, No. 4, p. 3.

Rosch, Paul, M.D. (1991, June). Salt, stress and hypertension. *Newsletter of the American Institute of Stress,* p. 7, and *Wall Street Journal,* (1991, June 3).

Rosch, Paul J. (1995, Summer). Getting the most out of leisure time. *Creative living, the Magazine of Life, Vol. 24, No. 3,* pp. 14-19.

Rosch, Paul, M.D. Townsend Letter for doctors. (1994, November). *American Institute of Stress Newsletter No. 3,* p. 5.

Rosch, Paul. (1990). High stress levels may cause excessive hair loss and some forms of baldness. *American Institute of Stress Newsletter.*

Rosch, Paul. (1991). Fatigue: Why is America so tired? *Newsletter AIS,* p. 3.

Rosch, Paul. (1991). Fitness prevents stress ills. *American Institute of Stress Newsletter, No. 12,* p. 5.

Rosch, Paul. (1991). Stress has been implicated in Chronic Fatigue Syndrome. *AIS Newsletter, No 8,* p. 5.

Rosch, Paul. (1991). The Stress Reducing Effects of Crying. *AIS Newsletter, No. 8,* p. 2. (Also, *Arthritis Today,* Oct. 1991).

Rosch, Paul. (1992). *American Institute of Stress, Stress in Children, No. 1,* p. 5.

Rosch, Paul. (1992). Commuter Audio Review. *AIS Newsletter,* p 7.

Rosch, Paul. (1992, April). *Archives of Internal Medicine, No. 8.*

Rosch, Paul. (1993, July 12). *AIS Newsletter, No 8,* p. 2.

Rosch, Paul. (1995). Cardiac Rehabilitation for Type A's. *AIS Newsletter, No. 3,* p. 4.

Rosch, Paul. (1995). Mental vs. Treadmill Stress Tests. *AIS Newsletter, No. 3,* p. 7. (Medical Tribune, May 5, 1994).

Rosch, Paul. (1995). Perfectionism and Poor Health. *AIS Newsletter, No 7,* p. 3.

Rosch, Paul. (1995). The Stress Reduction Effects of Music. (Based on Seventh International Montreux Congress on Stress, February 19-24, 1995). *AIS Newsletter, No 4,* pp. 1-4.

Rosch, Paul. (1990). Goodness of fit between person/environment important for job stress management. *American Institute of Stress Newsletter, Number 8,* p. 5.

Rosenbaum, J., (Ed.). (1997). Treatment of Panic Disorder: The State of the Art. *Journal of Clinical Psychiatry, Supplement 2, Vol. 58.*

Ross, Jerilyn. *Triumph over fear: A book of help and hope for people with anxiety, panic attacks and phobias.* Also US Air — Fearful fliers program. Phone (412) 366-8112.

Rudolph, David L., & McAuley, Edward. (1995). Self-efficacy and salivary cortisol responses to acute exercise in physically active and less active adults. *Journal of Sport and Exercise Psychology, 17,* pp. 206-213.

Sarkis, J. (1991, July). Near misses, 20/20 foresight. *Employee Assistance,* 13, 12, 21.

School stress – No. 1 cause of children's headaches. (1995). National Headache Foundation, Chicago, IL.

Schwartz, G.E. (1982). Stress management in occupational settings. In Washington, D.C. (1988). Toward a sociology of worksite health promotion: A few reactions and reflections. *Social science and medicine, 26,* pp. 569-575.

Schwartz, J., et. al., (1994, April 15). Society of Behavioral Medicine meeting. *Associated Press,* p. A3

Seligman, Martin. (1994, September). *American Health, 62.* University of Pennsylvania.

Sellers, Patricia. (1995, August). What's so good about failure? *Fortune Magazine,* pp. 107-110.

Seven stress-busters for air travel. (1995, November/December). *Car and Travel.* pp. 8-9.

Shatan, Jeremy. (June, 1995). Displaced aggression, contact sport as stress reliever. *Men's Health,* p. 40.

Sheehy finds new life after 50. (1995, July 6). Greensboro, NC. *News and Record,* p. D6.

Sheehy, Gail. (1995). *New passages.* Random House.

Simpson, Sarah. (2000, March). Staying sane in space. *Scientific American, Vol. 282 Issue 3,* p. 61, 2p., 1c.

Sommer, Bobbe, Ph.D., & Falstein, Mark. (1993). Psycho-cybernetics 2000. *Maxwell Maltz Psycho-Cybernetics Foundation, Inc.* Prentice Hall International Limited.

Spence, J. David. (1996, February). American Heart Association conference presenter at annual stroke conference.

Spielberger, Charles (with Gorush, R.L.; Lushene, P.R.; & Vagg Jacobs, G.). (1977). Self-evaluation questionnaire for anxiety. *Consulting Psychologist's Press.*

Standley, J.M. (1986: 23(2): 56-122). Music research in medical/dental treatment: Meta-analysis and clinical applications. *Journal of Music Therapy.* Spingte, R., & Droh, R. (Eds.): Music and Medicine. New York: Springer-Verlag.

Stern, Caryl. (1996, January 21). Who is old? *Parade Magazine,* p. 4-5.

Sternberg, Robert. (2000, Fall). *Wisdom as a form of giftedness. Vol. 44, No. 4,* p. 258. Yale University.

Stevo, Julius. (1991, March). Autonomic nervous dysfunction in essential hypertension. *Diabetes Care, Vol. 14, No. 3,* p. 249.

Stoddard, Alexandra. (1991). *Living beautifully together,* p. 48. New York: Avon Books. The Hearst Corporation, 1350 Avenue of the Americas, New York, NY 10019.

Stop taking your child to work. (1995, April). *Men's Health,* p. 54.

Stress distracts, after four hours significant decrease in attention. (1993, May). *Prevention,* p. 134.

Stress hurts arteries in some, study says. (1996, January 28). The Associated Press. San Antonio, TX.

Studying for and taking tests. [Brochure]. An excellent resource for parents is this 13-page booklet available from The Parent Institute, P.O. Box 7474, Fairfax Station, VA 22039-7474, Phone 1-800-756-5525 or <http://www.parent-institute.com>.

Swartz, M.N. (1991). Stress and the common cold. *New England Journal of Medicine, 325,* pp. 654-656.

Tanzer, Deborah, Ph.D., & Block, Jean Libman. (1972). *Why natural childbirth?,* pp. 35-36. Garden City, NY: Doubleday & Company, Inc.

Terman, Michael. (1990). Identification, assessment, and treatment of seasonality in mood disorders. *Psychopharmacology Bulletin. (New clinical drug evaluation unit issue) Volume 26, No. 1,* pp. 3-10.

Test-prep firms aim to prepare state's students. (2001, January 29). Greensboro, NC. *News and Record,* B4.

The Top Ten of Everything, p. 102. (1998). New York, New York: DK Publishing Co.

Timm, Paul R. (1990). Recharging your career. Crisp Publications, as mentioned in *Vitality Magazine,* p. 3, (1993, June).

Ubell, Earl M.D. (1995). Relaxation, it can be good for what ails you. *Parade magazine,* p. 14.

Unhappy and know it? Whine. Some Generation-Xers are said to notice life's inequities more vocally than others. (1995, December 26). Greensboro, NC. *News and Record.*

Verespej, Michael. (1990, March 19). Why managers fail. *Industry Week, Volume 239, Number 6,* p. 42.

Vincent, J.D. (1990). Stress kills brain cells. *The Biology of Emotions.* Cambridge, Mass.

Vos Savant, Marilyn & Fleischer, Leonore. (1990). *Brain building in just 12 weeks. (Exercising yourself smarter).* Bantam Books.

Wall Street Journal. <www.health.harvard.edu> email <peter_wehwein@hms.Harvard.edu>.

Weight gain and loss. (2001, March). *Harvard Health Letter from Harvard Medical School, Vol. 26, No. 5,* pp. 1-3.

Wigins, Beverly. (1995, January). Survey. Institute for research in social sciences, school of journalism and mass communication. University of North Carolina at Chapel Hill.

Williams, Redford, M.D. (1989). *The trusting heart: Great news about Type A behavior.* Random House, Inc.

Williams, Redford, & Williams, Virginia. (1993). *Anger Kills.* Times Books.

Williams, Redford. (1994, May 15). Duke University Medical Center. There is a very strong connection between hostility and all-cause death rates. Greensboro, NC. *News and Record, Vol. 104, No. 135,* A-1.

Zi, N. (1986). *The art of breathing.* New York: Bantam Books.

INDEX

A

ABC'S OF STRESS MANAGEMENT FOR CHILDREN, 170
ALBERT EINSTEIN, 72
ALCOHOL, 135
ALZHEIMER'S, 284
AMERICAN ASSOCIATION OF RETIRED PERSONS (AARP), 284
AMERICAN INSTITUTE OF STRESS, 254
AMERICANS' "BIG GUN" ATTITUDES OF ASTRONAUTS, 252
ANATOMICAL AND FUNCTIONAL GENDER DIFFERENCES… IN OUR BRAINS, 237
ANGER SPELLS DANGER, WITHOUT THE D, 266
ANTI-BOREDOM "WHOLE-BRAIN" CURRICULUM, 207
ANTI-STRESS SKILL-BUILDERS, 291
ANXIETY DISORDERS FOR ADHD, 185
ASTRONAUTS HANDLE STRESS, 249
ASTRONAUTS IN SPACE "TOOK THE DAY OFF," 249
ASTRONAUTS' SOURCES OF STRESS, 250
ATTENTION-DEFICIT HYPERACTIVITY DISORDER, A HANDBOOK FOR DIAGNOSIS AND TREATMENT, 192
ATTENTION-GETTER NOTES, 162
ATTITUDE AFFIRMATION, 163
AUSCHWITZ AND DACHAU CONCENTRATION CAMPS, 282
AUSTRALIAN NEIGHBORS: MEDITATE, 253
AUTOCRATIC RUSSIAN LEADERSHIP, 250
AVOIDING A NERVOUS BREAKDOWN WHEN YOUR COMPUTER HAS ONE, 20

B

BE TOUGH MINDED BUT TENDER-HEARTED., 176
BELLS AND WHISTLES, 162
BENEFITS OF A HIGH RQ, 28
BEST OF "BIOFEEDBACK" TRAINING, 190
BETTER THAN MONEY CAN BUY, DANZIGER, 263
BETTER TO BE HAPPY THAN RIGHT, 237
BLINDSIDED BY STRESS, 59
BODY/MIND DIVORCE OR DANCE? 129
BRAIN-BASED COMMUNICATION GAPS, 242
BREATHING CALMS DURING CHILDBIRTH, 81
BREATHING INSTRUCTIONS, 84
BULLIES, 179

C

CAFFEINE AND EXCESSIVE SUGAR INTAKE, 175
CARD-CARRYING OPTIMIST, 75
CAUSES OF TENSION HEADACHES, 274
CENTER OF THE UNIVERSE, 73
CERTIFICATION IN BIOFEEDBACK RELAXATION TRAINING, 86
CHANGE YOUR MIND TO CHANGE YOUR LIFE, 238
CHARACTER EDUCATION, 16
CHOICES FOR TAKING C.A.R.E. OF BUSINESS, 89
CHORAL WHINING, 73
CLOSING THE COMMUNICATION GAP, 44
COLORLESS ACHIEVER, 64
COLUMBIA UNIVERSITY STUDY, 202
COMMAND TO REST, 3,500 YEARS AGO, 64
COMMANDMENTS FOR PEOPLE WHO WORK WITH PEOPLE, 231
COMPLAINERS, (SEE WHINING), 100
COMPLAINING DOES RELIEVE STRESS, 100
COMPUTER GETS A LOBOTOMY, 21
CONCENTRATING ON THE "HERE AND NOW," 83, 274
CORPUS COLLASUM, 237
CORRECTIVITIS (OVER-CORRECTING COMPULSION), 243
CORTISOL, A STRESS HORMONE, CONVERTS CALORIES TO FAT, 187
COUNSELING, 68, 289
CROSSING YOUR "FAULT LINE," 74
CURBING SCHOOL VIOLENCE, 188
CURE FOR CORRECTIVITIS: TRY THE NAG APPROACH, 245

D

DEALING WITH DIVERSITY/HARASSMENT, 102
DIFFERENCES OFTEN CREATE SPARKS AND TENSION, 238

DIRECTOR OF THE NORTH CAROLINA WRITERS' NETWORK, 257
DON'T BE A "REACTIONARY," 99
DON'T BLEED UNTIL YOU ARE CUT, 269
DON'T COMPLAIN—TRAIN, 59
DON'T WORRY — WORK, 270
DOWNWARD COMPARE, 73
DRUG ABUSE IS ON THE RISE FOR CHILDREN, 168

E

EGOS OF THE AMERICAN ASTRONAUTS, 250
ELEANOR ROOSEVELT, 69
EMMY AWARD-WINNING WRITER, 255
"EMOTIONAL AMBUSHING," 50
"EMOTIONAL PACIFIERS," 277
EMOTIONAL TRUST FUND, 74
ENJOY SUNDAY MORE, 64
ENJOY THIS DAY, 281
EPIDEMIC NEED FOR STRESS MANAGEMENT FOR CHILDREN, 167
EXCELLENT SENSORY PERCEPTION, 83
EXTENDED WARRANTY, 21

F

FAILURE INTO SUCCESS, 143
FEMALES USE BOTH RIGHT AND LEFT BRAIN, 237
FIND A NEED AND FEED IT, 90
FIVE-MINUTE BRAIN SCAN, 240
FOCUS OF THE MIND, 254
FOCUS ON TODAY, 274
"FOODS THAT SOOTHE," 65
FOUNTAIN OF YOUTH, 286
FOUR C'S OF WORK: CONTROL, CHANGE, CONFLICT AND COMPLAINING, 89
FOUR RESPONSE STYLES, 38
FREEZE-FRAMER™, 232

G

GE CUTS BOTTOM TEN PERCENT, 54
GENIUS IS ETERNAL PATIENCE, 265
GET OR GIVE HELP, 273
GRIM HUMOR TO COPE, 70

H

HEADACHE IS THE MOST FREQUENT SINGLE COMPLAINT, 274
HIGHEST-RECORDED IQ, 27
HOLES IN THE BLOCK OF WOOD, 267
HOMEWORK SHEETS FOR THOSE IN COUNSELING SETTINGS, 289
HOW RQ AND IQ ARE LINKED, 29
HUMOR LIFTS MOODS/IMPROVES HEALTH, 152

I

"IF IT BLEEDS, IT LEADS," 77
"IN ONE EAR OUT THE OTHER," 101
"INFORMATION OVERLOAD STRESS," 11
INJECT HUMOR INTO YOUR LIFE, 152
INVENTORY OF STRESS RESPONSES, 36
IT'S NOT BETTER, BUT I AM, 285
IT'S TOO . . . IT'S TOO HOT, COLD, SLOW, EXPENSIVE 244

J

JLU, "JUST LIKE US," PRINCIPLE, 98
"JOB-READY" ARE BETTER 49
"JOB RUST OUT," 60
JOB-STRESS MANAGERS FOR TYPE A'S AND FOR ADULTS DIAGNOSED AS ADHD, 92
JOB-STRESS MANAGEMENT HABITS CHECKLIST, 55
JOIN THE PTA, 170
JUST LIKE US, 89

K

KAVA, 137

L

LA MAZE, 82
LEARNING DISABILITIES, 179
LEAVE A LEGACY, 255
LEFT BRAIN TAKES CARE OF BUSINESS, 63
LFT'S, "LOOK FORWARD TO'S," 69
LGE (LOEHR, GROPPEL, ETCHENBERRY) MENTALLY TOUGH CORPORATE TRAINING PROGRAMS, 71
LICENSED PSYCHOLOGIST, 86
LIFE IS 44% MORE STRESSFUL, 8
LIGHTNING ROD FOR COMPLAINERS, 101
LISTENING TO A STORY, 242

M

MAKE TODAY COUNT, 286
MALE AGGRESSION—FEMALE EXPRESSION, 241
MALE STRESS SYNDROME, 20
MALES NEED STRESS MANAGEMENT MORE, 186
MALES UNDER STRESS, AGGRESS, 186
MARS FLIGHT, A DYSFUNCTIONAL CREW COULD SPELL DISASTER, 252
MEAN SHALL INHERIT THE EARTH, 51
MEN FAINT: THE "NOCEBO" EFFECT, 11
MEN MAY ONLY BE "HALF-LISTENING," 242
MIGRAINE MONDAYS, 167
MISDIAGNOSING ANXIETY DISORDERS FOR ADHD, 184
MIXED MESSAGES ABOUT ACHIEVEMENT, 185
"MONDAY-NIGHT DELIGHT," 65
MONDAY STRESS IS BRAIN SHIFTING, 64
MONDAYS: HARDLY A FUN DAY, 63
MORE TEACHABLE MOMENTS, 188

N

NARROW THE COMMUNICATION GAP/REDUCE THE STRESS, 243
NATIONAL PUBLIC RADIO, (NPR), 137
NATIONAL SPACE BIOMEDICAL RESEARCH INSTITUTE, 249
NATIONAL TRANSPORTATION SAFETY BOARD, 145
NATIONAL WHINER'S DAY, 100
NATURAL HOMEOPATHIC REMEDIES, 137
NATURAL REMEDIES, 137
NAZI CONCENTRATION CAMP, 70
NEUROCHEMICAL LIES, 10
NEW ENGLAND CENTER FOR HEADACHES, 275
NEW ENGLAND JOURNAL OF MEDICINE, 187
NIELSON-RATED TV PERSONALITY, 254
NO WINE UNTIL IT'S TIME, 135
NUMBER ONE STRESSOR ON THE JOB, 90

O

OBSESSIVE-COMPULSIVE THINKING, 64
OLD FAITHFUL GEYSER, 38
OLYMPIC PRETRIAL COMPETITOR, 253
ORPHANED AT 55, BEING WIDOWED AT 75, 281

P

PADDLING DUCK, 38
PERFORMANCE ANXIETY, 29
PET YOUR PET, 171
PHYSICAL ABOUT STRESS, 129
PITY PARTIES, 272
POST-TRAUMATIC STRESS DISORDER, 141
PRESCHOOL COMPETITION, 169
PRESENTER PREPARATION -- DON'T SWEAT, 163
PRESIDENT BUSH, 16
PROFESSIONALS IN TRANSITION, 145
PUBLIC SPEAKING, 158
PUREST FORM OF STRESS, 254
PUSHING YOUR OWN RESET BUTTON, 59

R

RADIO PERSONALITY, 247, 253
RAISE SAT SCORES BY 100 POINTS, 204
RAISING TEST SCORES BY LOWERING TEST ANXIETY, 30
RELAXATION BREATHING, 82
RIGHT BRAIN AT THE WRONG TIME, 63
RIGHT BRAIN ENJOYS SPENDING, 63
RIGHT BRAIN STRESS SKILLS, 59
RQ (RELAX-A-BILITY QUOTIENT), 27
RQ TEST, 32

S

SAT, 1
SCHOOL MORNINGS, 180
SCHOOL PSYCHOLOGIST, 189
SCHOOL STRESS, 178, 185
SCHOOL STRESS AFFECTS UP TO 10%, 187
SEX AND STRESS: MALES… RESPOND TO ANXIETY WITH AGGRESSION, 43
SHARPEN YOUR LEFT BRAIN, 65
SHOOTER'S STRESS SYNDROME, 18
SLEEP AT THE SOUND, 278
"SMALL THOUGHTS VACCINE," 69
"SOMATOPSYCHIC," 129
SPORTS "BLOW-OFF" STEAM, 170
STAFF INFECTIONS -- NEGATIVE EMOTIONAL CONTAGION, 47
STRESS AND SUDDEN DEATH AT WORK, 68
"STRESS-BELLY," 5
STRESS CURES AT HOME, 167
STRESS IS FATTENING, 5

STRESS-MANAGEMENT FITNESS SCALE, 40
STRESS ROBS A DOZEN YEARS, 10
STRESS SQUELCHES YOUR SUCCESS, 141
STRESS STRANGLES PRODUCTIVITY, 51
STRESSES BETWEEN THE SEXES, 43
STRESSORS SHARED BY MEN AND WOMEN, 43
SURVIVORS IN THE BUSINESS ENVIRONMENT, 51

T

TACKLE TEST ANXIETY, 174
TEARS, 48
TECH-SUPPORT HEAVEN, 21
TEN MINUTE RESET, 59
TERRIFIC OR TERRIBLE TEENS, 177
TEST ANXIETY LOWERS TEST PERFORMANCE, 195
TESTOSTERONE POISONING, 238
THOUGHT MANAGEMENT, 254
THOUGHTS GENERATE EMOTIONS, 69
TIME MANAGEMENT FOR TYPE A'S AND ADHD, 92
TOP SPORTS PHOTOGRAPHER ADVISES, 253
TORTOISE AND HARE, 185
TOUGHNESS TRAINING FOR BUSINESS, 71
TRAINING NEEDS ASSESSMENT, 161
TYPE A HABITS ARE BEING CRYSTALLIZED, 187
TYPE A STUDENTS, 187

U

UNWANTED TEEN WEIGHT GAIN, 187
UNWHINING, 100, 123
URGENCY ADDICTION, 17

V

VALERIUM, 137
VALUES, 287
VERBALLY ABUSED, 47
VIETNAM, 254

W

W.A.L.K.E.R. PROGRAM, 189
WAKE FOREST UNIVERSITY, 5
WET PETS, 176
WHAT TEACHERS CAN DO?, 189
WHINING, 100
WHINERS' DAY (NATIONAL HOLIDAY), 100
WII-FM — WHAT'S IN IT FOR ME, 162
WORKSHOP-WORKSHEET CHECKLIST, 164
WORLD-CLASS LEADERS, 262
WORLD CONGRESS ON STRESS IN SWITZERLAND, 10
"WORRY HIT-RATE" 10%, 271
"WRITER'S MANTRA," 73

Y

YALE STUDY, 5

DON'T LET STRESS

SQUELCH

YOUR SUCCESS!